1008279935

"This volume is a long awaited, expert and updated series of scholarly efforts to inform clinicians and other stakeholders regarding the painfully neglected population of adopted individuals. I particularly appreciate the in-depth attention to the often disruptive psychological sequelae of adoption as these individuals face the separation/loss experiences associated with the challenges of emerging adulthood. Individuals with adoption histories are over-represented in the emerging adult population seeking and needing residential and other forms of intensive treatment."
—**Jesse Viner, MD**, *CEO & Chief Medical Officer, Yellowbrick Consultation & Treatment Center for Young Adults (Chicago, Ill.)*

"*Handbook on the Clinical Treatment of Adopted Adolescents and Young Adults* is a unique and wide-ranging exploration of the challenges faced by adoptees negotiating the critical developmental stages of Adolescence and Young Adulthood. Unusual in scope, it critiques historic, systemic, and legal aspects of adoption, all of which integrate with life histories and personal biology to impact identity development in adopted persons. Chapters illuminating the internal, experiential world of adoptees provide perspective on developmental issues faced by all adopted persons, whether clinically presenting or not. Advocating for a sorely needed "psychology of being adopted" and for expanded training in this specialized field, this volume is a must-read for any mental health clinician or health care practitioner who sees patients with an adoption history."
—**Susan C. Warshaw, EdD, ABPP**, *Editor in Chief of the Journal of Infant, Child and Adolescent Psychotherapy*

"There has been so much written about adoption that it is a striking scholarly accomplishment when a book brings a perspective that freshens the field and delivers on its promise to enhance assessment and treatment. Bertocci and colleagues weave their social work and psychological expertise and deep understanding of the field into an exploration of psychodynamic and systemic factors, simultaneously challenging the mental health of adoptees, using interdisciplinary and international research to bring new insights to bear on our understanding of adoptees' needs over time and place. Perhaps most important, they center the experience of adolescence and young adulthood, bridging the more common focus in research on early childhood trauma and challenge with an insistence on the well-trained clinicians' capacity to make a difference over the longer arc of youth."
—**Marsha Kline Pruett, PhD, M.S.L., ABPP**, *Maconda Brown O'Connor Professor, Smith College School for Social Work, Northampton, Mass.*

"This groundbreaking book addresses a crucial gap in our understanding of the intersection of adoption and adolescent development. The authors illuminate the critical challenges posed for mental health, healthcare, and social service professionals and organizations by the psychological dilemmas experienced by adopted youths and young adults as they attempt to consolidate their sense of self while coming to terms with the loss of their original parents and uncertainty about whether they can accept, and be accepted by, their adoptive parents and family. The book also highlights the parallel process of fragmentation that must be reckoned by service providers and organizations when their clients are youths who have been adopted, and essential implications that the combination of psychological and systemic fragmentation poses for psychotherapists across a variety of theoretical orientations. By bringing these complex issues to light, and making these often invisible adopted youths and their families fully visible, this book does them, and the professionals who work with them, a vital service."

Julian D. Ford, PhD, A.B.P.P., *Professor of Psychiatry and Law,*
Dir. Center for the Treatment of Developmental Trauma Disorders,
University of Connecticut Health Center

"This long overdue Handbook highlights how adopted individuals have unique presentations, needs, and experiences compared with their non-adopted peers. Focusing largely on the adolescent through early adulthood cohort, the authors stress that, as a group, these individuals are also extremely heterogeneous. In this context, their profiles cannot be easily summarized or generalized. From various perspectives, the authors set forth the premise that clinicians and professionals who work with this population need to have a comprehensive understanding of potential influences – e.g., developmental, familial, social, etc. – on these individuals' presentation during adolescence through early adulthood. In addition, they stress that adoptee-specific needs and experiences warrant consideration within larger systemic and societal domains so that adopted persons are able to be adequately assessed and receive appropriate care during the potentially turbulent 13-30 years of age and throughout their lives. The clinical and psychodynamic perspective of this Handbook is entirely consistent with my own lifelong experience providing comprehensive psychological evaluations using neuropsychological and projective instruments in hospital and private practice settings where adopted children, adolescents, and adults are seen. This is a must-read for those in the adoption, health and mental health fields."

James L. Rebeta, PhD, *Clinical Assistant Professor of Psychology in Psychiatry,*
New York-Presbyterian/Weill Cornell Medicine

"Adopted adolescents often have a difficult journey to adulthood with a desire to know who they are and the need to reconcile their experience of not being with their birth parents and being raised in a family that feels different. As they seek to grow into their genuine selves thay are confronted by a therapeutic and legal system that fails to understand their needs and their challenges. Bertocci, Deeg, and Mayers' *Handbook on the Clinical Treatment of Adopted Adolescents and Young Adult* provides a guide expressly developed to address their inner struggles of these teens and young adults. It is rich in clinical approaches and the voices of these overlooked and poorly served young people. Those of us who care for them and the treatment programs they utilize need to learn from them and the dedicated and thoughtful authors in this volume so that we can truly understand and help these young people become the adults they can be."

John Sargent, MD, *Professor of Psychiatry and Pediatrics,*
Tufts University School of Medicine

HANDBOOK ON THE CLINICAL TREATMENT OF ADOPTED ADOLESCENTS AND YOUNG ADULTS

This collection bridges the voices of international scholars and adopted persons to share knowledge about clinical practice with adopted people in adolescence and early adulthood.

Coming at a time when countries are beginning to focus on adoption reform, this handbook is the first to address not only the external, systemic contributions to their developmental complexities but also the underlying, internal meanings of being adopted as children become adolescents and mature into adulthood. It explains how adopted clients differ from those not adopted and emphasizes the need for clinical research on adopted people in this older age group. Exploring how clinicians can understand their client's clinical needs, it offers specific protocols and frameworks for assessment and necessary modifications in language and treatment. With a foreword by Miriam Steele, chapters examine the legal and sociopolitical cultures, policies, and practices in which adoption is embedded, calling for broad systemic change.

Embracing theoretical, conceptual, and global perspectives, this handbook is written for clinicians in all disciplines, at all tiers of practice, administration, and training, identifying the key roles they can potentially play in expanding and better focusing our understanding of the psychology of being adopted.

Doris Bertocci, LCSW, is in private practice in New York after a long career in college mental health treating young adults at Columbia University. She had previously worked with birth mothers and adoption agencies and, in recent years, has been active in adoption reform. She continues to work in the interface of mental health, adoption, family law, and child custody litigation.

Christopher F. Deeg, PhD, is a licensed clinical psychologist with over 30 years' experience treating adopted persons of all ages and those related to them. He is trained in cognitive behavioral treatment, interpersonal therapy, psychoanalysis, and psychoanalytic psychotherapy. He has several publications on the psychology and treatment of adopted persons.

Linda Mayers, PhD, is a licensed clinical psychologist and psychoanalyst in private practice in New York City and has worked for most of her career with adoptive families and adopted people of all ages. She is an adjunct associate professor at LaGuardia Community College, City University of New York. An ongoing interest is in the developmental complexities of adopted individuals throughout the life span.

COVER IMAGE

The North Star is the brightest, most fixed, and most visible star in the heavens. Since antiquity, it has been used for navigation across unknown space of earth and sea. When one is lost, literally or figuratively, the North Star represents the direction to gaze in order to be centered in the universe – to determine where one has been, where one is presently located, and the direction to proceed in order to find one's way.

The psychology of *being* adopted recognizes the *internal* sense of loss, and of being lost, that is typically reported by adopted people. This pertains especially to those impacted by the closed adoption system that still prevails in many countries and that continues to be an impediment in the lives of many adopted adolescents and adults. For adopted persons seeking help from qualified psychotherapists, the North Star represents order out of chaos, direction out of confusion, and realization of all that remains constant and available to them as they work toward centering themselves in their integrative process.

Similarly, this handbook represents a source to which the health-care, mental health, and many allied fields can turn in order to better understand and respond to the ongoing needs of adopted adolescents and young adults.

HANDBOOK ON THE CLINICAL TREATMENT OF ADOPTED ADOLESCENTS AND YOUNG ADULTS

Edited by Doris Bertocci, Christopher F. Deeg and Linda Mayers

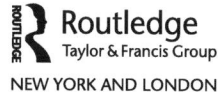

NEW YORK AND LONDON

Designed cover image: © Getty Images

First published 2024
by Routledge
605 Third Avenue, New York, NY 10158

and by Routledge
4 Park Square, Milton Park, Abingdon, Oxon, OX14 4RN

Routledge is an imprint of the Taylor & Francis Group, an informa business

© 2024 selection and editorial matter Doris Bertocci, Christopher F. Deeg and Linda Mayers; individual chapters, the contributors

The right of Doris Bertocci, Christopher F. Deeg and Linda Mayers to be identified as the authors of the editorial material, and of the authors for their individual chapters, has been asserted in accordance with sections 77 and 78 of the Copyright, Designs and Patents Act 1988.

All rights reserved. No part of this book may be reprinted or reproduced or utilised in any form or by any electronic, mechanical, or other means, now known or hereafter invented, including photocopying and recording, or in any information storage or retrieval system, without permission in writing from the publishers.

Trademark notice: Product or corporate names may be trademarks or registered trademarks, and are used only for identification and explanation without intent to infringe.

Library of Congress Cataloging-in-Publication Data
Names: Bertocci, Doris, editor. | Deeg, Christopher F., editor. | Mayers, Linda, editor.
Title: Handbook on the clinical treatment of adopted adolescents and young adults / edited by Doris Bertocci, Christopher F. Deeg and Linda Mayers.
Description: New York, NY : Routledge, 2024. | Includes bibliographical references and index.
Identifiers: LCCN 2023005073 (print) | LCCN 2023005074 (ebook) | ISBN 9780367555382 (hardback) | ISBN 9780367558666 (paperback) | ISBN 9781003095507 (ebook)
Subjects: LCSH: Adopted children—Mental health. | Adopted children—Psychology. | Adoption—Psychological aspects. | Adolescent psychology.
Classification: LCC RJ507.A36 H36 2024 (print) | LCC RJ507.A36 (ebook) | DDC 362.82/98—dc23/eng/20230210
LC record available at https://lccn.loc.gov/2023005073
LC ebook record available at https://lccn.loc.gov/2023005074

ISBN: 978-0-367-55538-2 (hbk)
ISBN: 978-0-367-55866-6 (pbk)
ISBN: 978-1-003-09550-7 (ebk)

DOI: 10.4324/9781003095507

Typeset in Bembo
by Apex CoVantage, LLC

To all adopted persons throughout the world, particularly adolescents and young adults, in whose honor this handbook was conceived, gestated, and produced.
To the memory of all those in the twentieth century, and beyond, who worked toward enlightening us about the fragility and profound intricacies of early childhood development.
(in order of year of birth)
Arnold Gesell, 1880–1961
Jessie Taft, 1882–1960
Melanie Klein, 1882–1960
Rene Spitz, 1887–1974
Anna Freud, 1895–1982
Donald Winnicott, 1896–1971
Edith Jacobson, 1897–1978
Margaret Mahler, 1897–1985
John Bowlby, 1907–1990
Mary Ainsworth, 1913–1999
Selma Fraiberg, 1918–1981
Anni Bergman, 1919–2021
Fred Pine, 1931–2022

And to the cherished memory of the remarkable twentieth-century clinicians and writers who were national and international pioneers in the psychology of being adopted. As an advanced clinical specialty, however, it is identified for the first time in this book. From their own perspectives, disciplines, and nations, each made seminal contributions to the literature, simultaneously impacting the fields of adoption, child welfare, mental health, sociology, social work, pediatrics, education, and family law. In their own respective ways, they shared the same mission of standing firm against the false assumptions and inadequate psychological, social, medical, and legal thinking of their day, providing a clear and eloquent voice on behalf of the unique developmental challenges and psychological themes in the experience of adopted persons throughout their lives.

(Listed chronologically according to their first publication in the adoption field.)

Florence Clothier, United States (1939)
Margaret Kornitzer, United States (1952)
Jean M. Paton, United States (1954)
Marshall D. Schechter, United States (1960)
Lillian Peller (b. Austria, 1893), United States (1961)
Povl Toussieng (b. Denmark), United States (1962)
Alfred Kadushin, United States (1962)
H. J. Sants, United Kingdom (1964)
H. David Kirk (b. Germany), Canada (1964)
Alexina M. McWhinnie, Scotland, UK (1967)
Benson Jaffee, United States (1970)
David Fanshel, United States (1970)
Michael Bohman, Sweden (1971)
Soren Sigvardsson. Sweden (1971)
John Triseliotis (b. Cyprus), Scotland, UK (1973)
Jules Glenn, United States (1974)
Herbert Wieder, United States (1977)
Remi Cadoret, United States (1978)
Annette Baran, United States (1978)
Reuben Pannor, United States (1978)
Arthur Sorosky, United States (1978)
Janet L. Hoopes, United States (1982)
Robin Winkler, Australia and United States (1988)

THE EDITORS' MEMORIALS

We, the editors, have our own very personal connections with adoption. But in particular we dedicate this handbook to the memories of specific persons in our lives, without whom this handbook quite literally would not have been possible.

Doris Bertocci: "To Michael S. Porder, M.D., who eagerly awaited this book and for whom 'there are no words.'"

Christopher F. Deeg: "To my mothers and fathers."

Linda Mayers: "To my parents, Clara and Kenny Mayers, who wholeheartedly encouraged and supported the adoption of my son, David."

CONTENTS

Editor Profiles — xvii
List of Contributors — xix
Foreword — xxv
Miriam Steele, PhD

PART I
Introduction: The Impact of the Adoption, Legal, and Mental Health Systems on the Development of Adopted Adolescents and Young Adults — 1
Doris Bertocci, LCSW; Christopher F. Deeg, PhD; and Linda Mayers, PhD

1 The Larger Context of Systemic Factors in the Interface of Adoption, Mental Health, and Family Law: How They Relate to Clinical Practice — 15
Doris Bertocci, LCSW, and Linda Mayers, PhD

2 Where Are We Now? Trends and Observations in Adoption Study in the Netherlands — 39
Rene A. C. Hoksbergen, PhD

3 Challenging Adoption Narratives: Adult Adoptees Write Remembrance – Four Australian Case Studies — 57
Catherine Margaret Lynch, PhD, JD; Sue Green, PhD; and Alison Ingram, PhD (Cand.)

PART II
Developmental Complexities and Necessary Modifications for the Assessment — 77

4 Life Begins Before Adoption: A Guide to the Essential Demographic Factors in Assessment and Treatment — 79
   Doris Bertocci, LCSW

5 The Adoptive Family Narrative and Its Effects on the Adopted Person's Development — 107
   Steven L. Nickman, MD

6 Understanding the Inner World of the Adopted Person: A Psychoanalytic Conception of the Psychology of Adoption — 124
   Christopher F. Deeg, PhD

7 Birth Fathers in Adoption: Into the Light — 137
   Gary Clapton, PhD

8 Growing Up Adopted in India – Mental Health and Well-Being: Implications for Therapeutic and Clinical Practice — 154
   Meera Oke, PhD; Sahana Mitra, PhD; and Valerie O'Brien, PhD

PART III
Considerations in Medical Care — 177

9 Adoption Medicine: Special Considerations in Pediatric and Adolescent Medicine and Young Adult Medical Care — 179
   Elaine E. Schulte, MD, MPH, and Laurie C. Miller, MD

PART IV
The Spectrum of Search and Reunion — 199

10 Revisiting the Meaning of the Search — 201
    Doris Bertocci, LCSW

PART V
Complexities of Psychotherapeutic Treatment   231

11   Observations on Clinical Problems and the Need for Shifts in Perspectives   233
      Doris Bertocci, LCSW, and Linda Mayers, PhD

12   Notes on the Psychoanalytic Treatment of the Adopted Person   264
      Christopher F. Deeg, PhD

13   From Fragmented to Firm Foundations in Identity Formation: A Neurosequential Approach to the Treatment of Adopted Adolescents and Young Adults with Early Developmental Trauma   275
      Alan John Burnell, OBE, and Jay Vaughan, MBE

14   Similarities and Differences in Attachment Representations between Late-Adopted and Non-Adopted Adolescents: A Study from Italy   283
      Cecilia S. Pace, PhD; Stefania Muzi, PhD; Fabiola Bizzi, PhD; and Donatella Cavanna

15   Countertransference Challenges in Working with Adopted Adolescents: Notes of a Psychoanalyst in Private Practice   303
      Anna Balas, MD

PART VI
Epilogue   321

Index   *326*

EDITOR PROFILES

Doris Bertocci, LCSW, is currently in private clinical practice in New York after a long career in college mental health at Columbia University. Prior to this, she had worked with pregnant young women planning to place their babies for adoption, and with agencies handling the adoptions. Following her position as a clinician and administrator at Columbia, she developed a specialty in working with parents in child custody litigation, which served as an introduction to family law practice. Over the years, she has been active in developing the psychology of *being* adopted and in adoption reform efforts. The common thread in her three areas of specialty is the systemic treatment of minors as property without their own human rights. Ms. Bertocci co-authored with Marshall D. Schechter, MD, "The Meaning of the Search" in *The Psychology of Adoption* (Oxford Press, 1990). Recently, she developed a metropolitan New York–based online directory of senior clinicians specializing in adoption who provide interstate consultation regarding adopted adolescents and young adults and their families. The editors of this handbook became clinical consultants for the first psychiatric residential treatment program in the United States to develop an adoption-specific component within their overall program for young adults.

Christopher F. Deeg, PhD, is a licensed psychologist with over 30 years' experience treating adopted persons and those related to, or in relationship with, adopted persons. Dr. Deeg has training in cognitive behavioral, interpersonal therapy and advanced training in psychoanalysis and psychoanalytic psychotherapy. He is the author of several papers and a textbook chapter on the psychology of adoption and the treatment of adopted persons. Dr. Deeg's writings formulate a framework of the intrapsychic world of the adopted person based on the object relation of adopted self to birth parent. Previously, he was an adjunct assistant professor of psychology at

Editor Profiles

Hofstra University. Dr. Deeg maintains a private practice and also provides consultation to adoption agencies and families of adopted persons.

Linda Mayers, PhD, originally from Montreal, Canada, is in private practice in New York City. She is past director of training, and training and supervising analyst of the Institute of the Postgraduate Psychoanalytic Society; adjunct associate professor at LaGuardia Community College, City University of New York; former director of Continuing Education, faculty and supervisor at Washington Square Institute; faculty and senior supervisor at the Postgraduate Center for Mental Health; former adjunct clinical professor at City University, Teachers College, Columbia University, and Yeshiva University. She is a member of the editorial board of *Journal of Infant, Child and Adolescent Psychotherapy* and editorial reader for *International Forum of Psychoanalysis*. She is a founding member of Psychoanalysis, Art and Creativity, a member organization of the International Society for Art and Psychology. Dr. Mayers has published in the psychology of adoption (co-editor and author of an article for "The Adoption Journey," *Psychoanalytic Inquiry*, vol. 30 (1), January–February 2010, Routledge) art and psychoanalysis, tattoos, the history of mental illness, and infant–parent disturbances. She is in the New York–based directory of senior practitioners specializing in adoption, offering online consultation and treatment. She is an adoptive mother of a young adult.

CONTRIBUTORS

Anna Balas, MD, is a psychiatrist and psychoanalyst for adults, adolescents, and children, in private practice in New York City. She is an associate professor on the faculty of Weill Cornell Department of Psychiatry, where she teaches psychiatric residents, and she is a training and supervising psychoanalyst at the New York Psychoanalytic Society and Institute, where she teaches and writes about psychic trauma, healthy and pathological narcissism, and resiliency. She has a particular interest in trauma and emigration and in working with adoptive parents around psychological aspects of adoption, alternative reproductive technologies, and divorce.

Doris Bertocci, LCSW, is currently in private clinical practice in New York after a long career in college mental health at Columbia University. She developed a specialty in working with parents in child custody litigation, which served as an introduction to family law practice. Over the years, she has also been active in adoption reform efforts pertaining to the sealed adoption record and to developing the psychology of adoptive status. The common thread in her three areas of specialty is the systemic treatment of minors as property without their own human rights. Ms. Bertocci co-authored with Marshall D. Schechter, MD, "The Meaning of the Search," a chapter in *The Psychology of Adoption* (Oxford Press, 1990). More recently she developed a metropolitan New York–based online directory of senior clinicians specializing in adoption who provide interstate (USA) consultation regarding adopted adolescents and adults and their families, as well as treatment for state residents. In 2021, they became clinical consultants for the first psychiatric residential treatment program in the United States to develop an adoption-specific component within their overall program for young adults. They are available internationally to consult with health-care professionals. From Ms. Bertocci's long university-based experience handling high-risk assessments and hospital admissions of students, she has a particular concern about adopted adolescents and young adults admitted to hospitals and intensive treatment programs where the significance of being adopted is not recognized or addressed.

Fabiola Bizzi, PhD, is a researcher at the Department of Educational Science of the University of Genoa, Italy. She is also a clinical psychologist and psychotherapist. She received her BSc in psychology and PhD in psychology, anthropology, and cognitive sciences at the University of Genoa (with merit certificate). She is a full member of the Italian Association of Psychology. Her research interests concern assessment methods and clinical applications of attachment theory, including attachment-based intervention, family relationships, developmental psycopathology, and emotion regulation. Since 2015, she has published 34 contributions on Scopus.

Alan John Burnell has a degree in psychology and social administration from the University of Wales and an advanced postgraduate diploma in treatment of children and families. He is a qualified social worker with 40 years' experience. Alan is the co-founder of Family Futures, which is an adoption agency and independent (private) foster care agency in the United Kingdom (UK) specializing in an interdisciplinary assessment and treatment program for traumatized children and young people who have been removed from their families of origin. Alan John Burnell and Jay Vaughan developed neurophysiological psychotherapy (NPP), which is a neurosequential-, neurological-, and physiological-based psychotherapy for the treatment of children and young people with developmental trauma.

Donatella Cavanna is a full professor of dynamic psychology and adult psychopathology at the University of Genoa, Italy. Currently, she is retired but continues to teach dynamic psychology and adult psychopathology at the University of Genoa. She was the director of the Anthropological Science Department of the University of Genoa. She is a full member of the Italian Association of Psychology and is a member of the editorial Board of *Psicologia Clinica dello Sviluppo* (Clinical Psychology of Development). She has 30 years of experience in working with adoptive families from an attachment perspective. Her research interests are attachment theory and research, adoptive parenting, family relationships, and development of personality. Since 2007, she has published 44 contributions on Scopus.

Gary Clapton, PhD, is an honorary fellow in social work at the University of Edinburgh. He holds a PhD in social work. His doctoral thesis was on birth fathers in adoption. Dr. Clapton qualified as a social worker in 1977 and has practiced for 40 years in the field of children and families. He attained a readership in social work at the University of Edinburgh in 2019, where he has taught and researched since 2003. His main interests and specialties include children and family social work practice, fathers and fatherhood, and adoption as it affects adults. He is also widely published on other topics, such as moral panics.

Contributors

Christopher F. Deeg, PhD, is a licensed psychologist with over 30 years' experience treating adopted persons and those related to, or in relationship with, adopted persons. Dr. Deeg has training in cognitive-behavioral, interpersonal therapy and advanced training in psychoanalysis and psychoanalytic psychotherapy. He is the author of several papers and a textbook chapter on the psychology of adoption and the treatment of adopted persons. Dr. Deeg's writings formulate a framework of the intrapsychic world of the adopted person based on the object relation of adopted self to birth parent. Previously, he was an adjunct assistant professor of psychology at Hofstra University. Dr. Deeg maintains a private practice and also provides consultation to adopted persons and their families, and to adoption agencies, pediatricians, and mental health professionals. He is listed in a metropolitan New York–based directory of qualified senior psychotherapists who can provide teleconsultation both nationally (USA) and internationally.

Sue Green, PhD, is a psychologist and adoptee who has been involved in the Australian adoption community for over 37 years. She was actively involved in getting changes to the *Victorian Adoption Act* (1984), which gave adoptees access to their adoption records and original birth certificates. In response to the Victorian state government apology for past and forced adoption practices, she developed a two-day competency-based training program and manual, *Working with Loss and Trauma Related to Past and Forced Adoption Practices* (2nd ed. 2017), which has been delivered to over 350 social workers, psychologists, and counselors. Sue has presented at conferences and run numerous workshops in adoption-related complexity and has been published by the Australian Psychological Society in *Working with Adopted People* (2014). She was also involved in the inquiry into *Responses to historical forced adoption in Victoria* (2022), which recommended access to free mental health services for those affected by historical adoption and further training for professionals. Sue maintains a small clinical practice providing therapeutic services to adoptees.

Rene A.C. Hoksbergen, PhD, has been a professor on the faculty of social sciences, Utrecht University, specializing in adoption, since 1984. He studied social psychology, pedagogics, and mathematical statistics at the University of Amsterdam prior to receiving his doctorate in 1972. He has held various posts in the fields of education and adoption and written or co-authored 35 books on adoption, adult education, modern procreation, and adolescence, some having been translated into English and German. He has also authored hundreds of articles in several journals of various countries, and he continues to counsel adoptees and adoptive parents in his clinical practice.

Alison Ingram is a theater practitioner of 40 years' experience. She trained with the American émigré to Australia Hayes Gordon, OBE, OA, founder of the Ensemble Theatre and the Ensemble Studios Acting School, Sydney. Alison studied Shakespeare at the Royal Academy of Dramatic Art, London (1990 and 1994), receiving an invitation in 1995 from New York–based theater company The Shakespeare Project Inc. to perform, direct, and develop theater programs for at-risk teens. She is nearing completion of her theater and performance doctoral research. A play, "*Infans,* VOIC'D: A History Play in Five Acts," was developed with six research participants, an ensemble of seven Australian-born adult adoptees placed under the closed record system. The play, performed in Melbourne, bears testimony to the lifelong impact of being adopted.

Catherine Margaret Lynch, PhD, JD, is a practicing Australian lawyer and founding member and vice president of Adoptee Rights Australia Inc. She researches current mother–baby separation practices in child protection, local and intercountry adoption, and surrogacy, and her work foregrounds not the users of adoption systems and reproductive technologies but the people used or created by them. She is part of the global abolitionist movement to stop mother–baby separation practices because of their intrinsic cruelty. Her publications include the chapter "The Symbol of the Separated Mother and Child in Peter Carey's True History of the Kelly Gang" (*Australia: Who Cares?* David Callahan (ed.) Perth: Network Books, 2007) and articles and book reviews in *Australian Studies* (British Australian Studies Association, 2006), the *Australian Journal of Adoption* (National Library of Australia, 2011 and 2012), and *Dissent* (Sydney Uni. Law Society, 2013). Her most recent chapter, "Putting Children First; What Adoption Can Teach Us About Surrogacy" in *Towards the Abolition of Surrogate Motherhood*, Marie-Josèphe Devillers and Ana-Luana Stoicea-Deram (eds.) (2021), has been published for the International Coalition for the Abolition of Surrogate Motherhood in English (Spinifex Press) and French (L'échappée) and is soon to be published in Spanish.

Linda Mayers, PhD, originally from Montreal, Canada, is in private practice in New York City. She is a past director of training, training, and supervising analyst of the Institute of the Postgraduate Psychoanalytic Society; an adjunct associate professor at LaGuardia Community College, City University of New York; a former director of continuing education, faculty, and supervisor at Washington Square Institute; a faculty, senior supervisor, and former president of the Professional Board of the Postgraduate Center for Mental Health; and a former adjunct clinical professor at City University, Teachers College–Columbia University, and Yeshiva University. She is a member of the editorial board of *Journal of Infant, Child and Adolescent Psychotherapy* and editorial reader, *International Forum of Psychoanalysis*. She is a founding member of Psychoanalysis, Art and Creativity, a member organization of the International Society for Art and Psychology. Dr. Mayers has published in the psychology of adoption (co-editor and author of an article for the Adoption Journey, Psychoanalytic Inquiry, Vol. 30, Number 1, January–February 2010, Routledge), art and psychoanalysis, tattoos, the history of mental illness, and infant–parent disturbances. She is in the metropolitan New York–based directory of senior psychotherapists specializing in adoption and offering online teleconsultation nationally and internationally. She is an adoptive mother of a young adult son.

Contributors

Laurie C. Miller, MD, is a professor of pediatrics, adjunct professor of nutrition and of child development, Tufts University (Boston, MA, USA), and senior consultant to the National Center for Adoption and Permanency. She has published more than 120 peer-reviewed articles and more than 40 chapters related to pediatrics, international child health, and international adoption and two books (*Handbook of International Adoption Medicine*, Oxford University Press, and *Encyclopedia of Adoption* [with C. Adamic], Facts on File). She is currently a visiting professor in the Department of Child Psychiatry at Ste. Anne's Hospital (adoption consultation service) and the International Adoption Clinic at Necker Hospital in Paris, France.

Stefania Muzi, PhD, PsyD candidate, is a post-doc research fellow in clinical psychology at the Department of Educational Science at the University of Genoa. She is also a clinical psychologist and an associated member of the Italian Association of Psychology (AIP). She received her PhD in social sciences at the Department of Educational Science at the University of Genoa, and her MA in clinical and community psychology. Her research interests concern assessment methods and mental health outcomes of attachment, emotion regulation, and adverse childhood experiences in adolescence; attachment-based intervention and applications; clinical outcomes of residential care, foster care, and adoption; and binge-eating disorder. Since 2017, she has published 21 contributions on Scopus.

Steven L. Nickman, MD, was educated at Princeton University and Duke Medical School. His pediatric training was at Montefiore Hospital in New York and the Children's Hospital of Philadelphia. He was trained in adult and child psychiatry at Massachusetts General Hospital and the Judge Baker Guidance Center, both in Boston. He is board-certified in pediatrics and psychiatry and an affiliate member of the Boston Psychoanalytic Society. Dr. Nickman was co-chair of the Adoption and Foster Care Committee of the American Academy of Child and Adolescent Psychiatry and co-leader of the Interdisciplinary Adoption Study Group in Boston. His clinical work includes over 50 years in private practice, 42 years at Massachusetts General Hospital (child psychiatry), 2 years at Boston Floating Hospital for Children, 19 years at the New Bedford Center for Human Services, and 4 years at the New England Home for Little Wanderers. He has worked with over 400 adoptees and their families, as well as having teaching responsibilities with child psychiatry trainees and early-career social workers and psychologists. He has an adopted son, now an adult, whose questions led to his strong interest in adoption.

Cecilia S. Pace, PhD (corresponding author), is an associate professor of clinical psychology at the Department of Educational Science at the University of Genoa. She is also a clinical psychologist and psychotherapist. She received her MA in clinical and community psychology, her PhD in dynamic, clinical, and developmental psychology, and her post-doctorate at Sapienza, University of Rome. She is a full member of the Italian Association of Psychology (AIP). She has 20 years of experience in working with adoptive families from an attachment perspective. Her research interests concern assessment methods and clinical applications of attachment theory, including attachment-based intervention, adoption, residential care, adolescents, adverse childhood experiences, emotion regulation, alexithymia, mental health outcomes, and eating disorders. Since 2009, she has published 48 contributions on Scopus.

Elaine E. Schulte, MD, MPH, is the vice chair, academic affairs and faculty development, and a professor of pediatrics, the Children's Hospital at Montefiore, Albert Einstein College of Medicine (Bronx, NY), and the medical director, Adoption Program. In the early 1990s, she started one of the first comprehensive adoption programs in the United States, providing pre-adoption consultation, post-adoption screening, and ongoing primary care. She has cared for thousands of adopted children/adolescents and their families. She served as a member of the American Academy of Pediatrics Executive Committee for the Council on Foster Care, Adoption, and Kinship Care. She is an adoptive parent.

Jay Vaughan, MBE, has a postgraduate diploma in dramatherapy and is a dyadic developmental psychotherapist, theraplay practitioner, and somatic experience practitioner. She has worked with adopted, fostered, and special guardianship children for over 30 years. She co-founded Family Futures and is a co-developer of the NPP model of assessment and treatment along with Alan John Burnell. Jay has a particular interest in body-based approaches and working with trauma in the nervous system as part of supporting children and young people in healing from trauma.

FOREWORD

This volume, *The Handbook on the Clinical Treatment of Adopted Adolescents and Young Adults*, edited by Doris Bertocci, Christopher F. Deeg, and Linda Mayers, is a unique contribution to the field of clinicians working with adopted children, adolescents, emerging adults, and beyond, as well as for developmental researchers. It is actually surprising that this volume counts as one of first and perhaps only compilation to focus on the specific features of the internal world of adopted older children, adolescents, and young adults. The volume provides a unique blend of perspectives which offer what the authors describe as "adoption-specific knowledge" that is essential for health and mental health professionals in their care of adopted young people. This knowledge base includes all that we know from empirical studies of adopted children, along with clinical explorations in the context of therapeutic relationships with adopted patients as they grow into adulthood. Both of these sources should go in the clinical toolbox of all clinicians, as they provide knowledge of the critical features of the experience of *being adopted* and its links with trauma, the development of identity, and the ways of understanding complex changes over time. These become integrated with the attachment relationship with the adoptive parents, as well as with the experience they may have in psychotherapy.

The permanent removal of a child from their family of origin is perhaps among the most significant traumatic forces impacting human development that exists. Given the gravity of its effect on children, it has also been found that adoption is the most effective solution available for repairing psychological difficulties for children who have suffered from early adversity. We also know that there are myriad routes taken when a child is relinquished from the care of birth parents to be fostered or adopted. Each child's path to adoption is unique, but there are commonalities among them which are imperative for clinicians to be familiar with so that they can acknowledge the significance of their role in their adopted patients' mental health.

Understanding the complexities inherent in the change from often-chaotic or insensitive care with birth or foster parents, which often is rife with repeated disruptions and impingements on their development, can ultimately help us clarify the factors associated with better outcomes over time. Meanwhile, the adoptive parents are charged with the unique task of taking on a new and different attachment relationship than perhaps one they had imagined.

An attachment theory and research perspective (Bowlby, 1969, 1973; Ainsworth et al., 1978) points to the power of the caregiving environment in the development of an "internal working model" of the adopted young person's self and attachment figure(s) which organizes thoughts and feelings regarding relationships and guides expectations regarding the nature of future interactions. The challenge for adults interacting with children and adolescents, whether they be birth parents, adoptive parents, or teachers, is to recognize that a young person's sense of self and others, of expectations and behavior, has developed out of many interactions with a range of caretakers whose functioning reflects their own internal working models. The representations in the minds of those who faced non-optimal caregiving won't necessarily be as smoothly functioning as the internal working models that are formed in the minds of youth lucky enough to have the sensitive and attuned caregiving that enables attachment security. Otherwise, erratic, chaotic, irrational, and often-aggressive behavior follows.

In our study of "Attachment Representations and Adoption Outcome" (Hodges & Steele, 2000; Steele et al., 2003; Hillman et al., 2020), we found compelling evidence for the influence of parental states of mind assessed with the Adult Attachment Interview (Main et al., 1985). The study highlighted the intergenerational transmission of attachment capacities in non-biologically related dyads by showing that, overall, most of the children exhibited an increase in positive attachment themes from the time of the initial placement. Most importantly, the children who were placed with parents who demonstrated autonomous, secure responses to the AAI were also able to show declines in the negative themes over time. This finding illuminates a critical feature of working with traumatized young people, namely, that **it is easier for them to take on new positive representations through carefully selected adoptive parents** than to ameliorate the negative or toxic representations, that is, through "trauma treatment," which otherwise continue to exert an influence.

While the use of evidence-based assessments such as the Adult Attachment Interview requires specialized training, it is crucial that clinicians working with clients within an adoption context be familiar with the extensive research base underlying the clinically rich material the Interview reveals, affording a unique window into the attachment system. The Interview is especially useful as it explores not only the probable experiences of the caregiving system(s) but also, and perhaps more importantly, the individual's current states of mind with regard to attachment. The Interview often "surprises the unconscious" by asking questions not usually asked, even in clinical contexts, such as "What would you do when you are upset as a child?" or "Why do you think your parents behaved as they did during your childhood?" The coding of the interviews assesses how loving, rejecting, derogating each of the caregivers was, as well as the overall coherence of the narrative. In addition to Main et al. (2003), we include a coding of "reflective functioning" (Fonagy et al., 1998) which has shown to be one of the most important markers for mental health, as it provides a window on the coming to terms with adversity, and it offers important indicators to the possibility of therapeutic engagement and outcome.

Aside from specific research findings that may help clinicians in their treatment, when it is in the context of treating those who are adopted, the health-care professional must start with this handbook as a critical introduction to the complexities in the treatment of adopted individuals of any age.

Miriam Steele, PhD, is the Alfred J. and Monette C. Marrow professor in psychology and co-director of the Center for Attachment Research at the New School for Social Research in New York City. She has authored over 120 peer-reviewed papers, including those that initiated the concept of "reflective functioning" as the underlying mechanism in intergenerational patterns of attachment in parents and their children, and the central catalyst for change in psychotherapeutic interventions. She has also been involved in the longitudinal study of attachment representations in families who adopted previously maltreated children and who were followed up in early and middle childhood, adolescence, and adulthood. She has been the honored recipient of the Bowlby-Ainsworth Award and the American Psychological Association Division 39 Research award.

Miriam Steele, PhD

Endnotes

Ainsworth, M.D.S., Blehar, M.C., Waters, E., & Wall, S. (1978). *Patterns of Attachment*. Hillsdale: Lawrence Erlbaum.

Bowlby, J. (1969). *Attachment and Loss, Vol 1, Attachment*. New York: Basic Books.

Bowlby, J. (1973). *Attachment and Loss, Vol 2, Separation, Anxiety and Anger*. New York: Basic Books.

Fonagy, P., Target, M., Steele, H., & Steele, M. (1998). *Reflective-Functioning Manual Version 5 for Application to Adult Attachment Interviews* (Unpublished manuscript).

Hillman, S., Hodges, J., Steele, M., Cirasola, A., Asquith, K., & Kaniuk, J. (2020). Assessing changes in the internal worlds of early- and late-adopted children using the Story Stem Assessment Profile (SSAP). *Adoption & Fostering*, 44(4), 377–396.

Hodges, J., & Steele, M. (2000). Effects of abuse on attachment representations: Narrative assessments of abused children. *Journal of Child Psychotherapy*, 26(3), 433–455.

Main, M., Goldwyn, R., & Hesse, E. (2003). *The Adult Attachment Interview: Scoring and Classification System, Version 7.2* (Unpublished manuscript). Berkeley, CA: University of California.

Main, M., Kaplan, N., & Cassidy, J. (1985). Security in infancy, childhood, and adulthood: A move to the representational level. In I. Bretherton, & E. Waters (Eds.), *Growing Points of Attachment Theory and Research. Monographs of the Society for Research in Child Development, 50* (1–2). Hoboken, NJ: Wiley, pp. 66–104.

Steele, M., Hodges, J., Kaniuk, J., Hillman, S., & Henderson, K. (2003). Attachment representations and adoption: Associations between maternal states of mind and emotion narratives in previously maltreated children. *Journal of Child Psychotherapy, 29*(2), 187–205.

Steele, M., Hodges, J., Kaniuk, J., Steele, H., Asquith, K., & Hillman, S. (2008). Forecasting outcomes in previously maltreated children: The use of the AAI in a longitudinal adoption study. In H. Steele, & M. Steele (Eds.), *Clinical Applications of the Adult Attachment Interview*. New York: Guildford Press.

PART I

Introduction

The Impact of the Adoption, Legal, and Mental Health Systems on the Development of Adopted Adolescents and Young Adults

Doris Bertocci, LCSW; Christopher F. Deeg, PhD; and Linda Mayers, PhD

The mission of this book is to introduce what the authors see as the reality and complexity in the lives of adopted adolescents and young adults. This specialized area of adoption has not been adequately understood because the health and mental health fields have limited their focus to younger children, with the expectation that any behavioral and/or emotional adjustments related to being adopted would be resolved before adolescence. Because many such assumptions of the adoption culture remain in the thinking of health-care professionals and psychotherapists, they continue to practice with outdated notions of what is involved developmentally, and for life, in being adopted. We are aware that recognition of our clinical perspective will likely require significant changes in the thinking of the adoption, health, and mental health fields, with many implications as well for the allied fields in social service, education, health sciences, and law. We believe that this recognition is long overdue.

Most importantly, this handbook brings in the voice of the adopted person from several sources, including a number of the authors who are adopted themselves and are also clinicians. The authors are familiar with the autobiographical publications of adopted people, which often include memories of their adolescence and young adulthood, as in Chapter 3 by three Australian authors who are adopted and are professionals in three different fields. We cite the most recent literature and research from the fields of adoption, child welfare, social service, social work, sociology, and clinical psychology, and our updated bibliographies provide a rich resource for further study. Finally, there are many adopted people and adoptive parents in our own families, and those of us who are primarily psychotherapists and physicians have extensive experience working with adopted people of all ages.

Most of the adoption literature on assessment and treatment focuses on adoptive families and their pre-adolescent children. It is intended primarily for a readership of adoptive parents and "adoption professionals," including the broad fields of child welfare and social service (Wrobel et al., 2020). This handbook, however, attempts to address the needs primarily of health and mental health professionals who provide services in diverse clinical settings where adopted patients may be seen more at random. These settings range from private treatment services, including private practice, to family therapy settings; hospital inpatient, outpatient, and intensive outpatient treatment programs; and services offering clinical specialties, such as for anxiety disorders or depression, eating disorders, dual diagnosis, trauma, and attachment. Clinicians in these settings are generally not trained to know the complexities in the psychology of *being adopted*, for which reason they are inclined to minimize its significance and to proceed with the usual conventional treatment. In the hope of changing this thinking, this handbook is offered as a clinical introduction to the psychology of *being adopted*, with particular reference to adolescence and young adulthood. Their treatment has been neglected in research, scholarship, and training, at all tiers of the mental health disciplines.

Our chapters have the goal of not only deepening and expanding practitioners' understanding of the psychology of being adopted, but also woven throughout the chapters are the authors' recommendations for the many modifications needed in the general practices of health and mental health professionals. Regardless of how the patient/client conceptualizes and understands the concerns they bring to us as mental health professionals, and regardless of whether these concerns have any relationship to being adopted, we believe that the treatment of adopted persons is a complex clinical specialty. The authors explain why, especially regarding those in the designated 13-30 age range. This requires that psychotherapists work from a broader but also more in-depth and adoption-specific knowledge base that begins with this handbook. It also requires health-care professionals to be prepared to commit the additional time needed for addressing adopted clients' unique needs – and for acquiring the knowledge base needed in order to provide the highly skilled psychotherapy that they deserve.

The editors want to share one of our fundamental positions at the outset: there is nothing "pathological" about being adopted. Further, clinicians trained in the traditional mental health disciplines do not "pathologize adoption." Our authors try to identify ways that therapists can help adopted persons learn alternate but healthy, or potentially healthier, ways to respond to their non-normative circumstances. And for professionals working in the overlap of adoption, health, mental health, and law, we try to identify more effective ways to work with, or on behalf of, adopted clients while also addressing the serious systemic problems that need to change. For psychotherapists, regardless of the presenting problem, this requires modifications in evaluation and treatment that are based on an understanding of

Introduction

the *alternate development* of the adopted person. Most importantly, we believe *the pathology is in the systemic dysfunction*, in both domestic and international domains of adoption, that significantly impacts, and contributes to, the developmental challenges of adopted people as identified and discussed throughout the book. Further, we believe that by far most of their adjustments, complicated as they can be at times, do not reach the level of clinical significance. Also, in the specified age range, the mere fact that an adopted person has seen one or two psychotherapists does not serve research purposes of quantifying "psychopathology" in adopted patients. In fact, in the college and graduate school years, or when young adults have jobs in the USA, the UK, and the most western countries, therapy is fairly routine for age-appropriate concerns. Finally, we have no question but that adoptive placement, if handled by qualified professionals, is the best option over foster care and group/institutional settings, given the child's own particular circumstances. We also have much to say about the deficiencies and inertia of the legal system that contribute to the children's trauma.

We believe that, by definition, the psychology of *being* adopted requires inclusion of clinical perspectives that, depending on the goals of the client/patient, warrant a good deal more than "support" and "cognitive behavioral" or psychoeducational approaches to treatment. Psychodynamically informed clinical perspectives represented in this book bring in the dimension of the adopted person's *internal* life, that underlies outward behavior, which the health-care field and allied disciplines, and most adoption research, have not sufficiently understood or reflected in their work. At the same time, there is no presumption that what we have learned from the adopted people with whom we have worked clinically can be found to the same degree, or necessarily with the same themes or emphasis, as adopted persons in the general population: there is no one script by which adoption issues emerge or are to be addressed in treatment, and each adopted person is different from the other. Generally, there is no avoiding the impact of adoption despite the very best circumstances that an adoptive home can offer. But when adopted youth and their parents seek treatment, engagement requires psychotherapists to learn "the language of adoption," as it will come up and need clarification within treatment, but they also need training in special considerations in *therapeutic process* when treating adopted patients.

Primarily, this book provides an in-depth understanding of the adopted person's experience *from birth* in responding to "events," external and internal, not experienced by the non-adopted population. This relates to the meanings they ascribe to these experiences and, overall, to their *alternate* development in many areas over time, which begins with the permanent separation from their birth mother, typically at a critical developmental time. Although generally dismissed by the health-care and mental health fields, the significance of this particular "event" is beginning to have the support of neonatology and the most recent neurobiological research. We add the further observation that, granting the many challenges in their own development, most foster children (in-care) have not experienced this "primal wound" (Verrier, 1993) within the critical first few months of life. Yet those working in foster care, not trained to understand the complexities of being adopted, typically think of adopted youth as "the lucky ones."

The Paths to Adoption

To understand the psychology of *being* adopted, it is necessary to have a basic knowledge of the primary paths taken to adopting a child, and of the common clinical issues for adopted individuals that relate to each pathway.

Other than through stepparent adoptions, in North America children enter adoptive families through four primary sources, not the commonly referenced three:

1. The majority of placements are through the child welfare system (a.k.a. child protection systems), that is, through foster care, handled by an insufficient, poorly compensated workforce with limited training typically trying to manage large caseloads. The children have generally had traumatic experiences, such as abuse, neglect, or abandonment, that brought them to the attention of child welfare and legal authorities. Before being adopted, most spent some time in one or several foster homes or in a group care/residential setting. The law's inertia in legalizing their adoptions, if this becomes the plan, and the long wait involved for the child contribute enormously to the child's stress. Funding for child placement services within public welfare departments is the responsibility of the government, but it has usually been unwilling to provide sufficient support for the hiring of qualified staff as recommended in this book.
2. The second route for adoption was the most common through much of the twentieth century, that is, professionally staffed, often clinically trained, private adoption agencies that established and followed high professional standards for selection of parents who wanted to adopt as a presumed protection for the child. However, since the latter part of the twentieth century, this option has become very limited because of social changes allowing more birth mothers to keep their babies and also because of inadequate financial support for their professionalized services. As a result, most private adoption agencies either closed or shifted to handling foster care. When adults whom they had originally placed return seeking information from their records, private agencies typically offer very limited, if any, service. This is at a time that the adopted person is most vulnerable and has the greatest need for adoption-knowledgeable professional services. The question needs to be raised whether such perfunctory practice would meet the criteria for unethical practice. This question is raised on the grounds that, for many adopted persons, it does great harm emotionally because of the intensity of the impact at such a time.
3. With the much-preferred youngest children (infants and babies) rarely being available for adoption, there was the rise in international adoptive placements, which peaked in 2004. This has continued to decline precipitously, largely

because countries did respond to the important research findings about the resulting difficulties for the children and shifted to trying to find families within their own country to adopt them. But the decline is also related to child trafficking even in subtle forms, adoption corruption, and/or the failure to comply with the 1993 Hague Convention on Intercountry Adoption for countries that are signatories to it. It is time for greater accountability. One of the overall themes of this book is that the role of adoption placement resources continues to be primarily recruiting adoptive parents and placing children rather than developing ongoing treatment programs and other services for adoptive families and adopted persons, even for traumatized children, which are particularly needed for minority families (Fong & McRoy, 2016; Jackson & Samuels, 2019).

4. In the 1980s and 1990s, potential adoptive parents in the United States came to perceive the professional adoption agencies as excessively rigid and narrow in their requirements. And so, the fourth route for finding babies became the placement of personal ads in the media intended for women with unwanted pregnancies, and the procurement of lawyers to draw up a legal contract. This practice, "private" or "independent" adoption (not to be confused with private agency adoption), has greatly expanded into the twenty-first century, while the prior standards and requirements intended to protect the child have been replaced by only the most general legal guidelines, as lawyers tend to prefer. In the popular press in the USA, they are referred to as "baby brokers." In effect, the lawyer represents only the adults seeking to adopt, while the child is provided no representation of its own or protection by a child development professional. As long as the home study can be outsourced, not necessarily to well-qualified people, lawyers do not see it as a conflict of interest. It is not the child who is paying the bill. Meanwhile, the birth mother is given little assistance with her decision, which might delay the actual adoption process, or with the follow-up care she may need. The lawyers represent only the people adopting.

It is noteworthy that in the United States, the professional adoption literature reports research results focused only on the first three sources for finding a child to adopt, while there are no known statistics or studies on private/independent adoptions, where we have reason to believe that the risks for the children are likely to be greatest. We are aware that any inquiry into this common "pathway" in the United States would meet great resistance from adoption lawyers, who stand to benefit substantially from the current system where it is allowed. Based on anecdotal reports within the United States, the impact of these private (legally handled) adoptions has significant consequences for the adopted person's mental health. Some countries prohibit it, for good reason: A prominent psychiatric intensive treatment program for young adults in the United States, which has the usual disproportionate number of adopted patients, estimates that half of them are from international adoptions and the other half had been placed privately through lawyers. We cannot know to what extent these estimates would also be found in other programs, because it has never been studied. This handbook identifies multiple areas begging for clinical research, including the context of residential and hospital programs, a crucial variable being the sources of their patients' adoptions.

In our experience, adoptive families and adopted persons have been frequently and directly failed by the traditional mental health field, because it has been unwilling to acknowledge or learn about the complexities of the psychological needs of this subgroup of the population. It typically justifies its position on the basis of this subgroup being relatively small in numbers. By contrast, in medicine, unique and exceptionally complex cases in small numbers tend to generate great interest. Instead, adopted patients are often misdiagnosed, for example, as having borderline conditions, when it is the way they try to explain their external circumstances and their attempts to survive them that give this impression. For example, they may use odd wording, such as "I have never known who I am," or "when I look in a mirror I just see a blank," that is most likely a (false) red flag diagnostically. These are actually typical symptoms of mild dissociation related to early developmental trauma. However, anecdotally, a consensus of some clinicians who are adopted themselves is that "being adopted can be a very 'borderline' experience." With what we now know about the complexities in treating adopted clients, "best practices" would call for therapists to have advanced training *before* taking on an adopted client to treat, yet therapists typically believe they already know enough. Psychotherapy of adopted patients/clients often results in adoption issues being ignored or minimized, misinterpreted as something else, or misunderstood as being no different from those of any other patient or family (e.g., *generic* trauma and attachment). In the minds of society and of health/mental health care, treatment is most often focused only on helping with the parenting of pre-adolescent children and on treating the child, or on emphasizing family therapy as the primary and most important treatment modality, even when the child is an adolescent.

In short, at the present time, the mental health field's understanding of the adopted person has been arrested in childhood, with adolescence little more than an afterthought, and with young adulthood nowhere on the radar. We maintain that because of the profound physical and psychological changes that are ushered in by adolescence, the fullest impact and complexity of *being* adopted is usually in adolescence and young adulthood, not in earlier childhood.

The Three Fundamental Areas of Developmental Challenge

The psychology of *being* adopted at any age involves three fundamental areas of complexity, and in many cases potential difficulty, in the adopted person's development:

1. Traumatic loss related to the separation from (severance of) the birth mother, followed in many cases by subsequent losses due to disruptions and changes in caretakers prior to adoptive placement.

Introduction

2. Disruptions in forming and maintaining attachments that are likely to take a toll prior to placement but also post-placement, typically in the form of anxious or ambivalent attachments, or difficulties around trust, that can remain a problem into adolescence and adulthood. This rarely meets the criteria for RAD (reactive attachment disorder), although, unfortunately, too often therapists associate it with adopted children.
3. Complexities in the adopted person's struggle to develop an organized, coherent personal identity while, in the limited understanding of the mental health field, "identity" remains little more than a label. Therapists are not trained to understand what the struggle is about.

Those of our authors who are psychodynamically trained clinicians emphasize the powerful impact of underlying intrapsychic and unconscious phenomena that are understood to be integral to the psychology of being adopted, operating within all three areas of vulnerability. This form of treatment takes many years to learn in order to accomplish the enduring changes that many adopted persons seek, while "adoption professionals" have more immediate goals in the counseling services they customarily provide families and children. The latter are offered in entirely different settings (social service) from clinical services provided through the mental health field. For example, Christopher F. Deeg's two chapters explain, from a psychoanalytic perspective of treating the adopted patient, how the intrapsychic encoding of the representation of the birth mother interacts with the representation of the adopted self throughout the life cycle and critically determines identity formation as well as the adopted person's interpersonal relationships. Dr. Deeg explains further that the internalized relation of adopted self to birth mother is revived during treatment and becomes the central dynamic of the adopted person's psychotherapy. Overall, from a clinical perspective, the editors contend that meeting the full needs of many adopted adolescents and adults – if they are skillfully and thoroughly evaluated – requires much more than the customary skills of social workers and counselors who provide support and important psychoeducation at a cognitive level, address intra-familial needs (e.g., birth parents, foster parents, and adoptive parents), and perhaps suggest additional resources.

All the clinical complexities addressed in this book, distinguishing the adopted person from the non-adopted, have always been *hidden in plain sight*. Yet the mental health field continues to dismiss the need for specialized training, and so therapists continue to treat their adopted patients no differently from any others. Of particular concern in this regard is the highly disproportionate number of adopted patients, especially adolescents, admitted to intensive treatment programs, hospitals, and residential settings, which generally provide little or no adoption-informed treatment or services for either the patient or the family and that typically make only the routine discharge plans. Or in the case of many residential programs, they do not hire sufficiently trained staff to provide the advanced level of treatment each adopted young person needs at a critical time in their development. In all cases, the programs are primarily group therapy, typically run by social workers or counselors. The perspective of this book is that such programs, including hospitals, do not meet the necessary standards for best practices in the treatment of their adopted patients, particularly in institutions/hospitals that have otherwise distinguished themselves. In particular, they are inadequately trained in the complexities and impact of early developmental trauma on the adopted patient, in its sequelae in adolescence and young adulthood, and in adoption-specialized protocols for evaluation and treatment of trauma (McSherry et al., 2022), attachment (see Foreword), and fragmented identity as addressed throughout this handbook. In the hospital acute-care setting, this becomes particularly salient for making appropriate discharge plans, but presently, hospitals do not give consideration to making arrangements for ongoing treatment with adoption-knowledgeable clinicians.

In summary, the combination of each child's innate traits along with factors relating to the birth parents, the pre-placement history, including any experiences in institutions or foster care, the handling of the adoptive placement, and the adoptive family all account for the significant diversity in the adopted population and for the many complexities in each adopted person's personality organization. These include the details and variations within each of the three major areas of vulnerability identified here, along with the great differences among adopted persons in resilience, in internal and external resources, and in various random fortunate or unfortunate factors. While adopted persons share many experiences that the non-adopted world would not likely understand, each adopted person is still very different from the non-adopted and also from each other.

Topics Important to Clinical Evaluation and Treatment

Chapters following our **Introduction** lay the groundwork with a review of the many systemic problems that contribute to adopted persons' developmental challenges (Chapter 1), followed by an updated account by Rene Hoksbergen, a prominent researcher and therapist from the Netherlands. He reflects back on his long career in the adoption field and concludes with his concerns about the direction in which the international demand for young babies is going. He discusses his observations on past and current adoption placement practices which he believes are not handled by sufficiently trained personnel, whose work continues to be based on assumptions, belief systems, and practices of an earlier era. At the same time, the authors recognize that adoption workers continue to struggle against governmental neglect in providing adequate financial resources for the full range of services needed in order to protect the most vulnerable, namely, *the children*, and to assist their families over time. This problem is echoed in other chapters.

But further, the editors question the appropriateness of public welfare departments, mandated to arrange concrete services for the financially disadvantaged but also to monitor limits in benefits, handling adoptive placements at all. This is because very different roles and far different training and more advanced skills are required in order to give priority to the needs of the most vulnerable, traumatized children. A high level of clinical skill is also necessary for the process of screening potential parents that is both sensitive and professionally astute, as concluded in the chapter by Dr. Hoksbergen. The editors argue for active advocacy through a joint effort between the adoption and child health-care fields, not public welfare, for closer affiliations with each other and for the return of the highly professionalized adoption services where the importance of clinical training was recognized. However, this will require sufficient funding sources in order to provide both immediate and ongoing services for all who seek their help. This is the ethical and moral responsibility of all levels of government and, in turn, of the adoption and mental health fields.

The section that follows, **Developmental Complexities and Modifications in Assessment**, addresses the areas in which the adopted child's development differs significantly from that of the non-adopted child, with sequelae that become particularly complex and intense in adolescence. These include health, interpersonal, intra-familial, and sexual concerns that do not pertain either to younger children or to their non-adopted peers. Of particular note for therapists are the special considerations warranting an extended evaluation process. This would allow health and mental health practitioners to consider the benefit of additional diagnostic tests in order to identify developmental "fault lines" and to make more suitable and better-focused treatment plans. We emphasize that the developmental struggles are particularly intensified in adolescence and into young adulthood because the usual decisions about school, work, family relationships, sexuality, and choices of close personal relationships – that can have so many long-term consequences – are often infiltrated by adoption themes that carry particular risks. These might include re-enactments of abandonment themes in interpersonal relationships, poor choices of long-term partners, or avoidance of potentially life-enhancing experiences due to enduring struggles with low self-esteem, such as inability to accept a promising job in another location because of early neuropsychologically based problems with separation anxiety.

The section on developmental complexities is followed by Chapter 9 on **adoption medicine** as it relates to adopted adolescents and young adults, by two prominent American pediatricians in this relatively new medical specialty. Drs. Schulte and Miller have extensive clinical and administrative experience in adoption medicine domestically and internationally, and their work has included significant numbers of adolescents, including college students. Our perspective as editors, however, is that adoption medicine, which currently focuses primarily on new parents and adopted children under 3 years of age, should consider expanding to include adolescent mental health services because of the great need for specialists in the care of adopted adolescents generally.

"The Spectrum of Search and Reunion" serves as an updated account of the adopted person's search for birth relatives. The point is made, and already established in the literature, that this is both common and *normative for adopted persons*. However, contrary to claims in numerous references in the literature (Wrobel et al.,

2014; Godon-Decoteau & Ramsey, 2020), from a clinical perspective, the search is far beyond "normal curiosity," a notion that the cognitive perspective uses from common language so as to "normalize" it, but without understanding its actual significance. In contrast, the psychodynamic perspective informs us about the complexity of the adopted person's intrapsychic life, and although the search is still common and *normative for adopted individuals*, treatment in most cases needs to be based on a psychodynamic understanding of the underlying meanings to the adopted person. At the simplest level, the adopted individual is trying to understand their place in the world, how they came to be in it, how safe they are in being understood and protected, and how it relates to their concept and uncertainty about achieving a complete personal identity and a personal future. The search is also typically motivated *internally* by the adopted person's sense, conscious or unconscious, of being blocked in their development unless and until they can satisfy their craving to know about *and experience* their birth family and the reasons for their placement. These chapters attempt to explain the underlying needs, some of which derive from human instinct, that compel so many to engage in the search, along with suggested therapeutic responses to them if any aspect of search or meeting birth relatives ("reunion") comes up in treatment. These chapters also note that, regardless of what may be learned through a completed search, findings from the limited research, and also from massive anecdotal reports, from many countries, are that the completed search does meet the adopted person's internal needs significantly, and usually permanently (Chapter 10).

The final section of the book, **"Complexities of Psychotherapeutic Treatment,"** addresses considerations that need to be made in evaluation and treatment of adopted adolescents and young adults, including specialized interventions for more detailed evaluations, and specialized treatment approaches, such as use of the neurosequential model to address arrests in brain development, as discussed by our British authors in Chapter 13. Overall, the editors maintain that although other treatment modalities, such as those for trauma or attachment problems, may be helpful at particular junctures, treatment is not completed without incorporating these specific approaches into a fuller adoption-informed treatment plan, or at least inquiry, regarding the fuller scope of what the adopted patient may want in the future. That is, one cannot treat the trauma and consider the treatment completed. Since specialized training is required, priority now needs to be given to the development of advanced clinical training programs for all areas of the mental health field, particularly the traditional disciplines, including family therapy. At the same time, these will need to be developed within different countries to meet their own treatment conceptualizations, customs, and needs.

The Continuing Systemic Problems

Clinical social work brings to the mental health field the contention that a clinical understanding of the psychology of the adopted person requires a broader knowledge base regarding the larger system within which adoption operates. Our authors from

Introduction

India (Chapter 8) present their "ecological perspective" that incorporates systemic resources in work with the familiar "adoption triad" (adopted person, birth parents, adoptive parents). Their co-author from Ireland, a clinical social worker, adds her Western perspective. Clinical social work, as represented in this book, integrates its clinical perspective, which has typically included psychodynamic training, into its long history in the adoption field, along with its specialties in the full life span, family systems and intergenerational concerns, and systemic dynamics at a "macro level." As the twenty-first century approached, all these, along with its longstanding alliance with psychiatry, became particularly important in understanding the psychology of adoption, which automatically involves the long time frame of multiple families. This unique combination along with the knowledge base of other fields, such as education and special education, have added their own research results and perspectives. But most puzzling are the absent voices of those in developmental psychology.

At the same time, the editors and authors maintain that it is necessary to integrate the many *external* factors cited in the literature with a deeper understanding of the *internal* life and psychodynamics of being an adopted person in an adoptive family. However, until the present time, focus has still been primarily from the perspective of meeting the desires and needs of the adoptive *parents*. Into the twenty-first century, we have seen an increased blending of inquiry in clinical and counseling psychology, clinical social work, marriage and family treatment, psychiatry, and psychoanalysis. However, this integration of thought has not always come easily, and the focus has continued to be primarily on helping the adoptive family with adopted children to work together as a cohesive unit, but with little attention given to learning about the internal life and challenges for the adopted person her/himself.

Sociopolitically, much has changed in the twenty-first century. In Western countries, the typical birth mother/parent is more likely not a teen but an older woman who is parenting other children, with multiple psychosocial problems and limited resources. The law's contribution to her dilemma is that, as in other areas of family law, biological fathers are not involved or held responsible for helping in the child's support. The emphasis supported by legal practice is on foster care, while minimal attempts are made to "rehabilitate" the birth mother, that is, to assist her with stabilizing her life, regardless of whether there may even be such a possibility. In low-resource countries, the birth mother and the child are at risk due to the lack of access to adequate services and sometimes due to outright exploitation. Countries differ in their requirements for record-keeping and in the information that they make available to the adoptive parents. This means there are many variations in what information may or may not be available to the adopted adult at a time that they feel a need to have this information, perhaps also to search for their birth family, in order to consolidate their personal identity. This includes learning of any risks to their own health at a time in their life that, in some cases, becomes critical. The first chapter presents one such case of an adopted triplet whose treatment had to be conducted without knowledge of the significant inheritable disease in the birth family, resulting in his suicide.

Introduction

Regardless of whether the placement service is handled through a professional private adoption agency or through a welfare department or an international placement organization, or simply by a lawyer and a contract, the adoption field has never had a policy of taking ongoing responsibility for helping the adoptive family and the adopted person – particularly an adolescent in the throes of anxiety, bewilderment, and angry conflict – obtain adequate, adoption-knowledgeable services as may be needed over time. Questions need to be asked about why adoption reform over the past half century has come, by far, from grassroots rather than from the adoption field itself.

Conclusion

All adopted clients/patients vary enormously in their resilience and capacity for self-reflection in trying to understand themselves, their families, their relationships, and the relevance of their earlier histories to their current concerns. However, all adopted persons deserve careful consideration of the timing and form/s of treatment most suited to the integrative process they need to undergo as they grow up and mature into full adulthood. Adopted young adults in particular need to be able to make an informed decision about this, which obligates the therapist to provide an accurate explanation of their options from the beginning. Overall, this handbook attempts to bring together the relevant findings from the existing research and contributes reports of recent research in areas that have implications for clinical practice.

We are challenging the medical and mental health fields to consider the experiences and special needs of the individual who *should have been seen* as the primary recipient of adoption services **the adopted person her/himself** – but never was. Partly because of society's inclination to idealize adoption rather than understand it, the health-care field, along with its allies specifically in mental health, education, law, public health, and social service, is not accustomed to contemplating the many complications throughout life that have been the difficult experiences of many adopted people. There are ideas and recommendations throughout the book for greatly needed *clinically focused* research.

Finally, the editors of this volume, all with long clinical careers founded in psychodynamic perspectives, note the difficulty and strong reluctance of the mental health field not only to acknowledge the profound developmental differences between adopted and non-adopted clients but also to "think outside the box" beyond the early childhood years and beyond the traditional training within their discipline. Clinicians especially are challenged to contemplate the underlying psychodynamics in the mental health field itself of minimizing the complexities in being adopted, and to reflect in particular on the strong resistance within themselves.

Ultimately, the issues addressed in this book, and any progress in adoption reform, depend on a commitment to fundamental children's rights and, when children become adults, to their enduring human rights.

Introduction

Note 1: Within the text we include verbatim quotes from adopted people that capture the adopted person's unique reactions to various topics in the text, typically comments that would never be heard from those who are not adopted.

Note 2: In the context of discussing clinical treatment, the authors refer to adopted persons as "clients" or "patients" interchangeably, aware that these terms may vary according to the therapeutic setting. Also, without in any way underestimating the importance of kinship adoptive placements, most chapters refer to the special considerations in non-kinship adoption.

Endnotes

Fong, R., & McRoy, R. Eds. (2016). *Transracial and Intercountry Adoptions: Cultural Guidance for Professionals.* New York: Columbia University Press.

Godon-Decoteau, D., & Ramsey, P. (2020) Transracial adoptees: The rewards and challenges of searching for their birth families. In G.M. Wrobel, E. Helder, & E. Marr (Eds.), *The Routledge Handbook of Adoption.* London & New York: Routledge, pp. 238–252.

Jackson, K.F., & Samuels, G.M. (2019). *Multiracial Cultural Attunement.* Washington, DC NASW Press.

McSherry, D., Samuels, G., &. Brodzinsky, D., Eds. (2022). Exploring the relationship between adoption and trauma for children who are adopted from care: A longitudinal case study perspective. *Special Issue of Child Abuse and Neglect,* 130 (2), 105623.

Verrier, N. (1993). *The Primal Wound: Understanding the Adopted Child.* Baltimore, MD: Gateway Press, Inc.

Wrobel, G.M., Grotevant, H.D., Samek, D.R., & Von Korff, L. (2014). Adoptees' curiosity and information seeking about birth parents in emerging adulthood: Context, motivation, and behavior. *International Journal of Behavioral Development,* 37 (5), 441–450.

Wrobel, G.M., Helder, E., & Marr, E. Eds. (2020). *The Routledge Handbook of Adoption.* London & New York: Routledge.

1

THE LARGER CONTEXT OF SYSTEMIC FACTORS IN THE INTERFACE OF ADOPTION, MENTAL HEALTH, AND FAMILY LAW: HOW THEY RELATE TO CLINICAL PRACTICE

Doris Bertocci, LCSW, and Linda Mayers, PhD

Introduction

This chapter reviews some of the most fundamental systemic problems that impact the life of every adopted person and that are part of the adoption-specific information base from which psychotherapists need to work if they treat adopted clients, particularly those within the age span that is the focus of this book. While much is derived from our experience within the United States, many of the themes apply internationally as well. After briefly reviewing some of the legal issues and practices relating to adoptive placements, and some inconvenient truths that impact mental health care, discussion leads to a specific, recent case in the United States of multiple systemic blunders that eventually led to tragic results. This story has continued to reverberate in recent years in adoption and mental health discourse, at least in the United States. Extracted from this case are many common and ongoing themes representing the enduring dysfunctions in the adoption, child welfare, and legal systems at large. In the experience of clinicians with substantial knowledge about the psychology of adoption, there is the puzzling question about why mental health practitioners generally have not shown themselves to be particularly motivated to learn about the unique psychology of *being* adopted or about the treatment complexities involved, even when training opportunities are offered to them. This may partly derive from an adoption culture that, based on its historical contention that adopted children are, for the most part, "not very different from biological children," has felt no need to be concerned about the adopted person's fuller development into adolescence and adulthood. The limited interest within the mental health field, especially since the 1980s, has been referred to as its "conspiracy of silence" (Henderson, 2007).

In the thinking of mental health generally, adopted individuals continue to be simply – and simplistically – included among larger groups with seemingly common features, such as children in foster care, children with trauma, children with attachment problems, "acting out youth," adolescents and young adults with borderline features, etc. The field resists recognizing that although treatment of adopted persons requires many modifications in order to work skillfully with their developmental differences, it is a unique and challenging opportunity that no other patients can provide. Thus, within the overall clinical field presently, adopted patients/clients are denied any identity of their own (irony intended) by not being recognized as a subgroup distinguished by multiple complexities that, in many cases, include neurobiological changes resulting from early developmental trauma (Bick et al., 2017). For example, from a clinical perspective, it can be assumed that the adopted person may have at least "implicit memories" of other family members in their intrapsychic life, many say somatically as well, of not only the birth mother but also of early caretakers, siblings, and others from their earliest experiences. The mental health field, particularly the traditional disciplines, has not been trained to work with these complexities or to know the special considerations in history-taking, language, differential diagnosis, and treatment *process*. At the same time, counselors and most adoption professionals are not trained to work at an in-depth level with clients' internal (intrapsychic) lives. Overall, since each discipline working within the overlap of adoption and mental health tends to focus only on its own parameters for practice, there is insufficient interdisciplinary collaboration in this field, i.e., what the practitioner does not already know or understand may be considered unnecessary to learn. Regardless, there is growing consensus that treatment of the adopted person requires the inclusion of the adoption-specific components of the adopted client's life experience as addressed in this book. However, there is no consensus on the significance of psychodynamically based treatment to address the underlying (subconscious and unconscious) dynamics and conflicts within the adopted person and the adoptive family (Chapters 11 and 15). But from a clinical perspective, this is the "mother lode" of all that "in-depth" treatment that can work with in order to help the patient with the complexities of both their sexuality and their integration process.

Highly trained adoption placement professionals understand the meanings of *psychological* parenting. This refers to the importance of adoption workers being able to identify the nuances and consistent capacities of parent-applicants for emotional attunement with children over time and to the importance of keeping the transition period as short as possible in order to minimize the risk for the child of complex and enduring trauma (Goldstein et al., 1973; Taub, 1984; Spinak, 2007). But as one of the important themes of this handbook although not recognized by the adoption culture, given what is at stake for the child, advanced clinical skills are needed for evaluating all parent-applicants without depending on superficial interview formats, questionnaires, or testing protocols. The problem into the twenty-first century is that the meager financial support, resulting in the loss of most of the highly professionalized adoption agencies, reflects the degree to which children are devalued, especially those who are minorities (Fong & McRoy, 2016; Jackson & Samuels, 2019). Over the decades, incalculable numbers of children have been paying the price for the large-scale governmental neglect internationally. This includes high-resource countries like the United States that do not consider their own "self-interest" to include the provision of appropriate, dependable care for their most vulnerable citizens – their children.

The Role of Legal Processes

The impasses in permanency planning in the United States (Pertman, 2011) are largely and increasingly due to several factors within the legal system:

a. In the United States, even in family law, it is not in the legal culture to take into account the special needs of children, particularly those with early trauma, or to make legal decisions from a longitudinal perspective. Fundamentally, the child is viewed as collateral damage resulting from adult problems, about which judges hold hearings and eventually render decisions. Further, the judiciary is accustomed, as it deems necessary, to deferring decisions over months and even years. This also applies in other areas of family law, such as in child custody litigation. When children are involved and they are forced to wait indefinitely, for judicial decisions this likely means significant trauma that can profoundly impact their development even into adulthood.
b. As an integral complicating factor, inadequate staffing of the judiciary in the United States, which is the responsibility of the state legislature, results in a high volume and backlog of cases for judicial review and determination. Also, inadequate training of the judiciary, along with expedience, are often key factors in the quality of decisions made. In addition to those cases that involve adoption proceedings are the high numbers of young children consigned to "long-term temporary," sometimes very inadequate, care that may involve serial foster arrangements for months and years. Regardless of attempts to place a limit on the child's time in foster care, its oversight and enforcement have been seriously lacking.
c. Family court practices, which are based more on concepts of probate (property) law rather than special considerations for children, tend to yield to formulaic biases favoring "reunification of the family," regardless of whether it is actually in the "best interests of the child." In many cases, it is not, but like "shared custody" decisions, it is simply easiest and most expedient for the judge. Presently, in pre-adoption proceedings, judicial dilemmas keep many children in protracted foster

care in order to allow a sub-group of birth mothers extensive time to be "rehabilitated," regardless of the likelihood of this even being possible. The legal system does not see the need to include highly trained forensic evaluators as a means of both expediting and ensuring the best informed decisions on the child's behalf.

At the same time, family court practices and lawyers handling private adoptions fail to ensure skilled services for the birth mother regarding her decision (Madden et al., 2020). For example, if lack of financial resources is the primary reason a birth mother believes she cannot raise her child, as in other contexts, in the United States the law makes no effort to enlist and maintain financial support from the birth father. In a highly capitalistic society, the counterforce to providing appropriate help for the birth mother has always been the greater priority of accommodating the high demand for babies to adopt. Overall, if the judiciary were willing to be guided by the child's needs for permanency and placed with professionally screened adoptive parents, a time-limited structure needs to be installed for providing *professional* assistance to the birth mother in making a realistic plan that is sensitive to the child's needs, while also enforcing a time limit of weeks or months, not years, for termination of parental rights. On ethical grounds, the legislative system *must* attend to the short staffing of the judiciary in family law, enforce shorter time limits for children in foster care, but also ensure adequate financial support for continued *professional* oversight of children's care.

d. Long delays in international placements continue to be a problem for several reasons that vary from country to country and from political situation to political situation. These include the toxic combination of sociopolitically based national self-interest, and sometimes indifference to the needs and rights of children that may be partially based on cultural norms. It is certainly evident and likely where conservative values prevail, resulting in inadequate funding for the highly professionalized services required for protecting all children. Finally, adoption placement services have never taken responsibility for either providing or advocating for the adoptive family's access to affordable ongoing services with well-trained practitioners, not only "post-adoption," but also over subsequent years (Grotevant, 2020). This reflects the adoption culture's enduring perspective that, once the child is placed in an adoptive home, their job is done.

The Relevance for Therapists of Adoptive Placement Information

Into the twenty-first century, most paths or pathways to adoption (see Introduction) have increasingly been placing older and more developmentally challenged children, often out of foster care, while still not providing or transitioning the adoptive families to affordable, highly skilled ongoing post-adoption services (Barth & Miller, 2000; Welsh et al., 2007). One of the common misunderstandings of psychotherapists relates to the presumed rigor of pre-placement home studies. There is great inconsistency in training and skill for this part of the placement process, so much so that it warrants posing the long-overdue question of whether welfare departments, focused on financial and concrete services, are the appropriate setting for determining the future lives of vulnerable children, rather than highly professionalized child health-care settings. Clinicians know from their experience, treating internationally placed youth, that there are similar problems of seriously inadequate practice in the handling of international placements, including the lack of provision of ongoing post-adoption services that is left to the community.

Of great concern, in the large number of private ("independent") adoptions in the United States, there are no requirements, as a protection for the child, either that lawyers be credentialed through a national organization that provides the additional training needed or that lawyers handling adoptions work in tandem with child development specialists credentialed by the state, and whose priority is the best interests of the child. The lack of any studies or statistics in the United States on private adoptions, or of their outcomes, is another reflection of the overall neglect of children in the social infrastructure of high-resource Western countries. Private adoption arrangements involving only a legal contract have become common in the United States since the latter part of the twentieth century because they have been a preferred and relatively convenient route for adults hoping to adopt, since many want to avoid the scrutiny of the private adoption agency sector. Parents who could afford the legal fees were increasingly able to procure babies through the internet or through hospital staff members with access to newborn infants, and they needed only a lawyer to handle a contract. Even currently, if the birth mother is given a purported "choice" by selecting from profiles of people the lawyer may propose, lawyers do not have the training or credentials necessary to provide adequate evaluations of potential parents, not to mention the fact that the potential parents are paying the lawyer's bill. Further, lawyers handling private adoptions deny the birth mother the independent support or assistance of a qualified specialist so that she can make the most informed decision possible about placing her child. The problem here is that, lawyers' claims to the contrary, they have a conflict of interest in representing only the adults and presuming to represent the child at the same time. As in the legal culture more generally they also want independence from collaboration with other professionals who are viewed as interfering with their prerogatives. Similarly, the potential adoptive parents feel entitled to this arrangement since they located the child in the first place, and they want their parenthood ensured as soon as possible.

In short, psychotherapists need to know that, regardless of the means of accessing a child, since the latter part of the twentieth century, the quality of services throughout the placement process depends on a far more random mix of skills, financial support, and legal procedures that still may have only the most superficial grasp of the needs of the child. Overall, the system involving the overlap of adoption and law is inconsistent from jurisdiction to jurisdiction and has continued to be more focused on the desires of the adults, while the child, who is provided no protection at all, is treated as a commodity over which adults must compete.

The relevance of this for mental health professionals is that they are not accustomed to thinking of anyone's life, family, or experience growing up being determined by so many random external factors. This, in fact, is a component in the psychology of being adopted, that is, the realization of the role of randomness in their lives, which may then lead to the common question, asked in various ways, "If even one of these factors had been different, what family would I have ended up in?" They are really asking, "Who would I have become?" The meaning of this question for the adopted person is complex, but it may also be overdetermined. As an example of the therapist's important role in providing some balance to an adopted client's perspective, it could be pointed out that a good deal of both the beginnings and the outcomes of many families' lives can actually be traced to one or more random factors or to "wild coincidence," such as in the way parents initially met. There is also the scientific fact that for the most part, conception itself is a random event. As pointed out by the American psychologist Robert Plomin, fellow of the Academy of Medical Sciences and of the British Academy (Appendix 1), the twentieth century was about the crucial role in human development of the environment, especially the family. As we enter the third decade of the twenty-first century, this is still the assumption, but Dr. Plomin alerts us that this will be the century of revelations from the science of genetics and epigenetics.

Thus, the mission of adoption personnel, as they have continued to define it, has been limited to recruiting adoptive parents and handling the placement process, which they have referred to as the "rewarding" and "happy place" in the social service field. It is hard to sacrifice this pleasure in order to address the more complex adjustments that follow in the life of the *person* they placed. But in the larger picture of potential needs of the adoptive family and/or the adopted person a decade or more after placement, the term "post-adoption" no longer applies. This is because of the family's additional life experience with each other over time, that is, both the adoptive family and their adopted daughter or son, are in an entirely different place developmentally. Therefore, services would best be identified as "adoption knowledgeable," which refers to substance, as distinct from "adoption-sensitive," while also well-informed by the larger context of clinical findings from multiple areas relevant to the psychology of *being* adopted.

Further, from the beginning, it has never been agency practice to follow up their placements over time in order to offer assistance with any concerns the family may have, or with potential problems in the child's development – or to evaluate their own practices. This is based on the twentieth-century notion that outreach efforts would be intrusive but, further, that they were unnecessary, since adopted children were presumed to be little different from "biological" children anyway, so all should proceed "normally." This concept has been reflected in research that paradoxically has continued to compare "adopted" with "biological" children (Cohen et al., 1993; Bick & Dozier, 2010). The convenience of such language reflects the field's identification with the adoptive parents, which has pervaded adoption practice. As a derivative of this practice, adopted young adults from closed adoption have revealed variations on the fantasy that they must have origins other than biological, for example, perhaps they are "alien." Such a comment is entirely normative for adopted individuals, but any such reference a client may make to a therapist would likely result in diagnosis of borderline features. Some adopted youth have taken an interest in common fictional stories of seemingly ordinary children whose origins are concealed. Superman may be a "safe" fantasy for children born into their families, and it serves certain purposes psychologically. However, it has a clear reality when one is adopted. This duality of being either "born or adopted" could be a possible basis for anxiety for some adopted children, since prior to approximately their third year, they are not adequately equipped developmentally to comprehend a good deal of the adoption narrative. This pertains, even if explained in small amounts, with the risk of being confused or even *internally* overwhelmed by the narcissistic injury they must absorb (Chapter 5). But psychotherapists insufficiently trained in early childhood development are likely to dismiss the significance and meanings of the adoption narrative for the child.

> *There was never any reference in my family to pregnancy or birth, so I never even knew about it, but I knew what an agency was, because we had gone to one to get my little brother. When I was 4, I asked my mother where the agency got the babies from. After a long pause, she just said, "From seeds." But the only seeds I knew of were in packets for growing vegetables. I just guessed that when the time came, the babies were given to an adoption agency to find parents. I could never figure any of this out, so for a long time, I just gave up trying. The only thing I was sure of was that my mother didn't want to talk about it, so I learned not to ask. I never knew there was a birth parent until I was 13, when I found the agency papers in a file cabinet. Nothing was ever said about what "being born" meant. I had been told, "You're adopted," and finally I just decided to find out what they were talking about.*

This comment is important for its revelation that some adoptive family narratives, especially in the mid-twentieth century, omitted specific reference to the birth parents, unwittingly sparing the child from having to adjust at an early age to the concept of there having been another set of parents who decided not to keep her/him. In some cases, the adoptive parents choose to not tell their daughter or son about the adoption at all. These variations are the reason the clinical approach requires the therapist to follow the patient's lead rather than make typical assumptions, to "listen" for adoption themes and look for ways to pull the necessary threads, in order to explore the client's actual experience with learning about their adoption, along with the developmental timing of it and what it meant to them over the years.

The minimization of differences between being "born or adopted" have long served the adoption field as a marketing tool for attracting potential adoptive parents, even though the statistics, culture, and changes in adoption no longer justify this twentieth-century mindset. The quote earlier from an adopted young adult reflects the problems that many say they encountered if raised in families with difficulties in open communication about adoption (Brodzinsky, 2006; Thomas & Scharp, 2020). This especially pertained in the mid- to late twentieth century, before the development of psychoeducational programs for adoptive parents and popular literature on the complicated and sometimes-difficult considerations in adoptive parenting. There are two points here for therapists: First, even when adoptive parents have learned about the importance of "open communication about adoption" within the family, they still convey a great deal about their underlying feelings non-verbally. Second, since most adopted persons are no longer children, the therapist wants to learn about the common psychological issues for adopted adolescents and adults at different stages – and also about generational differences in the way adopted people have grown up. This includes the significant problem, for the development of adopted adults, especially males, that over a period of time in the twentieth century, fathers were much less involved directly in parenting children and in participating in parenting education, as reflected in the culture. There are still, in some parenting education programs, insufficient accommodations for the attendance of adoptive fathers. In our experience, a number of adopted people have expressed perceiving their mothers as more involved in various aspects of adoption and in their (the adopted person's) feelings and concerns about it, than their fathers. However, generational differences in these perceptions need to be considered.

The theme of cultural and institutional neglect is currently demonstrated by programs and services, such as in hospitals, intensive treatment programs, and various clinical specializations (e.g., trauma, major depression, and severe anxiety disorders) that do not express any interest in contributing to the adoption-specific clinical knowledge base by adjusting their patient databases to include adoptive status. In the United States, this includes the highest tiers of academically affiliated teaching hospitals with research programs. The identification of adoptive status in patient databases would be very useful for study at a future time, especially if correlated with differential diagnosis and with data on other variables, *including the source of the adoption placement*. At the very least, it is suggested that longer-term intensive treatment programs develop their own demographic and health questionnaire based on suggestions in this handbook or on some version of the author's questionnaire in the Addendum in Chapter 11. The authors also urge collaboration between treatment programs in data collection, analysis, and further study.

As one example, there is reason to believe that a disproportionate number of eating disorder patients may be adopted, given the convergence within both subgroups of difficulties relating to early trauma, especially sexual trauma, anxious attachment, preoccupation with body image, and low self-esteem. As a fundamental reminder, the two most basic neurophysiological functions required for human life postnatally are respiration and eating/nutrition. Studies linking eating disorders and adoptive status are rare (Holden, 1991), but a recent Swedish study found that internationally placed adopted adults, especially female, had significantly higher levels than the non-adopted of vomiting, loss of control with eating and preoccupation with food, and wish to be thin (Strand et al., 2018). Similar findings were recently reported by a team in a prominent American hospital studying subjects who were adopted adolescents and young adults (Rossman et al., 2020). In the United States, from many direct inquiries by one of the authors (DB) in outreach to eating disorder programs, including the most distinguished, none expressed an interest in learning more about the significance of adoptive status despite being advised that there is *still a need for significant modifications in their treatment.* As suggested earlier, one of the biggest handicaps in the mental health field generally, in both research and practice, is the reluctance to think outside the familiar bounds (limits) of each discipline's current knowledge base. This, in fact, constitutes one of the greatest of the systemic problems in all fields intersecting with adoption.

Finally, since human (child) rights should not vary according to the state or province of any country, the need for adoption-specific, highly professionalized and consistent standards for adoptive placement at a national and international level needs to be given priority, as urged in other publications by experts in the systemic problems in adoption (Palacios et al., 2019).

Forthcoming Changes in the Adoption Market with Implications for Practice

Because of the continually decreasing numbers of babies and very young children available for adoption, the circumstances of adoptive placements from the 1990s into the first two decades of the twenty-first century have become very different: the "adoption revolution" (Pertman, 2011) is increasingly complex, involving use of surrogates, now arranged through "concierge services" and commercialized on a global scale (Scherman et al., 2016; Rotabi & Bromfield, 2017); covert versions of child procurement in different countries (trafficking); and alternate forms of reproduction, that is, the rapidly developing market for *production* of babies rather than reproduction, such as artificial insemination, "gamete donors," and "donated embryos." Whether or not legal adoption is involved, this ensures much more to consider in the way of ethical practices (Leighton, 2013; Lynch, 2013), of genetic engineering (e.g., debates over whether people have rights to produce babies regardless of the means), qualifications of those planning to raise the child, complexities regarding the family narrative (explanation to the child), and the emotional impact on the children, especially in adolescence, when the confusion around sexuality and identity becomes prominent in their internal life. The actual experience of the person who has been conceived with assisted reproduction is only beginning to be studied, although to date it has not included a clinical perspective on their *internal* adjustment. Overall, as usual, adults' claimed entitlement to parenthood receives far more emphasis than the actual experience of the child over time whom the adults want to manufacture or acquire.

More typically, when eventually adopted, many young people have increasingly had to contend with the physical and emotional fallout from multiple pre-placement disadvantages, sometimes followed by a spectrum of difficult or complicated circumstances that may arise within the adoptive family or community, as well as inadequate interventions within both the health-care system (Chapter 9) and in education (Fishman, 2020). Always directly relevant is the inadequate financial assistance for special needs and minority/disadvantaged adoptive families. With the high numbers of adults in many countries seeking young children to adopt, it would be expected that they might become a stronger voice in advocating for adequately funded, higher-quality pre-placement care. For example, the United Nations is unwilling to fund any of the care of children in institutions or "baby homes" as they wait to be placed for adoption. In the United States, the court must provide better oversight to shorten the time children wait in "temporary" foster care, expedite the legal arrangements for adoption, and provide funding for ongoing services for the family. However, the impact of world events on global economies along with mounting conservative sociopolitical trends make reforms based on the needs and human rights of the child very unlikely.

The Great American Uproar Over a Nature–Nurture Study

The twentieth century witnessed a shift from the prior century's preoccupation with the importance of "bloodlines" to secure a child's "legitimate" place within its family to the gradual acceptance of adoption as a means of providing children for infertile married couples and a stable homelife for children who were destitute, or taken from mothers who wanted to keep them but were not provided assistance or support for raising them. From there came the attempt to reconcile the notion of the child as a "tabula rasa" with studies of temperament, preliminary genetic studies of vulnerability to disease, and eventually, of personality. It was found that, upon entering the world, the child is hardly a "blank slate," but she/he arrives with a wealth of genetically encoded traits, many, but by no means all, of which are potentially subject to modification by the environment (Appendix 1).

In 1961, the opportunity presented itself, or actually was taken, for identical triplet boys to be placed for adoption through a well-known American adoption agency in New York (Hoffman & Oppenheim, 2019; Spitz, 2019). Further, they were secretly placed, the adoptive parents not informed that the child was one of identical triplets, in three different adoptive homes representing three different socioeconomic classes in order to study developmental differences throughout their childhoods. As usual, this study was ended before the subjects entered adolescence. Officially heading the study was the late Peter Neubauer, MD, an Austrian-born psychiatrist and psychoanalyst in New York City, in collaboration with the agency's consulting psychiatrist, the late Viola Bernard, MD. This was done with two given justifications (rationalizations): the greater ease for parents in raising only one child, along with each child having more attention, and with the increasing demand for babies to adopt, making this an opportunity to "spread out" the advantage to three different couples. These justifications concealed the real agenda of studying class differences in the boys' development. At the same time, there was the familiar notion in psychology, which had held a long fascination with the nature–nurture debate, that the only way to examine this riddle would be to study identical twins separated at birth (Neubauer & Neubauer, 1990; Bouchard, 2007; Segal, 2021). And so the triplet boys grew up separately, each unaware of their other brothers' existence, until the secret of their three different placements was exposed when they were 19, when coincidentally two of them met for the first time on the same college campus. This is an example of the role of randomness and coincidence that can take on special significance in the lives of adopted people. Media reports resulted in the third brother coming forward when he discovered that he had two brothers identical to himself.

There followed long years of all parties having to adjust to the shock, the profound sense of betrayal that only grew over the years, and the impact of legally sealed adoption records denying access to medical and psychiatric histories of the biological family – which in this case proved to be significant for a serious subtype of depression. There was also the self-serving, ongoing intrusion of the media accused of sensationalizing the story. Not long after the full extent of the study was revealed over the next decade, one of the triplets, who had been long treated for significant and intense fluctuations in depression but with no accessible information about the psychiatric history of his birth family, ended his life at the age of 34. Whatever other factors may have been involved, suicide was likely the only control that he felt he had over his own life.

We know anecdotally that this is a subconscious dynamic that is not uncommon in the fantasy and thoughts of the adopted population, at least for those who have revealed this in treatment. From a clinical perspective, the authors maintain that it is especially critical for the therapist to know enough to ask about it, especially if the client makes any passing or seemingly benign or coded reference to suicide. For example, a seriously depressed adopted college student announced, "I don't want to be here anymore." While its meaning could have been variously interpreted as wanting to leave school, wanting to leave therapy, or wanting to leave the city, when questioned, the patient acknowledged that she meant ending her life. The vulnerability of some adopted persons to suicidal thoughts and impulses is addressed later in this chapter.

In 2018, a documentary film about the story of the triplets was released (Brook, 2018; *Three Identical Strangers*: IMDb.com, 2018; Sippel, 2018), revealing that the study involved not only a team of investigators but also a staff psychologist's intermittent home visits to obtain developmental data throughout the boys' childhood. Records of the data gathered cannot be released until 2065 and, meanwhile, remain in the safekeeping of Yale University, where Dr. Neubauer had had an affiliation. In response to revelations about the documentary throughout the media, the internet was in an uproar, while training institutes in psychotherapy and psychoanalysis held urgent meetings to discuss their alarm over what had happened to the boys and over the study itself, especially the active participation of well-known older colleagues with outstanding careers dedicated to children. This was aside from the fact that bioethics in research had not yet been established, along with the naïveté in those years about the limits of privacy and informed consent, even if any thought at all had been given to consent in this case. Of course, they also had the problem that if informed consent had been part of the preliminaries, undoubtedly the study would not have been possible. By the time the two remaining triplets were in their early 40s, the agency had closed under a cloud of multiple suspicions. In 2019, a "letter of protest" against the documentary was publicized from New York, with 52 signatories that were primarily prominent psychoanalysts objecting to the sensationalism of the story and to a number of unspecified historical and scientific inaccuracies in the documentary, resulting in the vilification of their colleagues (Spitz, 2019).

A Clinical Perspective on *Three Identical Strangers*

Without engaging in argument on any side, this story brings into relief a number of systemic themes throughout adoption, law, society and culture, and mental health:

1. *Three Identical Strangers*, an instance of deceptive adoption practices with broad repercussions, joins other exposes of cultural atrocities against children (Sinclair, 2007; King, 2012; Hentz, 2016; Redmond, 2018; Glaser, 2021), and indirectly against the birth parents, often accompanied by justifications on the basis of race, culture, and religion. This refers to the pervasive, malignant mindsets within different cultures and groups that have usurped power, such as the massive impact of entitlement and grandiosity of colonialism throughout the world, the abuse of power, and their shared indifference and underlying hostility toward certain large groups of children, as in the abductions and murders of indigenous children who have been designated lesser humans (Sinclair, 2007). Therefore, because of the inconvenience their existence represented, these children have been exploited and treated as property to be used or dispensed with, sold, stolen, or starved by the governmental entities in power. As another version of the sadistic, politically based indifference to the needs and rights of children and families, even at this writing, thousands of Ukranian children are being abducted in order to be raised by stranger adults "in the mother country."
2. The problem is that, regardless of their reputations in their respective fields, researchers and practitioners working in the overlap of adoption and mental health both benefit and are limited by the cultural mores, values, knowledge base, and assumptions of their times, including their own personal and professional biases.
3. The priority given then and now to the interests of adults wishing to adopt, by extension, includes the theme of some adults feeling narcissistically entitled to have one or more children regardless of their circumstances and/or capacities for *psychological* parenting (i.e., empathic attunement to the child over time) and regardless of the means for acquiring the child. Thus the ever-expanding industry of alternate reproduction, with its own versions of secrecy and sealed records

(Twine, 2015), exploitation of poor women for use as surrogates (Fronek, 2014; Scherman et al., 2016; Rotabi & Bromfield, 2017), and in some countries, exploitation of the system through covert forms of child trafficking, even in unrecognized forms domestically (e.g., procurement of infants from hospitals with the collusion of medical personnel), while there are no legalized protections for the child. There is also the developing complexity that the apparently limitless demands of human narcissism now extend to efforts to develop cloning techniques for the purpose of producing children who are genetically identical to one of the intended parents (Aloni, 2011; Leibetseder & Griffin, 2019). It is not yet known whether these techniques for the manufacture/creation of children may involve legal adoption by any of the parties. Regardless, according to Allen & Goldberg (2019), the current focus is on challenging conventional heteronormative entitlements. But in the process, an alternate version of entitlement is being announced and politicized, still with emphasis on the alleged rights of adults to have a child to raise. But this is with limited, if any, thought to the challenging developmental complexities for the children as they grow into adulthood, that is, to children's rights to be placed in the healthiest family setting possible. Of course, the devil is in the details of how this is to be defined. Future research would best be guided by many of the clinical and longitudinal perspectives in this book and by findings from forthcoming studies in the neurobiology and neuropsychology of early childhood development. In short, "how they fared" studies to date, including those focused on LGBTQ parents, are based on oversimplified variables, have limited numbers and sources of subjects (a significant problem in adoption research), and lack a deeper inquiry into the significant *internal* challenges, including medical, that often come in adolescence and young adulthood.

4. *Three Identical Strangers* epitomizes the cultural and historical theme of legitimizing "secrets and lies" in the name of some higher cause, such as scientific inquiry itself, and lack of consideration for either informed consent when a child is involved, or for the future needs of that child into adolescence and adulthood.
5. The lack of consideration for the longitudinal impacts of adoption practice, particularly regarding the claimed human rights of the adopted person to access accurate personal information about their biological origins, is still considered debatable, as in the argument of a prominent Canadian lawyer that the adopted person's wish to search is just a "social artifact" (Leckey, 2015).
6. The theme of exploitation of people when they are most vulnerable, especially birth mothers who were forced by systemic dysfunction (e.g., failure to require birth fathers to provide financial support for the child, acquiescence to the demands of the 'adoption market') to lose their children.
7. The lack of awareness within the clinical domain of mental health regarding the significant areas of vulnerability of adopted people, especially regarding the full spectrum of suicidal behavior (thoughts, impulses, attempts, or completed suicides). Although there was never a formal accounting from Dr. Neubauer or

his staff regarding the twins and the triplets placed separately for adoption (five sets of twins and the triplets), of the thirteen who were subjects, three (23%) are said to have suicided. Yet there has never been an attempt to understand the *internal meanings* of attempted or actual suicide in the adopted population. This vacuum of information must especially be brought to the attention of hospital and intensive treatment settings.

The Meanings of Suicide in the Adopted Population: The Need for Interdisciplinary Collaboration in Research to Inform Clinical Practice

A well-known American study published in *Pediatrics* (Slap et al., 2001) comparing 214 adopted adolescents with 6,363 adolescents living with a biological parent found that the proportion of adoptees (non-kinship) who attempted suicide was more than twice that of the non-adoptees. The study, unguided by any specialists in the psychology of adoption, and flawed by its very unbalanced number of subjects for comparison, concluded that there was no clarity about "the mechanism" that might account for the marked differences between the two groups of subjects. But from all that we know about the complexity and diversity in the adopted population, in their adoptive families, and in their pre-placement experiences, along with the multiple demographic and clinical factors needing to be included for such a study, the problem is in the simplistic notion of there being "a mechanism." Similarly, another American pediatric study which tends to be over-referenced because of its complete lack of generalizability (Keyes et al., 2013), in fact, used limited methodology, leaving its validity in serious question. It derived data through interviews with parents and with their adopted 18-year-olds (the median age), placed prior to age 2 through 3 Midwestern agencies; 74% involved international placements, the vast majority from South Korea. They found that the odds of a reported suicide attempt in adoptees were nearly four times greater than that of non-adoptees. Another finding for their adopted subjects was the higher rate of "childhood disruptive disorder" and the much higher rate of "family discord." No details were provided. There was also no data on the pre-placement experiences of the children, on the details of the reported suicide attempts, or on the underlying internal meanings to the patient either of being adopted or of attempting suicide. With so little important information available from these few studies, current claims about suicidal ideation and about the risk of suicide in the adopted population presently cannot be known. This is because of the lack of clinically focused research, such as within hospitals and intensive treatment programs. The lack of evidence to date raises serious ethical questions about the way the data is now being used and misused.

Similarly, a study of suicidal ideation in adopted youth (Festinger & Jaccard, 2012) asked few questions that would have meaning for clinicians at the "micro" level regarding the full spectrum of suicidal fantasies, intent, behaviors, and meanings. Full details would be needed of the subjects' histories and family relationships, as well as *internal meanings and contexts* for suicidal thoughts and impulses, and many other essential variables, including the sources of the adoptive placements (see Introduction). Overall, greater collaboration between sociological/social work studies and the clinical disciplines would help refine the questions being asked, the variables being cross-referenced, and the hypotheses being tested.

As another example, controlling for more variables than many American research efforts, Swedish studies of internationally adopted subjects (Hjern et al., 2002; Von Borczyskowski et al., 2006) found that, overall, adolescents and young adults were nearly four times as likely as the non-adopted to die from suicide, to attempt suicide, and to be hospitalized for a psychiatric disorder. The risks of suicide attempt or death were in descending order, the greatest for the internationally adopted, then the domestically adopted, then the non-adopted. However, without the critical details of the demographic data (Chapter 4) and psychiatric profiles of the adopted subjects, the numbers can serve only as general guidelines for further inquiry. Also, adopted subjects with suicidal ideation/attempts and adopted subjects hospitalized for a psychiatric disorder are two very different subgroups; any overlap was not mentioned.

Overall, on a more global scale, limits of the research methods, subject populations, and the lack of subsequent research on suicidal ideation and behavior of adopted adolescents and young adults warrant caution in interpretation. Also, in the United States, there are a large number of anecdotal reports throughout the adopted adult community of completed suicides by adopted people, some of them family members or friends (Appendix 3), but no such cases have ever been studied clinically.

In the aforementioned study by Festinger and Jaccard (2012), the authors represented an unusual amalgam of developmental psychology, clinical social work, and sociology, a combination we hope will be continued. Unlike the other studies of suicidal ideation in adopted subjects, it took into account the age at placement, finding that the most vulnerable had been placed at or over age 4. This is, of course, consistent with the findings of the first three years of life being the most critical in brain development (Schore, 2013; Perry, 2020) with respect to the three major developmental challenges for adopted persons (e.g., traumatic loss, insecure attachments, and fragmented identity). But Festinger and Jaccard also found that "depression decreases, on average, from adolescence to early young adulthood but then rebounds to higher levels during young adulthood" (ibid., p. 292). It could be speculated that this finding may be related to what we know about adolescence being a time, for many, of experimentation that includes more in the way of externalizing and potentially self-destructive behaviors which sometimes serve to counteract underlying depression. Examples would be difficulties in anger management and "moodiness" that are expressed behaviorally more than verbally, abuse of substances, self-harm, random sexual encounters, scattered thinking and poor judgment, inconsistent school achievement, and high-risk behaviors. This is supported by neurobiological research (Buss et al., 2012) which has found that it is only by the mid-20s that the myelinization of the brain's neurons is complete, allowing for more control over the earlier developing limbic system that controls emotional reactions. This may account for the more-impulsive acting-out behaviors in adolescence. But it may be a signal of more *internalized* turmoil to come in young adulthood.

The 20s are more likely to become a period of greater self-reflection, more retrospective, reflective, and critical thinking, improved internal control of impulses, and perhaps more conscious-level awareness of internalized conflict. But for adopted young adults, the important life decisions at this time re-invoke memories and feelings related to their birth families and important people from their early lives that they have lost (such as foster families and siblings), struggles in love relationships, and difficulty separating from their adoptive families, making it understandable that many will experience significant anxiety and depression, but without necessarily recognizing it. The problem comes when their therapists do not recognize it either.

Some of the psychodynamics explaining suicide may be related to the second individuation process (Blos, 1967) which generally occurs during adolescence, but in the case of some adopted individuals with delayed areas in adolescent development, it may extend to their 20s or beyond. Given their early histories, their challenges as emerging adults may rekindle unresolved losses and threats to their sense of security, along with their difficulty envisioning their future. This likely accounts, in some cases, for the "launching" into full adulthood being delayed or arrested. Based on anecdotal material, this is not uncommon in adopted persons, perhaps also relating to the impact of early developmental trauma on their *internal sense of time*.

> *How can I plan anything for my future when I can't even imagine having one? To counter common assumptions in both the health-care and social service fields about the "best age for placement," the impaired sense of time occurs as well in the case of adopted young adults placed soon after birth (see Chapter 4, Appendix 6).*

Inquiry into the *internal meanings of suicidal thoughts*, that is, what suicidal ideation represents psychodynamically, is particularly important not only in research efforts but also in intensive therapeutic treatment and partial hospitalization programs. Examples include suicide as the ultimate form of punishing themselves due to feeling defective or of having caused bad things to happen, feelings of hopelessness, subconsciously and simultaneously punishing both their birth parents, adoptive parents and themselves, ending the internal pain from which they have no hope of being freed, *taking the ultimate control they feel they do have over their own life*, or suicide based on the fantasy that it might result in their finally being able to meet their birth parents in the afterlife. Also needing more in-depth study are the sources and depth, in some cases, of their deep-seated rage over what happened to them (Perry & Winfrey, 2021), including details of their early histories and possibly inquiry into the meaning to them of feeling "abandoned again" by significant people in their lives (e.g., parental separation and divorce or illness and death).

It is important to note that in their view, their ongoing sense of abandonment may also include their prior therapists because of their seeming lack of attunement emotionally. This is all the more significant if the adopted person also experienced their adoptive parents as being poorly attuned and/or still carrying their internal wounds around "having to adopt."

> *They were basically very decent people who led ordinary lives, but emotionally I never counted on them to really be able to understand or help me.*

This not uncommon perception raises questions not about the adopted person's tenuous attachment, but more likely about the parents' (Buckwalter et al., 2017).

Anecdotally, many adopted adolescents and young adults say they experienced their many counselors and therapists in an ambivalent way, but particularly as having little in-depth understanding of what it means to be adopted. That is, even if a therapist occasionally had the words (i.e., a cognitive grasp of some issues and common cliches, typically using such terms as "sense of self" and "problems with identity"), they did not have the music, beginning with authentically attuned empathy that only comes through training and in-depth self-examination. One hypothesis for further study relates to the prior revelations from some of the adopted people who did commit suicide that they had given up their hope that therapy could ever help them, because they had found their many treatment experiences so inadequate (Appendix 3).

> *I was adopted through a lawyer. My mother was a manic-depressive who was always angry and fighting. My father had left a year after I was placed. The therapists I saw since I was 5 never brought up the subject of adoption and only focused on my mother's illness. For a while, I imagined maybe my birth mother would come back for me, but around my pre-teen years, the reality set in that she wasn't coming back. I began to act out through self-harm, drugs, and suicide attempts.*

Inconvenient Truths for Psychotherapists from Systemic and Clinical Perspectives

Presently, we are left with primarily anecdotal information from large numbers of adopted young adults, many of whom, had they been studied when they were younger, would likely have scored very high on all *external* criteria typically used in social work/sociological research for determining "good adjustment," "adequate school achievement," "satisfaction with adoption," and "overall wellness." However, the authors believe that such broad-stroke criteria may misrepresent their *internal* experience, regardless of whether it is viewed as having any relationship to their being adopted.

Studies comparing adopted with non-adopted children seen in psychiatric outpatient clinical settings, beginning with Marshall Schechter (1960), have found that adopted children in treatment were disproportionately represented (15% in the Schechter study). As stated elsewhere in this chapter, it is important to remember that in the United States, the estimated proportion of children under 18 in non-kinship adoption is 2.5%, whereas the proportion of adopted adolescents seen in hospital settings is estimated by staff to be in the 25–40% range (Brodzinsky et al., 2016). Yet no American hospital, again including the top tier, has taken any interest in studying this.

In the outpatient clinical setting, adopted adolescents and young adults have revealed information that has also never been studied. This includes a good deal of intensely personal, ongoing, sometimes subtle, but in some cases very painful, symptoms and personality struggles that may or may not reach clinical significance. Common examples are difficulties with avoidance and procrastination; feeling unable to change behaviors and attitudes that have continued from their younger ages; low self-esteem, memory deficits, or difficulty concentrating that they believe to have interfered with their studies; certain inhibitions or variants of social phobias that they struggle with; and psychosomatic symptoms (e.g., gastrointestinal or pulmonary). The latter two turned out to be frequently referenced by subjects in the informal study of a large number of adopted adults by Schechter and Bertocci (1990). Yet within their adoptive families and communities, many have easily passed for what their social context would consider "normal," often referred to as "great kids" and "high achievers." This does not, however, necessarily spare them from the impact of narcissistic injuries:

> *After I got my graduate degree and a great job, I used to resent the fact that I worked so hard to get so far with my career, while my parents were the ones who usually got the credit. The fact is that I came this way.*

In short, we have learned that adopted young people can be expert at hiding the real stories of what they have experienced *internally*, typically not wanting to disturb or hurt their parents. Therapists need specialized skills to help the adopted client feel safe enough to explore them, which may include carefully addressing themes of shame and guilt. The most troubling example would be the hidden prevalence of suicidal ideation and attempts, the multiple layers of complexity they represent, and at times, therapists' insufficient skills in decoding their oblique references to it.

Overall, in the United States, it is not at all unusual for adolescents and young adults generally to see counselors and therapists for age-appropriate concerns. In the college and young adult years, at least in the US it is normative and even routine. Most importantly, the treatment experience of the adopted person in late adolescence into the 20s is not by itself any indication of a "psychiatric disorder."

Conclusion

The developmental struggles for adopted adolescents and young adults have not been on the radar of *either* the health/mental health care or adoption fields. Of particular concern regarding mental health is the lack of interest evident in current psychiatric hospital, residential, and intensive treatment programs, despite the typically disproportionate numbers of adopted adolescents and young adults whose treatment is not presently differentiated in any way from non-adopted patients. Much needed in the twenty-first century is the return of interest by psychiatry that characterized much of the twentieth century: Florence Clothier, Povl Toussieng, H. David Kirk, Michael Bohman, Jules Glenn, Herbert Wieder, Marshall Schechter, Remi Cadoret, Arthur Sorosky. Extending from this, the overall contention of this chapter is that, if anything about adoption is to be pathologized, it is the global neglect by the adoption and legal systems that continue to give priority to the wishes of adults, that resist being better informed and open to change that see no need to fund clinically trained professionals to handle the placements of children (Chapter 2), and that are unwilling to provide funding for ongoing health and mental health care, as needed over time, rendered by highly trained, adoption-informed psychotherapists and, depending on the circumstances, advanced clinicians.

Also, health-care providers are advised to listen for the nuances and infinite variations on universal human themes and motives, many of which are not so noble after all, and that may be details in the adopted person's experience that need to be explored. The problems with existing adoption studies are noted, emphasizing the importance of researchers in certain areas being better informed about the complexities of the psychology of adoption. As appropriate to the timing and context in treatment, therapists can look for opportunities to reassure their adopted clients that, given their particular circumstances, they are far from being alone.

Endnotes

Allen, K.R., & Goldberg, A.E. (2019). Lesbian women disrupting gendered, heteronormative discourses of motherhood, marriage, and divorce. *Journal of Lesbian Studies*, 1–13.

Aloni, E. (2011). Cloning and the LGBTI family: Cautious optimism. *New York University Review of Law & Social Change*, 35 (1), 1–80.

Barth, R.P., & Miller, J.M. (2000). Building effective post-adoption services: What is the empirical foundation? *Family Relations*, 49 (4), 447–455.

Bick, J., & Dozier, M. (2010). Mothers' oxytocin production following close physical interactions with biological and non-biological children. *Developmental Psychobiology*, 52, 100–107.

Bick, J., Fox, N., Zeanah, C., & Nelson, C.A. (2017). Early deprivation, atypical brain development, and internalizing symptoms in later childhood. *Neuroscience*, 342, 140–153.

Blos, P. (1967). The second individuation process of adolescence. *Psychoanalytic Study of the Child*, 22, 162–186. https://doi.org/10.1080/00797308.1967.11822595

Bouchard, T.J. (2007). Genes and human psychological traits. In P. Carruthers, S. Laurence, & S. Stich (Eds.), *The Innate Mind: Foundations for the Future*, p. 3. Oxford: Oxford University Press.

Brodzinsky, D. (2006). Family structural openness and communication openness as predictors in the adjustment of adopted children. *Adoption Quarterly*, 9 (4), 1–18.

Brodzinsky, D., Santa, J., & Smith, S.L. (2016). Adopted youth in residential care: Prevalence rate and professional training needs. *Residential Treatment for Children and Youth*, 33 (2), 118–134.

Brodzinsky, D.M. (1993). Longterm outcomes in adoption. *The Future of Children*, 3 (1), 153–166. https://futureofchildren.princeton.edu

Brook, T. (2007/2012/2018). Film tells of secret study of triplets. *BBC News*. Three Identical Strangers at IMDb.com.

Buckwalter, K.D., Reed, D., & Mercer, D. (2017). Ghosts in the adoption: Uncovering parents' attachment and coping history. *Families in Society: The Journal of Contemporary Human Services*, 98 (3), 225–234.

Buss, C., Poggi Davis, E., Shahbaba, B., Pruessner, J.C., Head, K., & Sandman, C.A. (2012). Maternal cortisol over the course of pregnancy and subsequent child amygdala and hippocampus volumes and affective problems. *Proceedings of the National Academy of Sciences of the United States of America*, 109 (20), E1312–E1319. https://doi.org/10.1073/pnas.1201295109

Cohen, N., Coyne, J., & Duvall, J. (1993). Adopted and biological children in the clinic: Family, parental, and child characteristics. *Journal of Child Psychology & Psychiatry*, 34 (4), 545–562.

Festinger, T., & Jaccard, J. (2012). Suicidal thoughts in adopted versus non-adopted youth: A longitudinal analysis in adolescence, early young adulthood, and young adulthood. *Journal of the Society for Social Work and Research*, 3 (4), 280–295.

Fishman, F. (2020). Awareness of adoption at school. In G.M. Wrobel, E. Helder, & E. Marr (Eds.), *The Routledge Handbook of Adoption*, pp. 464–482. London & New York: Routledge.

Fong, R., & McRoy, R. (Eds). (2016). *Transracial and Intercountry Adoptions: Cultural Guidance for Professionals*. New York: Columbia University Press.

Fronek, P., Cuthbert, D., & Willing, I. (2014). Perfecting adoption? Reflections on the rise of commercial offshore surrogacy and family formation in Australia. In A. Hayes, & D. Higgins (Eds.), *Families, Policy, and the Law: Selected Essays on Contemporary Issues for Australia*, pp. 55–66. Melbourne: Longman Cheshire.

Glaser, G. (2021). *American Baby: A Mother, A Child, and the Shadow History of Adoption*. New York: Viking.

Goldstein, J., Freud, A., & Solnit, A. (1973). *Beyond the Best Interests of the Child*. New York: Free Press.

Grotevant, H.D. (2020). Open adoption. *The Routledge Handbook of Adoption*, pp. 266–277. London & New York: Routledge.

Grotevant, H.D., & Von Korff, L. (2011). Adoptive identity. In S.J. Schwartz, K. Luyckx, & V.L. Vignoles (Eds.), *Handbook of Identity Theory and Research*, pp. 585–601. New York: Springer.

Henderson, D.B. (2007). Why has the mental health community been silent on adoption issues? In R.A. Javier, A.L. Baden, F.A. Biafora, & A. Camacho-Gingerich (Eds.), *Handbook of Adoption: Implications for Researchers, Practitioners, and Families*, pp. 403–417. Thousand Oaks: Sage Publications.

Hentz, T.L. (Ed. & author) (2016). Stolen generations: Survivors of the Indian adoption projects and sixties scoop. In *Book 3: Lost Children of the Indian Adoption Projects*. Greenfield: Blue Band Books.

Hjern, A., Lindblad, F., & Vinnerljung, B. (2002). Suicide, psychiatric illness, and social maladjustment in intercountry adoptees in Sweden: A cohort study. *The Lancet*, 360 (9331), 443–448.

Hoffman, L., & Oppenheim, L. (2019). Three identical strangers and the twinning reaction: Clarifying history and lessons for today from Peter Neubauer's twins study. *Journal of the American Medical Association*, 322 (1), 10–12.

Holden, N.L. (1991). Adoption and eating disorders: A high-risk group? *British Journal of Psychiatry*, 158, 829–833.

IMDb.com. (2018, November 30). Three Identical Strangers. *IMDb*. www.imdb.com/title/tt7664504.

Jackson, K.F., & Samuels, G.M. (2019). *Multiracial Cultural Attunement*. Washington, DC: NASW Press.

Keyes, M.A., Malone, S.M., Sharma, A., Iacono, W.G., & McGue, M. (2013). Risk of suicide attempt in adopted and non-adopted offspring. *Pediatrics*, 132 (4), 639–646.

King, T. (2012). *The Inconvenient Indian: A Curious Account of Native People in North America*. Toronto: Doubleday Canada.

Leckey, R. (2015). Identity, law, and the right to dream (McGill Univ.). *Dalhousie Law Journal*, 38 (2), 525–547.

Leibetseder, D., & Griffin, G. (2019). States of reproduction: The co-production of queer and trans parenthood in three European countries. *Journal of Gender Studies*, 1–44. http://mc.manuscriptcentral.com/cjgs

Leighton, K. (2013). To criticize the right to know we must question the value of genetic relatedness. *American Journal of Bioethics*, 13 (5), 54–56.

Lynch, C. (2013). Doubting adoption legislation. *Dissent is the Sydney University Law Society Social Justice Journal*, 25–26.

Madden, E., Aguiniga, D.M., & Ryan, S. (2020). Birth mothers' options counseling and relinquishment experiences. In G.M. Wrobel, E. Helder, & E. Marr (Eds.), *The Routledge Handbook of Adoption*, pp. 219–237. London & New York: Routledge.

Merritt, D.H., & Ludeke, R.D. (2020). Post-adoption services: Needs and adoption type. In G.M. Wrobel, E. Helder, & E. Marr (Eds.), *The Routledge Handbook of Adoption*, pp. 483–492. London & New York: Routledge.

Neubauer, P., & Neubauer, A. (1990). *Nature's Thumbprint: The New Genetics of Personality*. Boston: Addison-Wesley Publishing Company.

Palacios, J., Adroher, S., Brodzinsky, D.M., Grotevant, H.D., Johnson, D.E., Juffer, F.M., & Tarren-Sweeney, M. (2019). Adoption in the service of child protection: An international interdisciplinary perspective. *Psychology, Public Policy, and Law*, 25, 57–72.

Perry, B.D. (2020). The neurosequential model: A developmentally sensitive, neuroscience informed approach to clinical problem-solving. In J. Mitchel, J. Tucci, & E. Tronick (Eds.), *The Handbook of Therapeutic Care for Children: Evidence-informed Approaches to Working with Traumatized Children and Adolescents in Foster, Kinship, and Adoptive Care*, pp. 137–156. London & Philadelphia: Jessica Kingsley.

Perry, B.D., & Winfrey, O. (2021). *What Happened to You? Conversations on Trauma, Resilience, and Healing*. New York: Flatiron Books.

Pertman, A. (2011). *Adoption Nation: How the Adoption Revolution is Transforming Our Families and America*. Boston: The Harvard Common Press.

Plomin, R. (2018, December 14). In the nature-nurture war, nature wins. *Observations, Scientific American*. https://blogs.scientificamerican.com/observations/in-the-nature-nurture-war-nature-wins/.

Redmond, P.J. (2018). *The Adoption Machine: The Dark History of Ireland's Mother and Baby Homes and the Inside Story of How 'Tuam 800' Became a Global Scandal*. Newbridge & Kildare: Irish Academic Press/Merrion Press.

Rossman, S.M., Eddy, K.T., Franko, D.L., Rose, J., DuBois, R., Weissman, R.S., Dierker, L.C., & Thomas, J.J. (2020). Behavioral symptoms of eating disorders among adopted adolescents and young adults in the US: Findings from the ADD Health Survey. *International Journal of Eating Disorders*, 53 (9), 1515–1525.

Rotabi, K., & Bromfield, N. (2017). *From Intercountry Adoption to Global Surrogacy: A Human Rights History and New Fertility Frontiers*. London & New York: Routledge.

Schechter, M.D. (1960). Observations on adopted children. *Archives of General Psychiatry*, 3, 21–32.

Schechter, M.D., & Bertocci, D. (1990). The meaning of the search. In D.M. Brodzinsky & M.D. Schechter (Eds.), *The Psychology of Adoption*, pp. 62–90. New York & Oxford: Oxford University Press.

Scherman, R., Misca, G., Rotabi, K., & Selman, P. (2016). Global commercial surrogacy and international adoption: Parallels and differences. *Adoption and Fostering*, 40 (1), 20–35.

Schore, A.N. (2013). Relational trauma, brain development, and dissociation. In J.D. Ford, & C.A. Courtois (Eds.), *Treating Complex Traumatic Stress Disorders in Children and Adolescents. Scientific Foundations in Therapeutic Models*, pp. 3–23. New York: The Guilford Press.

Segal, N.L. (2021). *Deliberately Divided: Inside the Controversial Study of Twins and Triplets Adopted Apart*. Lanham: Rowman & Littlefield.

Sinclair, R. (2007). Identity lost and found: Lessons from the sixties scoop. *First Peoples Child and Family Review: A Journal on Innovation and Best Practices in Aboriginal Child Welfare Administration, Research, Policy & Practice*, 3 (1), 65–82.

Sippel, D.M. (2018, July 27). Three identical strangers – an experienced adoptee's review questions and insights that others have missed. *Forbidden Family*. https://forbiddenfamily.com/2018/07/26/three-identical-strangers-an-experienced-adoptees-review-questions-and-insights-that-others-have-missed.

Slap, G., Goodman, E., & Huang, B. (2001). Adoption as a risk factor for attempted suicide during adolescence. *Pediatrics*, 108 (2), 1–8.

Spinak, J. (2007). When did lawyers for children stop reading Goldstein, Freud, & Solnit? Lessons from the twentieth century on best interests and the role of the child advocate. *American Bar Association, Family Law Quarterly*, 41, 393–411.

Spitz, E.H. (2019). Documentary danger: Reflections on 'Three Identical Strangers'. *Bulletin of the Columbia Center for Psychoanalytic Training and Research*, 1–8.

Strand, M., vonHausswolff-Juhlin, Y., Fredlund, P., & Lager, A.C.J. (2018). Symptoms of disordered eating among adult international adoptees: A population-based cohort study. *European Eating Disorders Review*, 27 (3).

Taub, N. (1984). Assessing the impact of Goldstein, Freud, & Solnit's Proposals: An introductory overview. *NYU Review of Law & Social Change*, XII, 485–494.

Thomas, L.J., & Scharp, K. (2020). *Communications about Adoption in Families*.

Twine, F.W. (2015). Outsourcing the Womb: Race, class, and gestational surrogacy in a global market (2nd ed.). In *Framing 21st Century Social Issues*, pp. 1–89. London: Routledge.

Von Borczyskowski, A., Hjern, A., Lindblad, F., & Vinnerljung, B. (2006). Suicidal behavior in national and international adult adoptees. *Social Psychiatry and Psychiatric Epidemiology*, 41 (2), 95–102.

Welsh, J.A., Viana, A.G., Petrill, S.A., & Mathias, M.D. (2007). Interventions for internationally adopted children and families: A review of the literature. *Child and Adolescent Social Work Journal*, 24 (3), 285–311.

Wrobel, G.M., Helder, E., & Marr, E., Eds. (2018). *The Routledge Handbook of Adoption*, pp. 253–265. New York: Three Identical Strangers, IMDb.com.

APPENDIX

1. Robert Plomin, PhD, writes that for most of the twentieth century, environmental factors were referred to as *nurture* because the family was thought of as all-important and crucial in determining who we become. However, genetic research has shown that this is not the case.

   In fact, he has recently stated that we would essentially be the same person if we had been adopted at birth and raised in a different family (Plomin, 2018). He acknowledges that environmental influences are certainly important and account, he estimates, for about half of the differences between us. However, they are largely unsystematic, unstable, and idiosyncratic, that is, random.
   He continues to say that the nature–nurture war is over and that nature wins.
   The only missing element in life development in the context of this book, and oddly missing in developmental psychology, is the neurobiological (prenatally) and neuropsychological (postnatally) impact of permanent separation from the birth mother. The universally cited conceptualizations of the life stages by Erik Erikson begin with trust vs. mistrust and autonomy vs. shame and doubt. But for most adopted persons, placed early, life as they experienced it began with amputation (primary loss).

2. In three papers, one on long term adoption outcomes (Brodzinsky, 1993), another on complexities for the adopted person of integrating a personal identity (Grotevant & Von Korff, 2011), and the third describing post-adoption services (Merritt & Ludeke, 2020), the options discussed for adopting children do not include the option of private/independent adoptions handled by lawyers. Yet since the latter part of the twenty-first century, for those who could afford them, private adoptions have become a preferred means for the parents, while lucrative

for the lawyers, and we believe it is now a significant proportion of adoptions in the United States. But there has been no effort to include them as their own "pathway" in adoption statistics, and there are no studies of their numbers (statistics), practices, or outcomes.

3. This chapter is written in memory of Carla, a friend of one of the authors (DB), who stated that, despite many efforts over the years, she could never find a psychotherapist who "really understood her as an adopted person." She had the misfortune of being born to a biracial unmarried couple (one birth parent Japanese, the other Caucasian) who were college students in the United States shortly after the Second World War. Being half-Japanese, she was considered "unplaceable" but, at the age of 4, was adopted and raised by an older foster mother with grown children, whose husband remained in the shadows. As a young adult, exquisitely beautiful and interpersonally warm and engaging, she hid well the internal depression with which she had long struggled throughout her life, derived in part from her deep-seated conviction that no one could ever love her. Paradoxically, in addition to lacking a psychological father, her beauty became a disadvantage because her involvements with men in love relationships were always fraught with difficulties in "handling them." Her judgment was frequently impaired by her low self-esteem and by her difficulty determining what, in these relationships, and in life itself, was "real."

Because her adoption records were sealed, Carla searched for her birth parents in vain and was coldly dismissed by the welfare-based adoption service that had placed her, because her search for information was such a threat to them. She never recovered emotionally from being forced as a young teenager to place her own daughter born "out of wedlock" and her only biological relative for adoption. As she approached mid-life, losing all hope that her life could ever stabilize (i.e., that she could ever find either her birth mother or her daughter and, on another level, that she could ever be authentically loved by anyone), she withdrew from her uncaring world and, in the garage, took her own life. Carla had left a note asking that she be remembered with white roses. She was found halfway up the stairs from the basement, suggesting that at the very end, she had changed her mind. Her white car's license plate read "ULUVME."

2
WHERE ARE WE NOW? TRENDS AND OBSERVATIONS IN ADOPTION STUDY IN THE NETHERLANDS

Rene A. C. Hoksbergen, PhD

Introduction

The concept of adoption is of Roman origin and in that society dealt only with creating the possibility of an heir, including a successor for the emperor. Strengthening the power and security of the Roman family was the primary goal. Today, the priority in adoption has been meeting the needs of adults wanting to adopt, and until recently, adoption placement organizations have wanted to give very young children to mostly involuntarily childless couples. Learning about the longer-term adjustments of adoptees from literature was not their issue or interest, so they did not engage in any follow-up studies of the adoptive families' adjustments, nor do they do this to the present time. Typically, these potential parents had hoped to adopt a young healthy child, imagining that this child would become attached to them, as other children normally do. They assumed that after an initial adjustment, the child would feel at home, safe, and happy with her/his new parents. This is the way the parents have been reassured by those who arranged adoptive placements since the 1940s, for which reason the adoptive parents have continued to be poorly prepared.

Since 1971, and up to the present time, I have been extensively occupied with the scientific and clinical approach with adoptees, adoptive parents, and other individuals who do not grow up with both biological parents (donor children a.o.). So far in the Western world, a lot of scientific research has been done about many basic aspects concerning intercountry adoption. On the whole, the outcome of the results of many of these studies, based on limited variables, seems to have been positive about the chances adoptees have for a satisfactory life with new parents in a

Table 2.1 Total Recorded Intercountry Adoptions, 1990–2019, Worldwide

Period	Number ICA Recorded
1990–1999	223,407
2000–2009	382,232
2010–2019	148,865

Note: The 60% decline of intercountry adoption in only the last ten years in all 24 Western countries is very substantial.

society that is typically very different from the child's origins. However, increasingly since the 1980s, important basic questions have also been raised. I refer especially to Nancy Verrier's *The Primal Wound: Understanding the Adopted Child* (1993), in which she exposes the effects of separation from the birth mother on adopted children and their inclination to testing-out behavior as they grow up.

Increasingly, I came to reach the conclusion that adoption – in the meaning and intention that Western society has given it – is a myth. This is because the idealized and untested proposition has been that the adoptive family is essentially the same, or very similar to, the presumably healthy and overall content biological family. But this is not at all founded. In fact, there are many complications, both in the emotional development of the adopted person and in the common adoption practices, that psychotherapists have not been trained to understand, because these two topics must be considered together. In the United Kingdom and the United States, the focus of research and clinical work has been on the adopted child's experience with traumatic loss and on making secure attachments, whereas my own work has focused on the adoptee's struggle with her/his identity, especially in adolescence. All these are greatly magnified for the adoptee who is placed internationally and/or interracially. But the other dimension that is part of the difficulty has to do with the naïveté of all adoption placement organizations, in particular, the innocence and lack of adequate preparation provided the adoptive parents, the insufficiency of financial support from governmental services, and the lack of ongoing services for the adoptive family.

Showing and discussing the historical development of adoption in the Netherlands between 1956 and 2021, we notice how all the experiences of adoptees and adoptive parents fundamentally changed the view on adoption in Dutch society and elsewhere. We see that foreign adoption in the Netherlands is almost disappearing, with almost 1,600 in 1980, declining to 75 in 2021 (Table 2.3 later). Looking at some general figures worldwide given by British researcher Peter Selman (2022b), it is clear that the substantial Dutch adoption decline is not unique (Table 2.1).

Memorable Cases from Practice

I offer three examples out of my clinical practice that are typical of what I have encountered in my work with families and adoptees who were internationally placed. With all three, the main psychological problems started when they were in their adolescence, when I was approached by the adoptive parents. In fact, the adoptee's struggle with their identity was the main issue. Adoptive parents often find this very hard to deal with, but it was also difficult for me as their therapist. The questions or conclusions arrived at are as follows:

1. "Why am I adopted in Holland?"

Two years ago, Dutch adoptive parents approached me with a rather-difficult question about their two adopted children, both born in China. One of them is John, a boy of about 16 years of age and adopted when he was only a few months old. We do not know anything about the birth mother. The boy is intelligent, does well at school, and is rather popular among his peers. But at home, things are complicated. On the whole, his behavior is within the norm for his age. However, he often has violent discussions, especially with his father, about being brought to Holland and adopted by them. It does not help that the father tells him that it is the adoption organization which decides where an adoptee goes.

The boy does not want to grow up and stay in Holland but would prefer to grow up and stay in the USA. At his young age, he has already visited, together with his parents, quite a few countries, also his country of birth, and two years ago, the whole family spent some weeks in the USA just for some sightseeing. His parents are very open regarding his background but really struggle with the way he came to them, seeming to have been randomly given to them by the Chinese official organization and the recognized adoption organization which provided babies only to parents in the Netherlands. This discussion in the family goes on. One of my suggestions to the parents was to send him for some time to a summer school in the States to see what life really is like over there, also to help John make contacts with other adoptees from China. I reassured the parents that this struggle of adopted adolescents who were placed from foreign countries is very common. So far, the parents seem to feel somewhat better. They accept the struggle of their son and have noticed that keeping him busy with the efforts of daily life seems to help. Perhaps it does, but the need might remain. We also discuss how well their son has been doing in school because he is highly talented and is serious about his studies. I then thought that perhaps I should discuss the issue directly with the young man himself.

2. "I don't belong here. I revoke the adoption."

The next example is of Peter, born in South Korea and now 42 years of age. His situation is completely different, but he is also very much concerned with the struggle with his identity, demonstrating that these concerns become especially important in young adulthood and continue in later years. His parents did understand his feelings of not belonging to anyone, anywhere. Because he was so preoccupied with his identity, and fueled by his anger, his narcissistic demands intensified to the point that he became a behavioral problem at work and was fired. (I agreed with their finding.)

Peter's adoptive parents already had a son born to them, quite a few years older than Peter, and could not have another child biologically. They very much wanted to adopt a girl and applied through the largest official Dutch adoptive placement organization. But the only way the organization was willing to grant their wish for a girl was to require that they adopt two children together, a girl of 3 and her brother, around 2 years of age. These two children had already been offered to candidate adoptive parents in three other countries but were not accepted because the two children had to be adopted together. However, Peter's Dutch parents had to agree to these terms; otherwise, they would not get any adopted child at all. Hesitating, because they only wanted to adopt a girl, the parents accepted the offer and adopted the two children.

When Peter was 30 years of age, the entire adoptive family – the two adult children from Korea and their biological son – went to Korea. There was a Korean intermediary who told them they had received information from the birth parents, who wanted to see the adult children. The adoptive parents had promised this arrangement, if it were possible, and they hoped that their relationship with their two adopted "children" would improve a bit. Peter learned that his birth father had died two years after his birth due to an accident. Peter said how much he would have loved to have seen him and spoken to him, as he saw himself more as Korean than Dutch. His adoptive father tried to tell him more about the reasons he was given up for adoption. Peter was told that he will be the last descendant in the Korean family of his father. Communication with his birth mother is difficult because she understands only Korean and she did not react in a positive way on Peter's first and also second meeting two years later. She was more eager to speak with her daughter and did not seem very interested in Peter's wishes. Peter stayed several days with his birth mother, and they travelled together to shops, visited uncles and aunts, and tried to find the grave of his birth father. But to his disappointment, she could not even find it. In effect, because Peter was male, neither his adoptive nor birth parents fully accepted him.

In discussions about the past, the adoptive parents had made it clear to Peter that originally they only wanted to adopt his sister, but that they were required to adopt him along with her. Somehow, they tried to hide their different feelings for their adopted children but did not succeed. One of the effects of this fact of life from a very young age was his struggle with thoughts and feelings, like, "Do I have to accept these people as my parents, and why do I have to do so?" For adoptees whose adoptive parents were at best ambivalent about having them as children in their family, this is one of their complex and difficult psychological problems. Their feeling not truly wanted, which they always can sense, and therefore feeling a certain distance from their adoptive parents, becomes part of their identity struggle. They desperately want to feel fully wanted, but if it is not by either their adoptive parents or their birth parents, where does this leave them?

Many years later, while in Korea, Peter struggled to communicate with his Korean family to get feelings of being accepted as one of the members of the family. He wanted this especially from his father's family, as his mother behaved in a strange and less-reliable way and he parted from her with the decision that he did not want to see her anymore. But the relationship with the brother of his father was much better because he could speak English and saw Peter as truly belonging to the Korean family. An important question for Peter was whether to see himself as Dutch or more as Korean. He told me that he never would be a true Dutchman but also never a true Korean. Peter had to struggle with the communication problem that many, or most, internationally placed adoptees encounter if they actually meet their birth families in person. They must face the difficulty of finally seeing them physically but of being unable to share feelings openly. Conversation, for instance, might only be possible with a translator or spokesman. Adoptees know that they need to accept this and find a way for a mutual discussion through a mediator. They also have to accommodate the fact that the birth family may not be what they had hoped for, and to find a way to accept whatever they learn. This is more difficult for some adoptees than for others.

When Peter returned from his second trip to see his Korean birth family, he decided that he did not want to see his adoptive parents anymore. He did not feel any relationship with them, especially not with his adoptive father, who was much more involved emotionally with Peter's sister. In the end, he managed to revoke the adoption when he was 40 years of age. Adoptees are able to do this in Holland through a court decision. This cannot be organized easily, and there are also age limits. But in this case, the situation was clear. For many years, Peter had not wanted to have any contact with his adoptive parents. He changed his name to his original Korean name. Peter feels much better now but has decided to live in Holland for the time being. He hopes to be able to build up strong ongoing relationships in both Holland and Korea and find work that suits him. He is writing an autobiography now (I am helping him), and he thinks perhaps in the near future he may find someone to live with.

3. A case of an adoption that did not work.

Birgit was born in Austria in 1975. She was born to an unmarried 17-year-old girl who could not care for her at all (being in prison) but also did not want to. After some months, Birgit was given to a German children's institution and then offered for adoption. At the age of almost 2, she was adopted by a childless couple in Holland. From the beginning, she avoided and sometimes rejected the adoptive mother. In contrast, the relationship with the adoptive father seemed much better. Still, Birgit could have difficult moods, like becoming very angry about nothing and reacting with tantrums when people asked her simple things. She was intelligent and did well at school and was also musically talented. But in puberty, Birgit became more and more closed off. She had only one friend but kept her at a certain distance as well, and the same would happen with any young man approaching her with interest. She didn't like showing her affection to anybody.

Rene A. C. Hoksbergen, PhD

When Birgit was about 21, she approached an adoption specialist for some assistance in finding her birth mother, and after some difficulty, she succeeded. Birgit met her and fell into her arms, having no problem in showing affection in this way, and the birth mother reacted positively. Birgit continued to meet with her birth mother. However, after some years, her birth mother was not so warm emotionally anymore and would not tell her about the birth father. The birth mother tried to enlist Birgit for financial help because her socioeconomic situation was still very limited. Birgit tried to help her, but soon this relationship became a burden. She now felt in between two families but without any closeness with either. The relationship with her adoptive parents remained stable, and Birgit was always welcome, but she did not want to visit them very often, because she had never developed any attachment to them. But also, her parents had never gotten professional help with their disappointment. Sometimes, adoptive parents feel very ashamed when there are intense emotional problems in their family.

But for some years, Birgit was in psychotherapy for herself to deal with her feelings of loneliness and loss. Although she had a job that was satisfactory, she remained unhappy with her life, felt lonely, yet also disinterested in finding someone as a life partner. I had known Birgit over many years, as she sometimes just wanted to talk to me as her counselor. She talked of feeling rejected by her birth mother, while knowing nothing at all about her birth father. She certainly felt psychologically homeless and unable to find any resolution. I later learned from her adoptive parents that when she was in her late 30s, Birgit had committed suicide by swallowing pills. Her parents had felt helpless because Birgit had remained so distant from them. In a letter Birgit had left her parents, she told them she knew that they had done their utmost and did not reproach them at all. Her severe psychic homelessness was obvious, and she viewed suicide as her only way out of her pain.

Some Retrospective Thoughts

Are these cases the exception? A Swedish cohort study titled *Suicidal behavior in national and international adult adoptees* might offer some information (Borczyskowski et al., 2006). A total of 6,065 international adoptees were compared to 7,340 domestic adoptees and 1,274,312 non-adoptees, all born between 1963 and 1973, and followed up until 2002. Cox regression method was used in multivariate analyses to compare risks for suicide death and suicide attempt. The findings were that *international* adoptees had clearly a 4.5 times greater risk for a suicide attempt than non-adoptees (95% confidence interval 3.7–5.5). For death by suicide, adoptees were at 3.6 times greater risk after adjustments for sex, age, and socioeconomic factors (2.6–5.2). *National* (domestic) adoptees also had increased risk, although it was lower than for international adoptees: suicide attempts were 2.8 times greater risk (2.2–3.5), and suicide death 2.5 times greater (1.8–3.3). The conclusion of the researchers was that clinicians should be aware that an increased risk for suicide and suicide attempts in international adoptees especially is a topic that should be of great interest and concern to child and adult psychiatry.

The reasons for these differences? In 2005, David A. Brent and J. John Mann published their study *Family genetic studies, suicide, and suicidal behavior*. Reviewed were extant adoption, twin, and family studies of suicide and suicidal behavior. Their main conclusion was that suicidal behavior may be highly familial (heritable). This means that for adoptees, the higher risk for suicide and suicide attempts could be partly genetic, aside from relating to difficult life events, like early neglect, losing the birth parents, and continuing to have to deal with the loss of their original identity.

The given examples of the lives of John, Peter, and Birgit show us that a feeling of *psychic homelessness* was perhaps the most decisive factor because they did not feel they belonged either in the country where they were placed or with their adoptive parents. They felt fundamentally homeless (Hoksbergen, 1999, 2021). Many studies have been done on adopted children and their parents. Most of them dealt with certain problem behaviors, like reactive attachment disorder (Hoksbergen & Ter Laak, 2007) as the effect of early deprivation (Bowlby, 1980), posttraumatic stress disorder, fetal alcohol spectrum disorders (Knuiman, 2015), and others. All these studies tell us something about the complexity of the phenomenon of adoption and the impact on vulnerable children. However, in none of the studies has the identity issue been given adequate attention.

International Adoption of Children in the Netherlands

Intercountry adoption dates to the mid-seventies and was by far the most popular form, but as we now know, it was also the most complex form. Altogether, up to 2021, there were more than 40,000 intercountry adoptions. Interracial, as well as international, adoptions began in 1970, when the first children from South Korea arrived. Since that time, Dutch parents adopted children from about 50 countries and also from the USA, all under 1 year of age: in 2018, 23 adoptees; in 2019, 16; in 2020, 12. Most adopted children came from China (Table 2.2). In 2020, there were adopted children from Taiwan (17); Hungary and USA (12); Haiti (6); South Africa (6); Philippines, Lesotho, and Nigeria (4); Thailand and Burkina Faso (2); and Bulgaria (1). A total of 70 children. This small number is partly caused by the Corona pandemic.

Non-Relative Adoptions of Dutch-Born Children

The figures in Table 2.3 show that today there are hardly any Dutch non-relative adoptions. The main reasons for this fundamental change are:

- Giving up a child for adoption is, since the late eighties, very much against social norms and values and is not done anymore. The rare cases are mostly babies from young immigrant girls who experience significant psychosocial problems.

Table 2.2 Most Important Countries for Intercountry Adoptions in the Netherlands since 1971

Countries	Number of adoptions
China	7,000 (0 in 2020)
Colombia	5,500 (0 in 2019)
South Korea	4,147 (0 in 2004)
Sri Lanka	3,420 (0 in 2018)
India	3,060 (0 in 2017)
Indonesia	3,041 (0 in 1984)
Brazil	1,393 (0 in 2009)
Ethiopia	1,130 (0 in 2016)
Haiti	1,121
Taiwan	1,058
USA	600 (first child in 1993)

Source: (Adoption Center, 1996; Hoksbergen, 2021).

Note: Most children came from Asia. Political views changed in many sending countries (China, South Korea, Brazil), in the Muslim religion (Indonesia), and in the development of domestic adoption in most countries. It also resulted in a Dutch concern for the reliability of data about the proposed child for adoption.

- The financial system of society supports the unmarried mother financially so she can care for her family.
- International adoption as an option for parenthood became more acceptable beginning in the 1970s (Hoksbergen, 1998).

Since 1956, we can speak of almost 20,000 Dutch non-relative adoptions in a population of 11 million in 1956 and 17.4 million in 2020. Since the 1980s, all these adoptions are open. As soon as the adoptee is 18 years of age, they will get all available official information; with the consent of the biological parents also their addresses.

Complexities for Different Generations of Adoptive Parents

Domestic adoptions prior to but also following World War II occurred in what I am calling the first generation of adoptive families, the *traditional closed* generation. This is when adoption placement practices were particularly naïve, and we are now seeing the tragic results in adopted adults. Adoption at that time was primarily seen as a very private service for childless couples. Only a restricted group, perhaps 5–10%, of all involuntarily childless couples decided to adopt. As soon as the child was placed, the door was closed to outsiders. Adoption was just functional for the needs and wishes of these childless couples. The child should be told about being

Table 2.3 The Netherlands: In-Country and Foreign Adoptions, 1972–2021

	Domestic Adoptions	International Adoptions
1972	396	379
1974	214	626
1976	157	1,130
1978	144	1,211
1972–1979	total	7,173
1980	104	1,594
1982	77	1,045
1984	63	965
1986	63	1,198
1988	49	577
1980–1989	total	10,716
1990		830
1992		618
1994		
1996		
1998		
1990–1999	total	
2000	1,193	
2002	1,130	
2004	1,307	
2000–2004	total	
2006	816	
2008	767	
2010	706	
2005–2009	total	
2012	488	
2014	354	
2015		304
2016		214
2017		210
2018		156
2019		145
2020		70
2010–2020	total	3,575
2021		75 intercountry adoptions postponed
(Appendix 1)		
Total		
1972–2021	38,961	

Source: Ministerie van Justitie en Veiligheid. Adoptie (1972–2021)

adopted when 4 to 6 years of age. This fact of life should be de-emphasized. Quite a few children were never told, or only told once or twice at a young age. There was no specialized adoption service for the family. In the literature, the primary topic focused on Kirk's "rejection of difference" as a problem for adoptive parents (Kirk, 1964) because they had not been properly prepared for the differences between adopted children and those born to, and raised by, their parents. Problems had to be solved by the adoptive parents themselves.

Since World War II, the foreign or intercountry adoptions increased worldwide. In the Netherlands, television broadcasts about the wars in Southeast Asia in the fifties and sixties exerted great influence. It became apparent what these wars meant for hundreds of thousands of displaced children in Korea, Vietnam, and other countries. With the consent of the Dutch Minister of Legal Protection, private organizations started arranging adoptions from these countries. In the seventies, with a total of almost 9,000 international adoptions, there was much acceptance of adoption and a lot of enthusiasm of candidate-parents and leaders of adoptive organizations to help a child in need. But infertile couples no longer got priority, and about 40% already had children by birth. They believed in their parental capabilities and felt that they should try hard to raise and educate the child as "their own" child. This second generation of adoptive parents could be called the *open-idealistic* generation of adoptive parents.

Norms and values of society changed, and the need for much more openness was obvious (Pati, 2007). Parents had to adapt their attitude concerning adoption thoroughly. As a result of this change, three main effects can be noticed: Many more couples, including infertile couples, wanted to adopt a child. And although Western societies no longer accepted the idea of a woman relinquishing a child, intercountry and interracial adoption became the more normative solution. Social workers now recommended that adoptive parents be as open as possible regarding their child's background. Soon there were many thousands of people waiting to adopt a foreign child. But scientific research on the welfare of these children did not come until the latter part of the twentieth century and began with issues of attachment and acceptance of differences between members of the family (Kirk, 1953; Raynor, 1970; Cederblad, 1982; Feigelman & Silverman, 1983). Meanwhile, because of the increasing openness about adoption, some families were given two, three, or even four children, including those with special needs, such as physical and serious emotional problems. It was the time of the "rose-cloud" (roze-wolk), which lasted in the Netherlands at least 10 to 15 years. It was assumed that the child would be loving and fully accept the adoptive parents, who only needed to love the child. Besides, adoption was also openly recommended as the last possibility for these children to survive and develop normally. But until 1991, no consideration at all was given to services to help the adoptive family with the complications that they faced. In fact, this change did not come until 2021.

Meanwhile, beginning with the 1980s, the attitude of adoptive parents changed because of increased publications of research demonstrating that there were serious problems for the adoptive parents of an internationally adopted child, both in education and in interpersonal relationships for the child. Also, publications in the media came out about placement organizations' misrepresentations about the background and age of the child, about the reasons the child was being relinquished for adoption, and about financial deceit. The adoption seemed little more than a legal contract over the life of a human being not able to give any consent. All the prior assumptions of childless couples needed to be revised. Between 1988 and 1998, about half the number of adoptees were placed as compared to the years between 1974 and 1986 (Table 2.3). This resulted in the increasing awareness that adoption is often accompanied by complex organizational, physical, and psychological problems for the family, and the child's attachment capabilities were no longer a foregone conclusion (Egmond van, 1987; Hoksbergen, 1998; Rijk, 2008).

During this difficult and emotional process of social changes in society, it became evident that more childless couples would turn to other ways to get a child (fostering a child, artificial procreation, surrogate mothers). This became what I call the *economic-realistic* generation of adoptive parents. Meanwhile, from 1996 to 2004, the number of foreign adoptions in the Netherlands suddenly increased, almost up to the number of adoptions in the seventies. The main reason for this increase was adoption of children from China, most of them very young girls (the one-child policy). Almost 90% of these adopted children were under 2 years of age. It was believed that these young Chinese girls were easier to parent than adopted children from other countries. I call this the fourth generation of adoptive parents: *the prepared, optimistic, and demanding generation.* They were "prepared" because there was much more knowledge about adoption, owing to the large amount of international and Dutch research. Since 1991, those wanting to adopt were officially obliged to take a six-session preparation course of adoption. In 2004, there were 710 Chinese girls and 90 boys, the majority under 2 years of age, arriving in the Netherlands. More or less the same change occurred in other European countries and in the United States (Table 2.4). The year 2004 was, worldwide, the year of most adoptions from China: 13,412 children (Hoksbergen, 2021, p. 124; Selman, 2022b, 2022c).

The current generation of adoptive parents can be called the *generation conscious of contradictions* (or difficult choices), remaining childless being one of them, regarding the wish to acquire a child. Recently, the concerned Dutch minister decided to install an independent committee to investigate potential abuses related to intercountry adoption in the past, and also to install in 2022 a special center to re-appraise adoption practices. Adoptees will be helped to find the birth parents/family, and in case of emotional problems, they will be helped to find a qualified professional. After two years of research, the Joustra Report concluded the following:

> A very large group of adoptive parents have legally adopted children according to Dutch law. They trusted that the adoption was in order – an assumption which fits with the dominant social view. However, whether deliberately

or not, they too have contributed to the creation of an adoption market. There is also a group of potential adoptive parents whose involuntary childlessness and genuine desire to have children have been exploited for commercial gain. There were also some potential adoptive parents who wanted to adopt a child by any means necessary; their own desire to start a family was paramount. They deliberately pushed the boundaries, and in some cases they acted illegally. Although the children were often presented as orphans, many of them still had parents. Adoptees are often confronted with existential questions about how and why they were adopted, as well as questions about their origins and identity. When adoptees discover that their adoption involved abuses, this often triggers emotions such as anger or sadness. They may feel "trafficked" or "bought," and this can have an impact on their self-esteem. In turn, this fuels distrust and anger, directed not only at their birth parents or adoptive parents, but also at the Dutch and overseas governments and intermediaries from whom adoptees receive no support or understanding.

Some findings of the committee were not new at all. A lot of research had already been done, and since 1979, the author has been interviewed by TV reporters regarding complaints about the organization of intercountry adoption. It was clear that since the late-1970s, the task of the Dutch adoption organizations increasingly became meeting the demand for children by involuntarily childless couples. Although some intermediaries reported abuses, the organizations, just like the government, preferred to look the other way. After all, in their simple view, children in need and involuntarily childless couples were helped! The Dutch ministers did not decide to do anything at all against it until 2019. This change of the government was due to complaints from adult adoptees from several countries in Asia and South America about the way they were adopted and taken to the Netherlands. Questions about their identity are central now.

Complexities for Two Generations of Adoptees

Looking back at almost 70 years of adoption in the Netherlands, we can speak of two generations of adoptees, the first being those that were trapped, and many still are, in society's ignorance and selfishness. This could be called the *silent, closed* generation. Adoption was kept secret and was a taboo subject. Adoptees were mostly silent, an extension of their parents' isolation socially, although some are now writing their autobiographies. They are now able to tell us much more about their feelings, emotions, and judgments about their adoption. About 30,000 intercountry adoptees are 18 and older, and some Dutch adoptees are now over 60 years of age. The second generation of adoptees could be called the *open, active, and protesting* generation. They are very different psychologically from the earlier generation that had difficult attachments to their parents because the adoption system was so naïve in not properly screening applicants to adopt, and in not offering services for the parents and for the adoptive family as the child grew up. But for either generation, as they become adolescents and young adults, adoptees' questions about their identity are now their main focus (Hoksbergen & Van Dijkum, 2001).

As the adoptee grows through adolescence and young adulthood, he/she will increasingly realize what they have lost: birth parents and family name; country of origin with its history, culture, religion, and language; in the case of those adopted by lesbian/gay couples, missing a parent of the other sex, particularly if this has not been compensated for through another close relationship in the family. If the child differs racially from the adoptive parents, there are additional complexities. The child may feel emotionally distant from the parents as he/she grows up, often having to deal with guilt about it. This does not seem to be resolvable, unless questions about their background and birth parents can be answered, and until the adoptive parents can accept and understand their daughter/son's identity struggle and ambivalence.

More or less comparable effects are seen with donor children. Last April, Sprado and de Lange (2022), both donor children and half-sisters (by "accident"), and over 30 years of age, published their Schaduw Familie De zoektocht van donorkinderen: "Donor children, like adoptees, struggle with their identity and often need some help to find answers about their missing biological parent."

There are thousands of them in need of help, primarily psychological. In mid-2022 the Dutch minister decided to install a center of experts (expertise centrum), with the main tasks identified as helping adoptees access their records and all information available about their origins; support services to help them with this, regardless of their country of birth; and psychological services and any legal assistance.

Intercountry Adoption Worldwide on Its Way Out

The annual number of international adoptions worldwide peaked in 2004 at 45,452 to 23 receiving countries (Selman, 2015). Since then, numbers have fallen precipitously in most countries, including the Netherlands and the United States (Tables 2.3 earlier and Table 2.4, which follows):

The Naïveté in the Field of Adoption

Naïveté starts with the biological parents and concerned organizations in the country of origin that do not provide them with adequate information. Quite a few birth parents believe that the child, grown up in that faraway rich country, will never look back or want to see their biological parents or try to understand why they were sent far away for adoption. Social workers in the country of origin believed that keeping adoption files by the adoption organization in the country of origin for at least 100 years was not necessary at all. Similarly, in the receiving countries, the feeling was, "We help a child in need, and adoptive parents will love

Table 2.4 Number of Intercountry Adoptions, USA, 2005–2020

Year	Number ICA USA
2005	22,726
2006	20,675
2007	19,601
2008	17,449
2009	12,744
2010	11,058
2011	9,319
2012	8,667
2013	7,092
2014	6,438
2015	5,647
2016	5,370
2017	4,714
2018	4,059
2019	2,971
2020	1,622

Source: Bureau of Consular Affairs, US Department of State.

Note: Detailed figures for 23–25 countries are available on the HCCH website (see Selman (2022b). By 2020, the global total had fallen to 3,718, a decline of over 90%. In the Netherlands, the annual number fell from 1,307 in 2004 to 70 in 2020, a decrease of 95%, and in the USA, which had had the most international adoptions, numbers fell from 22,988 in 2004 to 1,622 in 2020, a decrease of 93% (Selman, 2022a). It seems that international adoption is likely to continue to fall and has almost ended.

that child as parents usually do." In Holland, the social workers who did the home study were not sufficiently educated to do this job because they did not know or care about all the complexities involved. Almost all aspirant adoptive parents got their approval to adopt.

Until 1991, there was no proper preparation course for aspirant adoptive parents at all. Up to today, there are hardly any treatment services to help adoptive families as the adopted child grows up. Sometimes two or more children of different ages were placed, and with special medical and/or educational problems, without any assistance offered over time. The Dutch adoption organizations were very naïve. The idea was, the parents eagerly want a child, so they will love the child a lot. After some problems in the beginning, everybody will be happy. Naïveté and poor judgment of almost all organizations concerned were the main characteristics of foreign adoption. Fortunately, some of this has changed now, but we still have to cope with the mistakes of the past. Let us look at another example.

An adoptive father of two children from Africa, now 21 and 25 years of age, wanted to share his experiences with other adoptive parents after his 20 years of adoption experience. His conclusions were:

> The impact on my life is enormous. I did not expect this at all.
> Never adopt two children together.
> If I had known this, I would never have adopted.

This adoptive couple had the genuine desire to have children, and he experienced the two boys immediately as his children. Their expressions, like "I love you very much," really meant something (Marrevee, 2022, p. 20–21, 23). He considered himself as a "born father," but after some years of experience, he started considering himself as a very naïve father. The education of the two little boys was very complicated, and his "being the father" was no reality at all. Feelings of being rejected by the older boy was one of the consequences of the father's possessive behavior. Finally, now 20 years later, he realized that he and his wife started their parenthood with the wrong expectations and beliefs. The grown boys, now young men, struggle to feel at home in the Netherlands and to find some balance in the relationship with their adoptive parents. But they have met their biological father and some relatives in Africa, although it was not successful because they assumed the young men were economically advantaged and therefore asked for money, but there were no feelings shown. These are some of the typical complications that internationally adopted young adults experience.

A Comment on Birth Parents

Until the beginning of this century, we also did not hear much about their birth parents, but this has fundamentally changed now. More and more angry birth mothers now tell their stories. The sadness and anger are about being forced, often by their own parents or by some authorities, to relinquish their child. The birth mothers were mostly under 20 years of age. Until 1965 (Bijstandswet, Social Security Act of Minister M. Klompé), they were financially dependent on their parents. All this has changed, and there are hardly any Dutch adoptions anymore because birth mothers are now helped financially so that they can keep their children.

Main Conclusions

International adoption is no longer seen as the first or primary solution for a child in need of a permanent home; other options are far preferable. But more and more we realize that if international adoption is the only option for the child, his/her original identity must be taken seriously, requiring greater effort to obtain facts and details that the adopted child may need later in life. This will help a great deal for the adopted person to build a healthy relationship with the adoptive family, feel at home in the new country, and become a person who is at peace with themselves and with their life. The child in need of a permanent home with loving, sensitive parents should be the primary focus, not the wish of adults to find a child. Hopefully, transnational adoption will be avoided altogether, meaning, very reduced numbers of placement organizations.

From a systemic perspective, the need remains for better efforts globally to ensure access to affordable reproductive education and birth prevention, as well as interventions to protect women and children who would otherwise be exploited.

Of greatest importance is the great need for clinical services for adopted adolescents and young adults who are in the midst of their greatest emotional struggles at a time there are unique demands on them having to do with their confusion about their identities. This requires much more than assistance with their efforts to search for information or to try to locate their birth families. It requires a willingness of government authorities to provide funding for a high level of advanced clinical trainings for counselors and psychotherapists, while helping adopted people obtain the kinds of qualified therapeutic services they need and deserve. Clinical skills, including training in early childhood development, are required for both handling the child's care and for determining who will have the personality features needed for adults to be selected as potentially very good, wise, and sensitive parents. Of course, the clinicians who should be handling this require higher salaries, which the state/welfare does not want to pay. This is always at the considerable expense of the children.

Most probably, we need an international colloquium, a coming together of adoption specialists, especially in psychology, psychiatry, social work, clinical social work, and those in the counseling fields. Perhaps soon, for the first time and at a crucial time for intended reforms, the Netherlands can host a conference with the primary program being the presentation of papers and meetings relating to the clinical issues in the evaluation and treatment of adopted people and their families. Another part of the agenda would be working in a preliminary way toward establishing higher and more uniform standards in the adoption field. These would include developing ideas for clinical trainings and for establishing better credentials for staff handling the placement of children for adoption – if we value our children, including adopted children, at all. For the sake of young people everywhere, it is urgent that all countries make a much greater investment in caring for their most vulnerable citizens, children and women.

Endnotes

Adoption Center. (1996). *Most Important Countries for Intercountry Adoptions in the Netherlands, 1970–1995*. Utrecht: University Adoption Center.

Borczyskowski, A., Hjern, A., & Lindblad, F. (2006). Suicidal behaviour in national and international adult adoptees. *Social Psychiatry and Psychiatric Epidemiology*, 41, 95–102. https://doi.org/10.1007/s00127-005-0974-2

Bowlby, J. (1980). *Attachment and Loss. Vol. 3: Loss, Sadness and Depression*. New York: Basic Books.

Brent, D.A., & Mann, J.J. (2005). Family genetic studies, suicide, and suicidal behavior. *American Journal of Medical Genetics Part C: Seminars in Medical Genetics*, 133C (1), 13–24.

Cederblad, M. (1982). *Children Adopted from Abroad and Coming to Sweden after Age Three.* Stockholm: NIA the Swedish National Board for Intercountry Adoption.

Egmond van, G. (1987). *Bodemloos bestaan. Problemen met adoptiekinderen* (Bottomless existence. Problems with adoptive children). Baarn: AMBO.

Feigelman, W., & Silverman, A. (1983). *Chosen Children. New Patterns of Adoptive Relationships.* New York: Praeger.

Hoksbergen, R.A.C. (1998). Changes in motivation for Adoption, value orientations and behavior in three generations of adoptive parents. *Adoption Quarterly*, 2, 37–56.

Hoksbergen, R.A.C. (1999). Psychic homelessness. In G. John, & M. Abbarno (Eds.), *The Ethics of Homelessness.* Leiden/Boston: Brill Rodopi, pp. 105–121.

Hoksbergen, R.A.C. (2021). Psychic homelessness in adoptees. In G.J.M. Abbarno (Ed.), *The Ethics of Homelessness: Philosophical Perspectives.* Leiden/Boston: Brill Rodopi, pp. 154–171.

Hoksbergen, R.A.C., & Ter Laak, J. (2007). Adult foreign adoptees: Reactive Attachment disorder may grow into psychic homelessness. *Journal of Social Distress and the Homeless*, 2 (4), 291–307.

Hoksbergen, R.A.C., & Van Dijkum, C. (2001). Trauma experienced by children adopted from abroad. *Adoption and Fostering*, 25 (2), 1–8.

Kirk, H.D. (1953). *Community Sentiments in Relation to Child Adoption.* Unpublished doctoral dissertation. Ithaca: Cornell University.

Kirk, H.D. (1964). *Shared Fate: A Theory and Method of Adoptive Relationships.* The Free Press of Glencoe.

Knuiman, S. (2015). *Development of Children Adopted from Poland. The Role of Early Life Risk Factors, Fetal Alcohol Spectrum Disorders and Parenting.* dissertation. Utrecht: Utrecht University.

Marrevee, R. (2022). *Vaderland: Het eerlijke verhaal van een adoptievader. (Fatherland. The honest Story of an Adoptive Father).* Schagen: Leessst.

Ministerie van Justitie en Veiligheid. Adoptie. 1972–2021. *Trends en analyse.* Ministry for Legal Protection. Adoption. Trends and Analysis. http://www.rijksoverheid.nl

Pati, J. (2007). *Adoption. Global Perspective and Ethical Issues.* New Delhi: Concept Publishing Company.

Raynor, L. (1970). *Adoption of Non-white Children. The Experience of a British Adoption Project.* London: G. Allen and Unwin.

Rijk, C.H.A.M. (2008). *Coping with the Effects of Deprivation. Development and Upbringing of Romanian Adoptees in the Netherlands.* Enschede: the Netherlands Print Partners Ipskampo BV. dissertation. Utrecht: Utrecht University.

Selman, P. (2015). *Global Statistics for Intercountry Adoption Worldwide: Receiving States and States of Origin, 2003–2013.* Newcastle upon Tyne: Newcastle University (More recent figures: Adoption Worldwide: 1980–2019).

Selman, P. (2022a). *Changes in Annual ICA-rates 2015–2020.* pfselman@yahoo.co.uk

Selman, P. (2022b). Global statistic for intercountry Adoption. *Receiving States and States of Origin 2004–2020.* https://assets.hcch.net/docs/a8fe9f19-23e6-40c2-855e-388e112bf1f5.pdf

Selman, P. (2022c). One million children moving: Seventy years of transnational adoption since the end of World War II. In S. Hackenesch (Ed.), *Adoption Across Race and Nation: US Histories and Legacies.* Ohio: Ohio State University Press.

Sprado, L., & de Lange, V. (2022). *Schaduw Familie De Zoektocht van donorkinderen (Shadow Family: The Search of Donor Children).* Schiedam: Scriptum.

Verrier, N.N. (1993). *The Primal Wound. Understanding the Adopted Child.* Baltimore: Gateway Press.

APPENDIX

1. On February 8, 2021, all Dutch foreign adoptions were postponed by the Minister for Legal Protection (Ministerie van Justitie en Veiligheid), due to the results of an independent committee, to investigate potential abuses related to intercountry adoption in the past.
2. For all years: Ministry of Legal Protection. Adoption. Trends and analysis. Figures before 1972 not available, also no statistics for in-country adoptions in 1992.

3
CHALLENGING ADOPTION NARRATIVES
Adult Adoptees Write Remembrance – Four Australian Case Studies

Catherine Margaret Lynch, PhD, JD; Sue Green, PhD; and Alison Ingram, PhD (Cand.)

Editors' Note

The authors of the following chapter, adopted adults, speak entirely from the perspective of "lived experience," much of which they believe was affected by their early trauma. It has been observed in the adoption literature that "the voice of the adoptee" has had little representation. Therefore, we believe this chapter is significant because the authors, as professionals in different fields, speak in their own voices. Their comments reflect the subjective experience of some adopted people and reveal common themes, or variations of them, that may come up in the treatment of an adopted person. What they have to say about their experiences with trauma also demonstrate the way multiple traumas can be conflated into particular themes, that is, trauma around separation from the birth mother soon after birth, trauma from discoveries of secrets and lies, trauma from experiences of neglect or abuse within the adoptive family, which the adoption placement field has not wanted to acknowledge, and finally, the cumulative effect of being deprived of full human rights into and throughout adulthood by a system that purports to be concerned about the "well-being of children" – when the real priority has been appealing to the large "market" of individuals wanting to adopt.

Most of the existing studies of trauma and attachment as topics are based on subjects who are not adopted, and further, the studies do not specifically address early developmental trauma (Bertocci, Chapter 1) and its often-profound sequelae. However, we are very pleased by the recent publication of a special edition of *Child Abuse and Neglect* that finally links trauma with adoption and that includes the voices of adopted authors (D. McSherry, G. Samuels, and D. Brodzinsky, eds., 2022) In

DOI: 10.4324/9781003095507-4

the following chapter, the authors' perspectives demonstrate the details and depth of information that can only be obtained directly from adopted people and that can never be accessed through standardized testing protocols, or even by questionnaires designed by researchers, unless they are informed by the psychology of *being* adopted. The editors acknowledge the difficulties of finding adopted subjects who are not "self-selected," as are the survey respondents in this chapter. Clinically focused studies are much needed, and they must provide more in the way of *clinical* detail than the generalized findings, concepts, and labels that characterize much of the current research literature.

The following chapter by Australian authors demonstrates the accumulation of trauma throughout the lives of many adopted people *in all countries* (Newman, 2011) whose experience with their adoptive families was less than optimal, for reasons that relate to the systemic problems discussed throughout the book. The reader will recognize in this chapter many personal details and expressions that are heard in the consulting room of psychotherapists. The authors' accounts serve as a reminder of the enduring impact of the sealed adoption record on a global scale. However, this is being treated in some of the current adoption literature as a problem of the past. That is, the extensive focus on open adoption over the last few decades remains limited to young children, and in the process, it has eclipsed the tragic legacy of closed adoption that endures generationally.

However, the implications are clear for psychotherapists treating adopted clients who are no longer children, especially adolescents and young adults: we know that serious difficulties for adopted people endure due to adoption practices of the past as well as the present. These include different forms of neglect and abuse within the adoptive family that adopted clients have revealed in treatment, but it has never been acknowledged by any of the systems interfacing with adoption, and the authors are correct that research is very slight (Matthews, 2020).

We honor countries like Australia that say they recognize their debt to adopted people by now offering to provide any treatment they may need. However, the authors of the following chapter point out that in reality, it is still very difficult for adopted Australians to access their records, and they say they still have not been provided the support through therapeutic treatment that their government had promised. We, as editors, add that, according to their limited description of coursework for the training intended for counselors and therapists, the amount of training being offered is negligible relative to the amount of study needed in order to be qualified to provide a clinical level of treatment. Clearly, the message has not gotten through.

The additionally complex development of adopted persons *over time* cannot be known or understood if adoption research is limited to pre-adolescent children. If adopted persons seek the help of psychotherapists, they cannot be adequately treated unless practitioners in all disciplines are willing to avail themselves of serious clinical training. And if researchers wish to contribute to clinical practice, they must work collaboratively with those who are knowledgeable about not only the psychology of adoption but also the psychology of *being* adopted.

Introduction by C. Lynch

In October 2021, taking advantage of the Australian "lockdown" mandated by Australian state governments as a response to the COVID-19 pandemic, which kept Australians in their homes, I circulated a post on Facebook inviting adopted people to respond to an emailed qualitative survey of their experience as an adopted person between the ages of 18 and 30. As an adoptee myself, I was aware of, and had experienced, that commonality in adoptee experience which was the inability to speak publicly about adoption, at least critically, as a young person. This silencing had a multitude of causes, including lack of knowledge of one's origin due to adoption laws and policies, taboo within adoptive families who made it known that the topic was uncomfortable and off-limits due to their own issues with infertility or their attitudes towards children born from single mothers, and prejudice and discrimination against adopted people, who were historically categorized as "bastards," "illegitimate," and/or "orphans" and somehow the object of blame, shame, or pity, with the accompanying expectation that they should be grateful for being saved by their adoptions. Even today, speaking publicly about one's adoption places a young person's closest family relationships at risk, and further, abandonment is understandably one of an adoptee's greatest fears, having already survived what would have been experienced as abandonment at or near to birth, when they were separated, forcibly or no, from their mothers. For babies, all adoptions are forced adoptions, because no baby wants to be permanently separated from their mother. And for most adoptees, the only safe time to speak about adoption is once the adoptive parents have passed away.

Knowing this, I opened the survey to respondents of all ages, tailoring the questions to capture the retrospective wisdom of older adoptees, who can clearly recall their experiences when young. My impetus came from my lived experience as an adoptee interacting with adoptees all over the world and hearing time and again the lament that nobody understood what it was like being adopted except other adoptees. And this "nobody" included therapists.

Survey Methodology

To assist in collating the data gathered from the four respondents, a further two authors, Alison Ingram and Dr. Sue Green, came on board to bring their lived experience as adoptees to the data analysis. This approach of inviting participation from people with lived experience is informed by Vojtila et al. (2021) and studies found in their references to research on the collaborative care model. Three of the respondents, Cheryl, Darryl, and Michael, are Australian adoptees in their early 50s. Only the fourth respondent, Anne, a "late discovery" adoptee, is in her 70s. All four respondents were taken from their mothers at, or very soon after, birth and adopted under the Australian "closed-records" system, which typically recorded any names given to such babies, and the name of their mothers (and occasionally the name of their fathers), but issued a post-adoption birth certificate listing a new name and the names of the adoptive parents, as if the baby were born to them. "As if born to" was the actual phrase taken from the governing legislation in Australia's states and territories and reflects the intention that adoptions were to be kept secret, and the adoptee forbidden access to their origins information for the duration of their lives. Michael was the only respondent who was not quickly delivered to the homes of adoptive parents. Born three and half months prematurely, he remained in the hospital and an institution for his first six months, and impacts on children who enter out of home care are well documented (D'Cruz & Gillingham, 2017; Lonne, 2013).

Together, the three authors informed our reading with the four-tiered conceptual framework developed by Winkler et al. (1988, pp. 7–15) to underpin post-adoption clinical practice. Researchers have noted that there has been a lack of awareness about adoption in the therapeutic field (O'Brien & Zamostny, 2003), and Green (2017) notes that it is left to writers who are both professionals and impacted by adoption themselves to bring professional attention to this undeveloped space.

It is a commonality in the experience of all our four respondents that they lived through the legislative changes in the 1990s that began to dismantle the closed-records system, legislating access to adoption records for adoptees over 18 years of age, providing the opportunity to search for families of origin. These changes did little for Anne, as she did not discover her adoption until she was in her 70s. This reminds us that even today there is no guarantee that a child will be told they are adopted (despite holding the lived "knowledge" of it in their bodies), and that the new "integrated" birth certificate available to adoptees in Victoria and New South Wales that is purported to include both the adoptive parent/s and the parent/s of origin still does nothing to ensure that adopted people are informed they are adopted. Adoptive parents may simply choose to provide the certificate version that lists only them as the parents. The secrecy of the closed-records system lingers on in modern adoption legislation and practice, continuing to infringe upon the human rights of adoptees to know who they are and where they come from.

The respondents' data has been organized into four key themes. Part 1 examines the respondents' remembered experience of adolescence and young adulthood with respect to the perceived impacts of mother loss at or near to birth as well as their experience of any search, contact, and/or reunion. Part 2 examines the respondents' remembered experience of growing up in their adoptive families during the same period, along with their broader experience in the macrocosm of society and its adoption system. Part 3 focuses specifically on adoptees' conceptions of self-worth and their negotiation of interpersonal relationships. Part 4 presents their attitudes toward their experiences seeing therapists, followed by suggestions for clinical treatment.

Part 1: The Adoptee in Their Family of Origin

A. Mother Loss

Permanent mother–baby separation causes a "trauma common to all adoptees" (Clothier, 1943, 222), and this is both implicit and made explicit in the responses of Cheryl, Darryl, and Michael, who claim that their permanent separation from their mothers at or near to birth was a traumatic experience that continued to cause them suffering between the ages of 18 and 30 years of age: "The trauma I experienced at birth by the abandonment of my family has had lifelong and quite a devastating impact on me" (Cheryl). Whether or not Cheryl's separation from her mother was an abandonment or, more likely, fell along the spectrum between coercion and force is a matter of fact that would have made little difference to the infant experience of that separation and loss. In this respect, the physiological impacts suffered by babies by the mother's permanent absence – unassuaged calling, searching and rooting behaviors, excessive crying, sleep disruption, refusal of food, and dysregulation of a multitude of biological systems – are experienced by all adoptees who are separated from their mothers at or near to birth, regardless of the consent of the mother to separation (Lynch, 2021, pp. 142–144). Cheryl claims the long-term impacts of mother loss soon after birth continued to be experienced by her between the ages of 18 and 30 years in symptoms of depression, panic attacks, and suicidality. Like Cheryl, Darryl makes a specific connection between the separation event near to birth as an early childhood trauma and his later experiences as an adolescent and young adult: "I think I experienced separation anxiety, which led to depression, complex PTSD, gastrointestinal issues, and later in life has led me to experiencing poor relationships and other mental health issues."

In contrast to Cheryl and Darryl, Michael was born prematurely and suffered immediate further traumas after separation, moving between a children's hospital and a mothers-and-babies home for the first six months of his life. He believes that the impact from his early cumulative traumas, untreated and unacknowledged, caused him to make "multiple suicide attempts with long-term abuse/use of alcohol and prescription medication" between the ages of 18 and 30 years. He believes that remaining with his mother would have mitigated some of the impacts of premature birth and hospitalization, and he writes broadly of himself as a young man: "If I had been given the option and choice to know my mother/father and the truth of my origins, it would have saved me a huge amount of pain and the ongoing trauma throughout my life."

The previous three respondents were aware during their adolescence and young adulthood that they were adopted, as they had been told in childhood, Cheryl and Michael claiming that they had "always known" and Darryl finding out when he was 14 years of age. An adoptee's discovery of their adoptive status, either by being told or discovering it for themselves, is another commonality in adoptee experience, but Anne, at 70 years of age, had the conscious knowledge of her adoptive status kept from her for most of her life. Anne was told she was adopted by her brother, the telling precipitated by the obscure chance discovery by her (adoptive) sister of a penciled notation in recently acquired paperwork relating to the latter's daughter (Appendix 1). Anne writes about her adoptive sister:

> *I was 70 when I accidentally found out. My sister had an out-of-wedlock baby when she was 16 and spent the next 50 years looking for her to no avail, with strict adoption laws in place. When the laws changed in 2000, her daughter found my sister with much joy all round. They were looking through the welfare papers when my sister noticed a penciled note in a margin saying, "Mother adopted, but they don't think she knows." My sister asked me what I knew; I was bewildered and rang our brother, who said, "Secret . . . Mum and Dad . . . I'll tell you what I know." It transpired he had known for 50 years but he and his wife had been sworn to secrecy by our parents. He was their natural child. There had been a stillborn baby boy, and my sister and I were adopted! Absolutely floored at the news!*

The adoptee author Betty Jean Lifton claims that "hearing one is not born to one's mother is a profound and unrecognized trauma" (1994, 63). If this is the case, then it is safe to say that Anne is responding to our survey in the midst of a new "cumulative trauma event" (Lifton, 1994) as she tries to process an almost entire life lived through a lens of secrets and lies created by others. Because she was unaware she was adopted between the ages of 18 and 30, Anne writes that she was "completely unaware and [had] absolutely no inkling, apart from occasional feelings of what [she] called 'apartness.'" Yet a feeling of "apartness" is another commonality expressed not only by adoptees but also by other people who have suffered lengthy separations from their mothers after birth, such as premature babies kept in the humidity cribs of the 1970s. Separating mothers and babies creates a psychological distance in the mind of the child that continues to manifest as loneliness later in life, the sense of being "separated" from the rest of humanity exacerbated by the diminished experience of intimacy after birth that is a hallmark of being mothered by an initial stranger. Anne writes of her mother's death: "[I was removed] before she saw me. As evidenced by her dying words at 91, 'Why won't they bring me my baby?'", her mother's words disturbing evidence of the lifelong impacts of trauma caused to mothers by the removal of their babies (Rickarby, 1995, 1998; Higgins et al., 2016).

B. Search, Contact, Reunion

The feelings of rejection that at least three of the respondents describe in relation to their mothers and families of origin were re-experienced and amplified in a further commonality in adoptee experience: the search journey. The search journey can have up to three components: search for origins information, contact with relatives, and reunion/reunion failure with the mother. Searching may unearth origin information that produce flashpoints of rejection, such as if files containing personal information are stated to be lost (as is the case of Darryl), if documents on file contain hurtful information (as in the case of Michael and Cheryl), if a veto on contact has been placed against the adoptee, or in the discovery that the mother or father has died (again, as in the case of Darryl). Contact may be rejected outright or involve initial cooperation, which is withdrawn at a later date, as in the case of Cheryl, who had both her parents change their minds about getting to know her. Reunion, which occurs when adoptees are reunited with their mothers, is always fraught, complicated as it is by the trauma suffered by both the mother and the adoptee and which often makes reunion too emotional and difficult to sustain over time.

Michael, Darryl, and Cheryl were all successful in identifying and contacting their mothers and/or other relatives between the ages of 18 and 30 years. But if the practical reality of reunion with one's mother "constitutes a major life crisis" (Goodwach, 2001, p. 73), then how much more devastating is the experience of finding one's mother already in the grave, knowing that it is your own family, society, and government which actively prevented your reunion. Of his mother, who "died before the law allowed [him] to know her," Darryl says, "I feel terrible for her. I feel like I didn't want to go. I feel stolen, and this abuse is endorsed by the government and the Salvation Army."

For Michael and Cheryl, the secondary rejection by their mother is brutal and undeniable. During his adolescence, Michael was able to contact his mother's first husband and then reach out to her by both telephone and email. Her refusal of any further contact had such an impact on him that it took him "two decades to find the courage to reach out and/or search for other family members." Twenty years is a long time to find courage to continue searching, and this gives some indication of the magnitude of feeling that such rejection reinforces and amplifies, building, as it does, on the early childhood experiences of mother loss and the attachment disruptions caused in the care system and hospitalizations. For Cheryl, the secondary rejection is something you never recover from: "When my mother rejected me at 28, it absolutely shattered me, and I have never, even to this day, recovered from that. Her rejection changed me." When her father also rejected her, asking her not to make contact again two months after initially providing her with background information and saying he would be available at any time, Cheryl entered a very lengthy depression and claims she became permanently changed.

> *When my mother rejected me, I was a young mother at that time with a toddler and a baby. I physically felt pain in my heart as my mother told me she wanted nothing to do with me. While undiagnosed, I suffered a deep depression for a number of years, into my third pregnancy and beyond. I also spent a lot of time after this rejection rejecting others, pushing people away and carrying a great deal of anger. Throughout this time, I also experienced*

suicidal ideation, which has occurred at various times in my life, commencing in my teenage years.

The impact of secondary rejection in the process of search, contact, or reunion should not be underestimated. A reunion with a mother and contact with family who express love and regret for the loss of their child/grandchild/relative, commitment to getting to know the adopted person and learning of the adopted person's life without them, and acknowledgment of the multiple traumas they have suffered would go an immeasurably long way in helping adult adoptees to heal, by enabling them to relegate the source of their traumas to something in the past, a relegation that can only make their present management of impacts easier in the knowledge that the worst is over. But for so many adopted people, their family of origin has its own unprocessed trauma, including that caused by the loss of a baby, that compromises their ability to understand the adopted adolescent or young person. If a young adopted person is looking to their family of origin for the understanding and intimacy that they felt they never got within their adoptive families, then they are likely to be devastatingly disappointed, and the testimony of at least three of the respondents illustrate this clearly.

Adopted people, biologically programmed to need their mothers' love, may look for a way to interpret the rejection by their families of origin as selflessly and compassionately as possible, and in line with this, adopted people in the media are often quoted as saying they are grateful to their natural mothers, or forgive them, telling them they did the right thing and they have had a good life. But the reality, especially once the "reunion honeymoon period" is over, is that adopted people can really struggle to sustain sympathy for their natural kin in the face of relentless rejection. In the following excerpt, Cheryl oscillates in her struggle to reconcile the truth of her origins, relating her shock, anger, understanding, and empathy, before ending with the plaintive question of her abandonment:

I always had the belief that my mother was young and unsupported. When I received my information, I discovered my mother and father were both aged 37 when I was born. That was a real surprise. I had to come to terms with the fact that my birth parents were mature, supposedly responsible adults and not young and vulnerable. . . . I was also shocked to discover I was the result of an affair – single mother and married father. This was difficult to come to terms with as it challenged my values. After being rejected, apart from depression, I also became internally angry. For many years, anger simmered away inside me.

I have often wondered about her mental health throughout her pregnancy with me. My older birth sibling can recall, as an 8-year-old, that our mother cried a lot. (He can't recall her being pregnant or giving birth.) . . . I believe the stigma of single motherhood and financial hardship are the reasons I was placed for adoption. Had my birth mother received support, my story may have been different. I was the consequence of two adults having an affair — I certainly was not the cause. I will never understand how a mother can carry a baby growing inside her, birth it, and then turn her back and walk away. When did it become okay to give your child away?

Adoptees must come to terms with repeated rejections, from birth until death, from the very people from whom they so desire connection, acceptance, and love – a desire so powerful that Lifton has compared it to "a religious search because it's an attempt to connect to forces larger than oneself" (1994, p. 128). Cheryl can still recall the powerful sense of loss she lived with between the ages of 18 and 30:

> During these ages, many things happened. I moved out of my adopted home, married, created my own home, and had two of my children in this time frame. So many changes and challenges. Additionally, as stated earlier, the laws changed, and I sought my information. I don't recall a time that my mother, in particular, has not been at the forefront of my mind. I feel like I've missed her my entire life.

Part 2: Relation to Adoptive Family

A. The Adoptive Family Microcosm

The all-pervasive governmental and societal pressure to classify adoption as an act of benevolence has the capacity to blind therapists to the very real trauma that adoptees can suffer growing up in adoptive households. This presents a third layer of trauma for adopted people, who, at the very least, may struggle as children to be understood by and to understand their closest family members (as in the case of all the respondents, including Anne), unable to relax in the mirroring of genetic familiarity, and at the very worst, may suffer from childhood abuse, as in the cases of both Darryl and Michael, in some extreme cases, even fighting for survival.

Cheryl describes her adoptive family as "racist, prejudiced, misogynistic, and sexist": "I grew and developed separate opinions to them, particularly through the ages of 18 to 30, while creating my own family and developing an independent identity."

> I don't ever recall there being any expressions of love either verbally or physically. . . . I feel disconnected, alone, and unfortunately, not worthy of love. The trauma I experienced, I have no doubt, has impacted the ability for me to accept their love. During my search and attempted reunion with my birth family, I received no support or understanding. In fact, in finding and uniting with two of my siblings, I haven't even shared this with my adoptive family, as I'm sure they would have no understanding and would offend me

by providing their opinions. I feel that my adoptive family is quite dysfunctional. . . . Adoption has never been about me. I was a commodity, and so was my mother. It was always about my adoptive parents and how difficult it was for them: "We had to go through so much to get you." I don't believe my adoptive parents have ever considered what my birth mother went through, and they have no idea or interest in how it has impacted my life.

Cheryl writes that her adoption was "never really discussed," but that she still received "the general narrative of being special and lucky." She mentions feeling her family was different, searching faces in crowds, looking for "mirroring," some familiarity, but that despite this, she was unaware at the time of her adolescence and young adulthood how much adoption was impacting her life:

With hindsight, I know that I have been seriously impacted and am now more aware of triggers. I still cannot control the onset of triggers, but I try to control my reaction to them. It's still very hard.

Cheryl rejects the idea that she was "chosen" and never felt "lucky." "I believe I was the next on the list. I was once told by my adoptive mother that I was 'nearly Aboriginal' – my adoptive parents had been offered Aboriginal [stolen generation; Appendix 1] babies before me."

Neither was adoption discussed in Darryl's adoptive family:

I suspected it, and I had asked several times prior to me discovering the truth. My skin was white; my adoptive parents were olive. I didn't think like them. I didn't feel what I should feel as a "family." I didn't feel wanted by my adoptive father. I felt isolated and had to be self-sufficient. The revelation changed my personality from an outgoing, creative extrovert to an inward-thinking, isolated individual. . . . . I was too white, so I really didn't match their skin tone. I didn't have their features or think like them, but I think this was invisible to most people. I felt I didn't fit in, and once I discovered I was adopted, I was unconsciously questioning why I was there with them at all.

Like Cheryl, Darryl received the same adoption narrative about being "chosen" and rejects it as a lie:

I was told by my adoptive mother that I was "chosen." This, too, turned out to be a lie. There was no choice. I was just the next fresh baby in line. . . . All this has made me more insular as a person. Negatively affected my relationships. Unsurprisingly, I have developed more mental health issues. . . . It showed me I had been lied to by my adoptive parents all my life. . . . It separated me from my true family and cheated me of my true existence. Laws restricted me from ever meeting my birth mother (she died before I could know her). . . . There wasn't really a

> reason I was adopted. . . . Their story neglected to tell me I was fostered for the first two years, which I only found out two years ago. This has led to some distance between my adoptive mother and me.

Despite all this, Darryl felt his adoptive mother always loved and wanted him, and in this he had a similar experience to Anne, who "felt accepted, well-treated, and loved" by her adoptive parents, despite feeling she was "not so much understood" by her adoptive mother. Darryl is able to take pride in what he has been able to achieve in his life, despite the treatment of his adoptive father, who was angry and sometimes violent toward him and who, not valuing education, pulled him out of school in year 10 so he could add to the family income.

> Nevertheless, I relied on my innate talents and obtained work, which developed into a salary where I was able to buy a house for all of us (at 19 years old). I never felt supported. I was never included in family decisions or even given reasons why we moved around so much even though this disrupted my childhood so significantly.

Darryl had issues with his stomach during his childhood but was never treated for it, and he suffers from osteochondritis dissecans (holes in both knees). His surgeons suspect this was a malformation due to a lack of nutrients in his teen years. He also reports abuse:

> At 10 years old, I was subject to physical abuse by my adoptive father. At 14 years old, I was subject to sexual abuse by an uncle (adoptive family). Later, this was dismissed by my adoptive mother.

Michael's adoptive family rarely discussed his adoption, yet he received the same formulaic reason and came to the same conclusion, as Cheryl and Darryl, that his adoptive parents had lied to him:

> I was chosen and special – this is false. I was unwanted even as an infant.

Like Cheryl, Michael writes that his adoptive family was a "typical WASP family – racist, classist family." "I was highly aware of their bigoted views and speech – made me sick to the stomach." Asked if he felt whether his adoptive parents were loving, loyal, and supportive, or that the adults involved in his adoption were empathic towards him and that his best interests were prioritized over adult interests, Michael replied, "Not in the slightest – and this is still the case. This includes both my biological parents and adoptive parents (and the majority of members of all families)." Michael writes, "I did not fit in my adoptive family – scapegoat child/bad seed," and he describes the way they acquired him in similar negative terms:

My adoptive parents originally tried to adopt through their local parish (Anglican Diocese of Newcastle); they were denied this request due to poor attendance. 2ND DRAW PRIZE IN A SHITTY LOTTERY.

Michael sums up his experience within the adoptive household as "decades of abuse." Although abuse within adoptive families may not be a commonality in adoptive experience, the pressures to view adoption as an act and state of benevolence seriously fail adoptees like Michael by preventing public recognition of a whole demographic of adoptee survivors of family abuse. To this day, there has been no research done on this cohort that the authors are aware of, anywhere in the world. (See Editors' Note.)

B. The Adoption System Macrocosm

Despite his treatment within his adoptive family, Michael shows considerable bravery in his broaching of his adoptive status to people beyond the adoptive family, during his childhood and adolescence. When people told Michael that he looked like his mom or dad, Michael would tell them that he was adopted: "It took me a while to understand why I was then looked upon with sadness and embarrassment and the subject changed."

This negative reaction by people outside the immediate adoptive family can be replicated throughout a broader society that resists and obstructs adoptees' search for information and kin and continues to discriminate against them (in some countries by maintaining a closed-records system that continues to deny them their basic civil and human rights to know themselves). When the laws changed in Australia and allowed adoptees to apply for their original (pre-adoptive) birth certificate, which contained their original name, if they had one, and the name of their mother, it became quickly evident to Cheryl, Darryl, and Michael that there was no immediate change toward adoptees in broader culture and society. Typically, adoptees find themselves confronted by obstructionist and paternalistic staff in adoption organizations, hospitals, courts, and government departments. According to Darryl, when he searched, he was told that key documents had been "lost in the Brisbane floods," and Cheryl found her documents heavily redacted: "Love it when a government employee can decide to redact my information as they see fit!"

Darryl describes his tendency, as a young man, to bury his feelings due to the hopelessness brought about by a closed-records system. The hope brought about by the opening of records led him to the truth of how that system failed him. Darryl lays blame for his trauma at the feet of the Queensland government's children's department, along with the Salvation Army: "[They] separated me from my true family and concealed my identity, leading to me developing mental health issues." He states that when he asked the state government for his medical records in his 20s, he "was fed lies." Not only this, but the government had also failed in its duty of care by not informing his mother, who had gone on to marry his father, that he had not been immediately adopted by his carer and was, in fact, fostered for two years before the adoption by his carers was finalized. This failure to keep his mother informed meant that she did not know, even though she had married his father, that she would be able to get him back. Later on, the government made no attempt to inform Darryl that his mother had died: "My birth mother had died of a cerebral hemorrhage at 30 years old, yet I was not told anything about this."

For Darryl, the lies and negligence he discovered kept multiplying. Searching again at age 30, he writes of "finding incorrect records that stated [he] was the inbred product of a rape. Records which couldn't be changed according to the government." Her mother had told staff that her pregnancy was from a rape by her first cousin, but Darryl discovered later that his father was actually her then long-time boyfriend.

> She named me after her long-term boyfriend, the true father. . ... I had been marked as "unfit" for adoption (due to a doctor's assessment relying on my mother's false declaration of paternity). The government had incorrectly marked me as an inbred, with probable developmental issues coming. I had to be evaluated periodically during the first two years.

Darryl goes on to state that his adoptive mother "was told she could exchange [him] for any other should [he] not pass the tests." Darryl's foster/adoptive mother could have returned him, and his mother reclaimed him, but this was prevented by a government who failed to inform his parents that he was not, as they thought, yet adopted: "This made me feel, later in life, that the government had neglected their paramount consideration: their duty of care for me."

Darryl believes the interests of the adoptive family were prioritized over all other interests:

> Obviously, adoption is only in the interests of the couple that wish to adopt, and no real assessment of their ability to parent children, or even their mental health, was ever undertaken. The only qualification at my birth was that they were married. The state's mechanisms certainly worked well to expedite the consent from my birth mother and whisk me away to a foster family, but due diligence was never conducted in my case, and my best interests, set by law, were disregarded by the government.

Part 3: Remembering Relationships: The Impact of Being Adopted on Self-Esteem

Reflecting on the impact of his adoptive status on his sense of self-worth and his relationships in adolescence and young adulthood (between the ages of 18 and 30 years), Darryl writes that through those years, "[he] certainly would have had undiagnosed mental health issues." "Now that I'm older, I plainly see the effects of C-PTSD, depression, stress, personality splitting, perfectionism, compulsion, rumination."

Deep down . . . I told myself I was worthy; it was their loss (my birth parents). I set out to overachieve and was driven by this. I was an individual and dressed like it. I had my own ideas. At school in the country, this was frowned upon by other children, and I was bullied terribly. However, once I turned 18, I was working in advertising, and creativity was valued. I was successful at a young age. In relationships, however, I felt subordinate, worthy, yet compliant. I had learned compliance through my childhood, not fitting in with my adoptive family, not wanting to rock the boat for fear of violence or abuse.

Darryl became a pleaser, expending a lot of energy making others, including his partner, happy, but not himself.

Minor altercations and disagreements in relationships have been seen by me as devastating attacks and loss of trust, leading to breakdown. I feel I can never get close to anybody. I feel like no one ever supports me. I have never married or had children, and I attribute this to the effects of my relinquishment and adoption. As for friendships, I can count on one hand my remaining close friends over the course of my 56 years on earth.

When Michael is asked if he felt his adoption had impacted his interpersonal relationships between the ages of 18 and 30, he replies, "Absolutely – fundamentally so." He writes that adoption had a "huge negative effect." "Always thought I was ugly (abject/other) as there was no one to reflect back to me who I looked like in any positive way," and that he "was terrified of a girlfriend falling pregnant." He repeats that it had a "huge impact," that he had "no self-care," was "highly co-dependent and self-sabotaging." He writes simply that "infant adoption is a human rights violation."

When Cheryl is asked if she felt her adoption impacted her interpersonal relationships between the ages of 18 and 30, she replied:

Absolutely. I have been with the same partner since I was 16. . . . At around the age of 18, while not aware at that time that I was doing it, I pushed him away, fighting and arguing with him. . . . I have very few friends. Part of me is okay with that, because I'm quite happy in my own company. I enjoy time on my own, and I am able to entertain myself. However, I worry that I will be a lonely old lady in the twilight of life. Certainly, in my late 20s, I was very angry. This quite likely impacted my ability to maintain or create friendships. I tend to be the doormat in friendships. A low self-worth has also impacted my ability to be intimate.

Asked if she felt that being adopted impacted her advancement in life, her ability to know herself, look after her own well-being, and provide for herself and others, including convincing employees to hire and retain her, Cheryl replied:

Adoption and, particularly, identity issues and a low self-worth have certainly impacted my advancement in life. Throughout my teenage years, all I could think about was being old enough and gaining enough independence to be able to move out of my adoptive home. I always knew this was the only way I could develop my identity. I didn't achieve this. I married young – this was a pathway out. I didn't receive the support and guidance I needed to advance my education. I was encouraged to get any job and not complete my schooling. A career or work life was never considered important. I can recall my husband (who was my boyfriend at that time) and my adoptive father discussing/arguing about whether I would work after having children. My father insisted that I would be a stay-at-home mom. He tried very hard to maintain or retain a strong control or discipline over me beyond my teen years, which led to difficulties in our relationship as I gained maturity and independence. . . . I have found a lack of confidence and low self-esteem have impacted my employment. . . . I often put myself down, without even realizing it. My needs are always secondary to others'. I am a people pleaser, and my role in life is to ensure others are happy.

Regarding self-perception, in terms of her appearance and body image, between the ages of 18 and 30, Cheryl had body image issues.

With the knowledge of the impact mirroring has on identity development, I now know how much this affected me. . ... My second two children are physically like me. It has been quite amazing to watch them and pick the similarities we have. Interestingly, since meeting my full biological brother and his children, I feel like I'm more accepting and more relaxed about my looks and body image. However, my self-worth has taken more of a bashing, and I believe that's because I feel even less worthy because I was the unkept sibling.

Anne resents that the closed-records system prevented her from knowing that her mother suffered from diabetes, a condition Anne was diagnosed with at 60 and which she might have prevented if she had known this genetic susceptibility which was not shared with anyone in her adoptive family. With retrospect, she is beginning to see the impact being adopted had on her during the formative years between the ages of 18 and 30: "I had low self-esteem generally and bit my nails until I was 62! I spent the whole time poring over photo albums, trying to find someone I resembled, as there definitely wasn't anyone in my immediate family. I concluded I must be a 'throwback' to an ancestor. Not an inkling that I might be adopted."

I had many boyfriends during those ages, but none long-lasting. I wondered why I seemed to want to escape at this stage of my life. Why was it that I could never stay with one group too long – no one fella, no one country? (I went overseas at 21 for three years.) I always had to move on. I seemed to require constant validation.

On reflection, my relationships were born out of my need to be wanted and to be liked, so when I got that attention, there was a quick high but always followed by an empty feeling and a need to move on. This was validated in a letter from a girlfriend about a particular boyfriend at that time: "I still get cheesed when I think what a rat he's been to you. There's been a few on my list, but you seem to have even more bad luck than anyone." Sadly, my sister and I both had unwanted pregnancies (genetic, I wonder?) in our teens. I had a termination, but she went to an unmarried mothers' home and her daughter was adopted. Adoption was arranged by our parents.

Part 4: Recommendations for Therapists

When Anne was asked how she felt the understanding of adoptees by professionals such as social workers, legal professionals, and health-care professionals could be improved, she wrote: "There should be a completely separate branch of all these institutions, as adopted people's problems are much different to others'." Darryl wrote that he saw relationship counselors at different stages of his first significant relationship:

Psychotherapists need to learn more about adoptees. It's surprising, seeing we are over-represented in suicide, criminal activity (risk-taking), addiction (self-soothing), that more medical professionals don't first ask whether a person was adopted. No one is taking data or statistics on adoption; therefore, adoptee therapy isn't addressed in any standard way. The science is there already, but our medical professionals don't join the dots. Adoptees have their own bucket. As for social workers, they never seem to learn from their past mistakes. Governments and lawmakers, too, repeat the sins of the past and don't fix laws that could reconcile some of these issues for adoptees. Humans haven't yet learned what happens when a baby is taken from its mother. This is not natural. Adoptees are the guinea pigs in an unscientific, unorganized, and destructive experiment that violates our human rights and discriminates against us. This experiment changes who we are, who our subsequent families are, for all time. It breaks connection with genetic history, an ancestry all humans are morally entitled to.

Like Darryl, Cheryl found there really was no specific support or counseling for adoptees available to her between the ages of 18 and 30, and she agrees that mental health professionals need more education about adoption's impacts, and she suggests the best way to get this education is to listen to adopted people. Michael felt health-care providers he came into contact with between the ages of 18 and 30 did not understand the impact of adoption and "generally had no idea. "I saw a grief counselor once – she broke down after I told her 'my story' and said she had never heard anything like it in the 23 years she had been in the field." But otherwise, he was offered no professional support: "I have seen countless therapists, and only one (an adoptee) has ever said what happened to me was wrong, as opposed to my reaction to it being 'wrong.'"

Summary and Conclusion: Therapeutic Implications

Presenting the responses of Darryl, Cheryl, Michael, and Anne was a more difficult process than we had expected, revealing, as it does, that being an adoptee entails multi-layered trauma. We found the stark reality of the respondents' lives as adoptees confronting in their challenges to societal presumptions about adoptee well-being. These searingly honest, brave, and insightful responses teach us what it can mean to people to be separated from their mothers, prevented from knowing their relatives and ancestry, and cut off from knowledge of self. One should consider how these meanings are different in the case of intercountry and transracial adoptions, where an adoptee may be further cut off from their language, culture, and country of origin.

Adoptee voices hold up a mirror to ourselves, revealing that only a part of humanity that has lost touch with itself could ever consider the feelings of a baby towards her or his mother as anything but love, and separation from her as anything but an attack on love itself if it is not absolutely necessary for the protection of the child. This may well be the most difficult part of a therapist's job: to negotiate a brutal truth that nobody wants to admit about a system that is purported to best serve children. The task of the therapist, then, is to assist in the adoptee's unlearning of that lesson caused by love's destruction, a task that must be achieved by adopted children who grow into adults while living within a "family of strangers," often the labor of their whole lives. We conclude that best practice in the clinical therapeutic treatment of adopted adolescents and young adults is to approach all adopted people as cumulative trauma survivors, assess them for trauma symptoms, and assume that their trauma is ongoing. Cheryl concludes:

> *I really appreciate the opportunity to participate. . . .. I have been very honest in answering questions and relating back to the ages of 18–30, and I have shared things I've never spoken about. It doesn't seem to matter my age (I'm now 53); adoption just keeps "attacking." I am so much more aware of my triggers these days but still find difficulty in controlling them and dealing with them. I think generally between the ages of 18 and 30, I was trying to form my identity, but that has been a lifelong journey, because, unfortunately, I tend to act the way I think people expect me to act in all kinds of situations. I spend all my time being hyper-vigilant, scanning, searching, and trying to work out how to act. We adoptees seem to be masters at being chameleons. I hate being adopted. I am waiting for both my mothers to pass so that I can explore adoption discharge. My goal is to be legally related to my siblings. I hate that I will have to*

go through a process and it will be up to someone with no lived experience to make a decision about this – and I may not achieve it. I hate that I live under a false birth certificate. It feels like my life is a lie.

Endnotes

Clothier, F. (1943). The psychology of the adopted child. *Mental Hygiene*, 27, 222–226.

D'Cruz, H., & Gillingham, P. (2017). Participatory research ideals and practice experience: Reflections and analysis. *Journal of Social Work*, 17(4), 434–452. https://doi.org/10.1177/1468017316644704

Gillard, J. (2013). *National Apology for Forced Adoptions.* www.ag.gov.au/sites/default/files/2020-03/Nationalapologyforforcedadoptions.PDF

Goodwach, R. (2001). Does reunion cure adoption? *Australian and New Zealand Family Therapy*, 2.

Green, S. (2017). *Working with Loss and Trauma Related to Past and Forced Adoption Practices* (2nd ed.). North Melbourne: VANISH (Victorian Adoption Network for Information and Self Help).

Higgins, D., Kenny, P., & Morley, S. (2016). *Forced Adoption National Practice Principles: Guidelines and Principles for Specialist Services for Australians Affected by Forced Adoption and Forced Family Separation Practices of the Past.* Melbourne: Australian Institute of Family Studies.

Jones, J., & Placek, P. (2017). *Adoption by the Numbers: A Comprehensive Report National Council of Adoption.* Alexandria: National Council for Adoption.

Kenny, P., Higgins, D.J., Soloff, C., & Sweid, R. (2012). *Past adoption Experiences: National Research Study on Services Responses to Past Adoption Practices.* Melbourne: Australian Institute of Family Studies. aifs.gov.au/publications/past-adoption-experiences

Lifton, B.J. (1994). *Journey of the Adopted Self: A Quest for Wholeness.* New York: Basic Books.

Lonne, R. (2013). Reshaping our protective systems: Issues and options. *Communities, Children and Families Australia*, 7(1), 9–20.

Lynch, C. (2022). *Pilot Study of Adopted People by Adopted People. A 35-Question Qualitative Survey to Gather Data that Can Be Used by Researchers and Therapists for Improving the Clinical Treatment of Adopted People Aged between 18–30 Years* [Unpublished manuscript].

Lynch, C. (2021). Putting children first; What adoption can teach us about surrogacy. In D. Marie-Josephe, & S.D. Ana-Luana (Eds.), *Towards the Abolition of Surrogate Motherhood.* Europe & Australia: The International Coalition for the Abolition of Surrogate Motherhood; Spinifex Press (Transl. (2022) in *Ventres A Louer; Une critique feministe de la gpa*, Paris: L'echappee).

Matthews, J.A.K. (2020). Maltreatment of adoptees in adoptive homes. In G.M. Wrobel, E. Helder, & E. Marr (Eds.), *The Routledge Handbook of Adoption.* London & New York: Routledge, pp. 321–333.

McSherry, D., Samuels, G., & Brodzinsky, D. Eds. (2022). Exploring the relationship between adoption and trauma for children who are adopted from care: A longitudinal case study perspective. *Special Edition of Child Abuse and Neglect*, 130 (2), 105623.

Newman, E. (2011). Challenges of identity for maori adoptees. *Australia Journal of Adoption*, 3 (2), 1–30.

O'Brien, K.M., & Zamostny, K.P. (2003). Understanding adoptive families: An integrative review of empirical research and future directions for counseling psychology. *The Counseling Psychologist*, 31(6), 679–710. https://doi.org/10.1177%2F0011000003258086

Rickarby, G. (1995). *Excerpts from Dr Geoff Rickarby's Submission and Testimony to the Standing Committee on Social Issues Inquiry into Past Adoption Practices.* www.originsnsw.com/nswinquiry2/id12.html

Rickarby, G. (1998). Testimony to the social issues committee. *First Interim Report of the New South Wales Parliamentary Inquiry into Adoption Practices* [Online]. www.parliament.nsw.gov.au/prod/parlment/Committee.nsf/0/a4730ea536ad3b20ca256cfd002a63c2/$FILE/02Sep98.pdf [accessed 9 January 2012].

Vojtila, L., Ashfaq, I., Ampofo, A., Dawson, D., & Selby, P. (2021). Engaging a person with lived experience of mental illness in a collaborative care model feasibility study. *Research Involvement and Engagement*, 7(5). https://doi.org/10.1186/s40900-020-00247-w

Winkler, R.C., Brown, D.W., Van Keppel, M., & Blanchard, A. (1988). *Clinical Practice in Adoption* (Psychology Practitioner Guidebooks). Oxford & New York: Pergamon Press.

APPENDIX

1. From the *Report of the National Inquiry into the Separation of Aboriginal and Torres Strait Islander Children from Their Families*.

This report is a tribute to the strength and struggles of many thousands of Aboriginal and Torres Strait Islander people affected by forcible removal. We acknowledge the hardships they endured and the sacrifices they made. We remember and lament all the children who will never come home.

We dedicate this report with thanks and admiration to those who found the strength to tell their stories to the Inquiry and to the generations of Aboriginal and Torres Strait Islander people separated from their families and communities (Commonwealth of Australia, 1997).

PART II

Developmental Complexities and Necessary Modifications for the Assessment

4
LIFE BEGINS BEFORE ADOPTION

A Guide to the Essential Demographic Factors in Assessment and Treatment

Doris Bertocci, LCSW

Introduction

With regard to the setbacks and challenges in their histories and personality development, adopted persons in non-kinship adoption have many more complexities in their lives compared with other persons, adopted or not, than the mental health field realizes. Psychotherapists need to take them into account before reaching a decision on differential diagnosis and treatment planning. For background, the therapist needs to bear in mind some important basic factors regarding persons in non-kinship adoptions:

- Like the non-adopted, their life begins at conception, the gestational processes that follow, and birth. However, most adopted persons placed traditionally in closed adoption, now adolescents and adults, have little or no information about details of their prenatal history, their birth, the postnatal events, or their pre-placement lives. This likely accounts for the reports of some adopted persons that they lack a sense of having a human bond (an inability to mentalize their birth/infancy or their birth parents; Appendix 1). They believe this deficit left them feeling vaguely "unconnected," vulnerable in the ongoing attachment process that began *in utero*, and fundamentally "different." Also to be considered are the *internal* responses within the child that follow final separation from the birth mother, whenever this occurs, although the mental health field dismisses its significance. However, in the current century, neurobiological and epigenetic research in numerous countries is beginning to support claims of alterations in the brain related to early-life stress, of which separation from the birth mother must be understood to be one example (Hofer, 2005; Ventura-Junca & Herrera, 2012; Melo, 2015; Berens et al., 2017).

Doris Bertocci, LCSW

I always have a sense of floating, but I can never land – deep inside, I don't feel really connected to anything.

Retrospectively, I think I've had some form of depression all my life.

- The experiences of adopted persons in both closed and "semi-open" adoption must be distinguished from those placed in open adoption, which has increasingly become the practice in North America since the latter part of the twentieth century. But sociologically based research has tended to treat adoption as being (only) about children. Further, as in the case, oddly, of developmental psychology, it has not demonstrated any interest in the *alternate* development of the adopted person or the enduring legacy of closed adoptions that continue to impact the life span of adopted people globally.
- Unlike the non-adopted, adopted persons have four parents, or three, but not two.

Even though I don't know anything about them [birth parents], I still think about them, especially on my birthday, and I wonder if they're thinking about me.

- Society, culture, laws, practices, and attitudes in the adoption culture internationally, often along with the birth mother herself, due to her stress and shame, have all colluded in minimizing information about the birth father, resulting in complexities in the development of the adopted person, particularly in adopted males (Chapter 7).

I've mostly wondered about my birth mother, because at least she knows she gave birth to me. But my birth father? He may not even know about me. And my parents were given no information about him. Either way, I would probably search for whichever one I thought cared about me more.

- The traditional, narrow focus on pre-adolescent children in the overlap of adoption and mental health has resulted in a failure to address the *alternate sexual development* of persons in non-kinship adoption. In adolescence, for many, this includes confusion about reproduction, identification with an infertile parent, unconscious repetition of unplanned pregnancy/impregnation, gender dysphoria, and anxiety about the potential for unwittingly having an intimate relationship with a biological relative.
- Treatment of adopted persons is especially benefited if the therapist has had a solid background in several years of generic clinical practice; inexperienced therapists may not understand its importance. Broader clinical exposure helps maintain an essential and more balanced understanding of whether and how adoption-related factors may be involved (Brinich, 1990).
- Therapists typically use the past tense when referring to adoptive status, such as the client "was adopted," as though it had been a discrete event at some earlier

time. (The therapist would not say, "He *was* Chinese.") The reason adoptive status needs to be thought of in the present tense is that internally, at least subtly and intermittently, adoptive status permeates much of development into and through adulthood.

- Therapists tend to identify far more with adults (the parents) while giving scant attention to the internal experience of the child, especially the neurobiological and neuropsychological significance of the child's final separation from the birth mother. Findings from neurobiology and neonatology run counter to the common assumption that when children are "gotten" for adoption, the younger the child, the better. But there is mounting empirical evidence, further, of the link between early stress and the increased risk of anxiety and other stress-related disorders in adopted adolescents (Cohen et al., 2013; Melo, 2015; Csaszar-Nagy & Bokkon, 2017; Berens et al., 2017; Bergman, 2019; Lipschutz & Bick, 2020). Yet studies of early trauma have rarely mentioned the adopted population distinguished from the non-adopted, particularly regarding the multiple *internal* sequelae for adopted adolescents and young adults. In short, the details of the pre-placement history provide a necessary background for considering whether the adopted person's neuropsychological development may be impacted into adolescence and adulthood.
- Young people have increasingly been adopted out of a foster care system that regards adoption as the goal or outcome rather than as the beginning of further complex developmental challenges, especially in adolescence, involving different psychodynamics in family life, different legal parameters, and different skill sets for therapists. A systemic problem is foster care personnel's misconception of adoption specialists as working with the "lucky ones," whom they may also see as competitors for meager financial resources. Of note from developmental and clinical perspectives, however, by being placed at older ages, foster children have generally been spared an early neuropsychological rupture at the time of being permanently separated from the birth mother.
- The majority of adopted persons are not children, and in particular areas, they do not follow the same developmental pathways as non-adopted persons at any life stage. Therapists need also to be reminded that improved practices in the adoption field since the 1980s, such as open adoption and programs in adoptive parenting, may not have benefited adopted adolescents and adults because they were placed before these practices were better developed. This is part of the enduring adverse legacy of closed adoptions in an era that would not acknowledge the complexities in raising adopted children.
- In the United States, where adoption statistics are very inadequate and often confused with data on stepparents who adopt, those in non-kinship adoption are believed to represent little more than 2% of the general child population, while in the UK this may be a smaller proportion, children being primarily "in care," defined as long-term or permanent foster arrangements for children who were with one or both birth parents until being later removed because conditions

warranted a permanent change in caretaking. In the UK, depending on the circumstances, there is often a plan similar to open adoption in the United States.
- Treatment of the adopted client requires that the therapist have not just a solid foundation in early childhood development but that the details be explored about the adoptive family narrative (Chapter 5). That is, the therapist needs to recognize that what the child "hears," understands, remembers, and imagines can be very different from what they were told, especially if the initial disclosure was *prior to the consolidation of memory, language, and attachment* (c. age 3). Thus, the "family narrative" may be different from the child's own developing personal narrative and understanding about "what happened to them" (Perry & Winfrey, 2021). Because of the mounting complexities *beyond* childhood, the clinical level of treatment of adopted adolescents and young adults needs to be recognized as an advanced specialty requiring a foundation in early developmental trauma and in personality development and defenses that may follow in adolescence and beyond.
- An understanding of the psychology of *being* adopted requires an interdisciplinary approach recognizing that quantitative social science research and qualitative clinical research constitute two halves of a whole. Presently, the relatively few published studies that might inform some areas of clinical practice are scattered across the adoption and mental health literature, making it very difficult for therapists to access the information they may seek in order to improve their skills. Examples of needed study would include complexities in engaging adopted clients in treatment, inquiry into practitioners' capacities for clinical empathy with the internal experience of the adopted client (Szalavitz & Perry, 2010), whether and how to include the parents in treatment of adopted adolescents, special considerations in differential diagnosis, comparisons of treatment modalities and approaches, and variations depending on pre-placement circumstances and age at/source of placement.
- The mental health field has not considered how adoptive status may be relevant and significant within various clinical domains, such as eating disorders, anxiety disorders, mood disorders, substance abuse/dual diagnosis, and alleged borderline disorders. For many adopted patients, these might be secondary parts of the differential diagnosis, but the more accurate primary disorder would be early developmental trauma.
- Most important, "different" does not, in any way, imply "pathological," but in the context of adjustment, it *does* mean "more complicated." This is consistent with the prevailing views over the past three decades regarding the multiple dimensions and full spectrum of all that come under "adoptee adjustment" (Brodzinsky, 1990). This does not apply only to the post-placement years, or only to pre-adolescent childhood, but applies to the full life span of the adopted person.

These points challenge the greatly oversimplified assumptions of the mental health field currently, many of which are based on fallacies within the adoption culture.

Also, there are ethical questions to be raised if the therapist treating an adopted client does not work from an adoption-specific knowledge base. The trainings currently offered for adoption professionals and other personnel in child welfare, social services, and counseling (Atkinson, 2020; Koh et al., 2020) were developed out of work with families and adopted *children*. Their skill sets include supportive strategies, cognitive restructuring and psychoeducational interventions, counseling with both birth families and adoptive families, and didactic training in childhood trauma and attachment. But from the clinical perspective of the more traditional mental health disciplines, very different curricula and vehicles for training are needed.

Preliminary Considerations for Treating the Adopted Client

When encountering an adopted client in psychotherapy, therapists in the mental health field tend to reflect the common societal assumption that the adopted person's life began the day they arrived in the adoptive home, as though whatever preceded placement no longer matters. Besides, the thinking goes, regardless of whatever the earlier circumstances may have been, once experiencing stability and consistent nurturing within the adoptive home, children can usually "catch up." This limited knowledge base may be reassuring, but it also operates as a defense, and it is not fully informed by the actual research findings (Rutter et al., 1998). Indeed, there is much in the literature to suggest that, for many children with significant pre-placement adversity, after some months or perhaps years, they have been able to achieve a good deal of the normal developmental tasks for a particular age (Van Ijzendoorn & Juffer, 2006). But usually not taken into account are the additional time, effort, and emotional energy required for the "catching up" process, for both the child and the parents.

Further, as mentioned earlier, studies suggest that for some children, there can be permanent changes neurobiologically (*in utero*) and neuropsychologically (postnatally) that impact subsequent personality development, symptoms (e.g., mood and anxiety disorders), behavior patterns, and mental health, some of which can continue into and throughout adulthood (Bowlby, 1969; Van der Vegt et al., 2009; Schore, 2013; Dekker et al., 2016). In the United States, the child welfare literature has focused on the emotional disruption experienced by increasing numbers of young children, primarily minorities in poor communities, subjected to serial foster placements over months and years, but this may be a different population than some of the subjects in western European studies. The emphasis here, however, is that review of the *externally imposed* circumstances and events needs to include the impact and *developmental timing* of these events and of the changes that the child experienced early in life (Johnson et al., 2020). These, in turn, can interfere with the adopted person's *internal life*, including possible changes in the brain, not only prior to placement but also potentially in their future development.

Doris Bertocci, LCSW

Therapists are generally unaware that some adopted persons have difficulty conceptualizing their biological origins because there is no information about them. An American scholar, writing about her own adoption and, as an adult, her belated discovery somatically of her early preverbal trauma, states that the births of her two children "reminded [her] body that [she] too was born" (Merritt, 2022, p. 5). For some, the absence of any information prior to adoptive placement is combined with the adoptive parents' difficulty discussing adoption topics. As mentioned in Chapter 15, it is common for parents and therapists to make incorrect assumptions, such as about what the adopted individual actually knows and understands about many details, including sexuality, pregnancy, and birth. This pervasively impacts development, especially body image and sexual identity:

> *Actually, I never realized I was born the way everybody else seemed to be – even as an adult, I only heard about my being "gotten," the way my dog was. My birthdays were always observed, but as a child, I never really knew what "birthday" meant – it was just a word. Each person in my family got to celebrate it once a year, but I never understood what it was really about.*

> *When I look in the mirror, I see a blank.*

The former is an excellent example of the common discrepancies between adult terminology and the ways adopted children understand the meanings of the words used. The latter, also sometimes encountered with adopted adolescents and young adults, is discussed in the psychoanalytically based writings of British clinicians Dalley and Kohon (2008):

> *The rapid bodily changes of puberty create an experience of alienation that is acutely felt by adolescents. . . . The adolescent has to take possession of a body which, by changing in drastic ways, confronts her or him with profound issues of identity.*
>
> (ibid., pp. 225–226)

Dalley and Kohon continue that as pubescent adopted youth see their body changing in size, shape, and color that are entirely new to them, for some it can become a somatic dissociative process in which they feel like a complete stranger to themselves (see also Chapter 15). In most cases, this should be understood as one of the unique and not uncommon adoption-specific experiences of those in non-kinship adoption and cannot be considered "abnormal."

> *I looked at my arms and my hands and didn't even recognize whose they were. It was like I had never seen them before.*

> *I waited and waited to see what my body would turn into, and it was scary, but I think I know how a butterfly feels when it comes out of the cocoon. Before it came out, it's like it had no clue what was coming.*

Life Begins Before Adoption

The physical body is a link to the birth parents, whom they may have never met, or of whom they may have no memory or internalized image, and whose loss must somehow be mourned in a new way at the time that the adopted person's reflective capacities and early memories become increasingly a part of their internal life. Part of this struggle for the adopted adolescent, typically, is their inability to see similarities to their adoptive relatives. For non-adopted people, these similarities provide automatic reassurance of their internalized sense of "connection" to the people they are related to, providing an inner sense of security in the world. This is said on the basis of clinical experience, although it has not been studied from a qualitative or clinical perspective – probably because it is taken for granted in the non-adopted world. It is speculated that, without this form of comfort and "rootedness," the adolescent may be left with an underlying anxiety or, as one expressed it, a feeling of being "suspended in time with no beginning." It is well-known from both the scholarly and psychoeducational literature how adopted persons from closed adoptions express their craving – for some, it is an obsession – to literally see (and feel) the features of birth relatives' faces, to know their coloring, touch their skin, and hear their voices. The author believes that this, of all the experiences that adopted searchers express the need to have, may explain why some are not satisfied with information, including medical information. They feel they must literally encounter birth relatives, especially the parents, directly and in person in order to experience closure after years of "wondering" and "looking" and needing actually to see, feel, and hear a human who is biologically related to them.

I'm always looking at faces in a crowd to see if anybody looks like me.

When I was 13, I saw a photo of the Statue of Liberty and thought how much her face resembled mine – she was never just a statue to me, because I imagined we must be related – even down to the frown that I discovered when I later saw a closeup of her face. In my mind I remember thanking the French people for sending her to us as a gift. When I finally found my birth mother 20 years later, I learned that her family was originally from the west coast of France. I was thrilled – but somehow not surprised.

Further, state Dalley and Kohon (2008), for some, "instincts and impulses reactivated from infancy may lead to disturbance that had not been evident during childhood and latency, but can emerge in adolescent sexual life" (ibid., p. 226).

To be sure we weren't actually related, I could only get involved with guys who were of another race than me – this didn't go over well with my parents.

At some point, the adopted person learns, at least intellectually, that their life and development began like anyone else's, at conception, with a full and unique genetic template in place physiologically, neurologically, and in temperament and personality organization. The adopted adolescent will benefit from the therapist's reassurance that this inheritance is never lost but remains within them, although shaped over time by both internal and external influences. This process continues well beyond adolescence – in fact, *throughout the first three decades of life*. In the 20s, there is still a good deal of change, experimentation, perhaps at times faulty judgment, and inconsistency in maturation. And a lot of glances in the mirror.

However, it can be noted that this would not apply in the case of children placed out of foster care at older ages. They most likely had the advantage of being with the biological mother, or perhaps another caretaker in the family, for at least some months after birth, regardless of the conditions or circumstances that later warranted separation from her. The final separation from the birth mother is followed by variable conditions and quality of care in the next placement, disruptions, length of time between birth and the adoptive placement, and number and quality of caretakers. Increasingly, more children are being placed at older ages, often due to lengthy legal delays and other forms of systemic inertia. There are also inadequacies in the services needed by the birth mother who is in conflict about her plans (Baden et al., 2013; Madden et al., 2020). If she is a young teenager, her own mother may not give her a choice – thus continues the birth mother's own long mourning for the child taken from her. Overall, for many children, these conditions and events, both external and internal, represent a "perfect storm" of multiple adversities for the child before even meeting their adoptive parents for the first time.

None of these circumstances apply to the generalized "at-risk" populations of youth, nor do they apply to the large sub-population of youth diagnosed with either "childhood trauma" or "complex trauma" as described in the literature (Courtois & Ford, 2013), although they certainly qualify as a subtype of the latter. As in the case of attachment disorders (Steele & Steele, 2018), which are believed likely to be over-diagnosed especially for the internationally adopted subgroup (Welsh et al., 2007), childhood trauma fills the literature, but there is at most only passing reference to the adoption-specific forms and sequelae of *early* traumatic loss, defined here as *trauma prior to the consolidation of memory, language, and attachment*, or approximately "the first thousand days" (Schore, 2001, 2013, 2015). Because these involve neuropsychological events that are believed to become encoded in the neurological development of the brain (Berens et al., 2017; Lipschutz & Bick, 2020), the author (DB) contends that due recognition needs to be given to Bessel van der Kolk's proposed diagnosis of developmental trauma disorder (van der Kolk, 2005, 2015). However, in the sub-population of children placed before the consolidation of language, memory, and attachment, about age 3, the author argues here that within the 0- to 3-year age span, the profound impact of severe and/or protracted trauma warrants the modified diagnosis of *early developmental trauma disorder*. This would provide a means of readily identifying the clinical complexities that apply to this subgroup of children (Szalavitz & Perry, 2010; Perry, 2019), although, as a formal diagnosis, specific criteria would need to be established. Also, references to "stress early in life" are too vague to be useful clinically and cannot be confused with severe and enduring trauma of the kind so many adopted individuals have experienced. This contradicts the assumptions of the adoption culture and, in turn, of many uninformed therapists, that is, that adopted children placed soon after birth have an advantage developmentally. There are far too many variables to account for in each situation to warrant such a generalization.

Some Inconvenient Truths for Mental Health Practitioners

Presently, as mentioned previously, the mental health field, particularly the traditional disciplines, but also pediatricians, tend to dismiss the significance of early developmental trauma in the lives of adopted children, especially in regard to claims of neurobiological trauma for the child at the final separation from the birth mother. This has continued despite the seminal discoveries of the twentieth-century pioneers in early childhood development of non-adopted children (Bowlby, 1969, 1973, and 1980; Winnecott, 1971; Mahler, 1975; Ainsworth et al., 1978; see also Dedication), despite the findings from many studies of the impact of "early adversities" on the development of adopted children (Juffer et al., 2011; Julian, 2020), and despite the more recent findings from the neuroscience of early trauma (Ventura-Junca & Herrera, 2012; Schore, 2013, 2015; Cohen et al., 2013; van der Kolk, 2015; Hambrick et al., 2019; Hambrick et al., 2019). All these observations and findings have a consistency with each other and continue to challenge the ongoing belief systems, hypotheses, research, and practices that remain entrenched in the current overlap of adoption and mental health practice. The adoption field is uncomfortable with the alleged impact of early neuropsychological or developmental problems because it would complicate their mission of recruiting adoptive parents. Mental health practitioners dismiss it because this serves as a defense from learning painful information (and from experiencing authentic empathy), but perhaps also because they question what they can do about it. The answer to the latter is that therapists need to update their knowledge base in early developmental trauma and in the psychology of adoptive status and, further, consider adding specialized assessments to the overall treatment plan. These might include consultation with adoption medicine (Chapter 9), psychological testing that includes projectives and/or attachment inventories, or a neurosequential *evaluation* (Perry, 2019; Chapter 15). However, to date, mental health practitioners continue to state that when treating adopted clients, they believe that what they already know is sufficient.

Thus, the vast majority of adoption research and published literature, popular and professional, has focused on pre-adolescent childhood (Brodzinsky & Schechter, 1990; Brodzinsky et al., 1998; Howard & Smith, 2003; Hart & Luckock, 2004; Brodzinsky & Palacios, 2005; Palacios & Brodzinsky, 2010; Welsh et al., 2007; Reinoso et al., 2012) and on special considerations in *parenting* adopted children, many from the public child welfare system, prior to adolescence (Groza & Rosenberg, 2001; Hindle & Shulman, 2008; Henry, 2012; Waterman et al., 2018; Roszia & Maxon, 2019). Pre-adolescent childhood is still the emphasis as well in our companion volume addressing the broad scope of adoption as a field (Wrobel et al., 2020). However, one of its authors, Megan Julian, refers to the "sleeper effects" of institutionalization, or of ongoing "developmental irregularities," that were "less apparent in early childhood, and more notable in adolescence, with most types of problems persisting into young adulthood" (ibid., p. 180).

Further, "developmental irregularities" do not occur only in cases of early severe deprivation or protracted neglect and abuse in the earliest years. Rather, the developmental adjustments of adopted people, the multiple challenges they face over time, the degree of their innate resilience in handling the additional challenges to follow are part of the *alternate* but *normative* developmental experience of being adopted. They are "irregular" only if compared with the non-adopted population. This pertains particularly to those within non-kinship families, and even more specifically for those from closed adoptions. This is because of the cumulative impact of external forces imposed on their lives that relate largely to practices in adoption and the law, and that put their resilience to the test as they grow toward adulthood. Yet at the present time in mental health practice, when adopted individuals seek therapy, psychotherapists do not treat them any differently than non-adopted clients: their being adopted remains little more than a footnote in their history. As an Israeli colleague admitted, "I wish I had had more specific knowledge when I had a brilliant patient who was adopted and there was stuff I didn't grasp. For me it was like a regular therapy" (personal communication).

I'm tired of always having to explain to therapists what it's like to be adopted – they still don't get it.

Therefore, another inconvenient truth in the overlap of adoption and mental health is that practitioners' lack of training poses clinical and ethical problems in treatment programs, particularly for trainees of any discipline who are assigned adopted patients to treat (Appendix 3). For therapists who believe they are "trauma informed" or who work in specialized trauma programs, another common and troubling problem is the false presumption that all forms of trauma are approximately the same in their impact psychologically and can therefore be treated with the same modalities or interventions that the therapist has been trained to use with generic trauma. The more intensive the treatment, such as in hospital-affiliated and residential programs and intensive outpatient services, the greater this problem becomes (Chapter 11).

Especially when the agreed-upon focus of treatment is on the client's working toward a fuller and deeper understanding of themselves, their relationships, and their personal development over time, and also on whether and how they may relate to other matters of concern, the therapist needs to start with review of the client's profile regarding the six demographic dyads discussed next. These important details relate to the nature of the client's adoption and what each factor may potentially involve clinically. The following represents the first attempt to bring together into a basic template (checklist) six fundamental demographic factors in the client's adoptive status, along with the significance of them for diagnostic and treatment purposes. The particulars can be pursued through the selective literature cited.

Distinguishing the Demographic Subsets of Adoptive Status

1. Kinship/Non-Kinship

In the US Census taken each decade, no accurate distinctions are made among minors in kinship adoption (e.g., adoption by members of the extended biological family), those adopted by stepparents, and those adopted by non-relatives who are not stepparents. The common figure given for those in non-kinship adoption has been around 2.5% (Kreider & Lofquist, 2014), but there is reason to question its accuracy into the twenty-first century when the data is derived from only the head of the household, and when there is no clarity in legal distinctions. A report from the 2010 Census states that 95% of children under 18 live with one or both biological parents, thereby including those adopted by stepparents. This leaves 5% living either in foster care or in non-kinship adoption. Therefore, when therapists treat young people in non-kinship adoption, they are generally unaware of what a very small proportion of the child population they represent – or of the complicated skill sets their treatment requires.

Statistical accuracy will continue to be a challenge, but for the purpose of health and mental health practice, much more is needed in the way of qualitative research that will help inform clinical practice. For example, to emphasize the complexities of the adopted person's *internal* life, therapists who are psychodynamically or psychoanalytically informed have speculated that multiple caretakers may result in multiple internal representations of "mother" (Brinich, 1980; Zilberstein, 2011), not to mention the additional internalized neurophysiological representations of the birth mother (Priel et al., 2012; Chapter 6). But the psychology of *being* adopted is not (only) about children. Obviously, the overall numbers of adopted people are greatly increased once the adult population is taken into account. The clinical significance for the evaluation is not only in the degree of disruption and change early in the child's life but also in the amount and nature of information about the birth family for the adopted child that may or may not be available and that may impact their inner sense of security, connection, and capacity for emotional closeness with other people into and throughout adulthood.

This is the reason for the common assumption that, whenever possible, the child's placement with kin is to be attempted in order for intra-familial details and potential emotional bonds within the family to be maintained. However, the reality of the problems impacting the child is threefold: the lack of ongoing financial support for families of kinship adoption for whom inadequate subsidies still mean ongoing, difficult struggle for the family; the simplistic and formulaic basis for legal decisions that automatically favor placement with kin; and the inadequate knowledge and skills of placement staff. The latter are typically overwhelmed welfare workers with limited or no education at a professional level who, because of the pressure of time and volume, may feel coerced to follow certain protocols in their actual practice. In their assessment of parent-applicants, they are also not trained to recognize or understand the "permanency" of certain disadvantages (e.g., severe characterological disorders, alcoholism) in members of the birth family with whom they think the child should remain. In short, growing up with members of the extended biological family is an advantage only if stability and well-attuned parenting can be consistently provided. When this is in doubt, the judiciary is still inclined to settle on kinship placements, while insufficient consideration has been given to the possible alternative of non-kinship open adoption as arranged in the United States (Baran et al., 1976; Siegel, 2012; Grotevant, 2020). In many cases, we assert, the requirement of the birth mother's consent needs to be reconsidered, but criteria would need to be established for the court to make this decision. If some form of open adoption was *mandated*, it would greatly shorten the time that the child must wait. But the system must rethink its priorities as to whose rights need to prevail, and it must be prepared to ensure professional oversight for such an arrangement.

As a generalization in non-kinship adoption, it is primarily in adolescence and young adulthood that missing information becomes a particularly vexing problem for many because it represents lack of control over many personal matters, in great contrast to their non-adopted peers.

> *I never knew if I could be considering a serious relationship with a biological relative.*
>
> *When I've tried to find out certain things about my past, I get a different story from each person I've asked.*
>
> *In college, my application for a passport was rejected because all I had was a small slip of paper [the amended birth certificate] stating I was born to my adoptive parents. Aside from it being a lie, I was shocked, feeling like I was being held hostage, restricted in where I could travel, for the rest of my life.*

Because of the greater complexities of growing up in non-kinship adoption, this is the primary focus of this chapter.

2. Closed/Open Adoption

The adopted person's access, or lack of access, to information about the birth family and, in some cases, occasional direct access is the primary distinguishing feature of closed vs. open adoption. The increased amount of research and publications on open adoption since the 1980s to the present time (Baran et al., 1976; Berry, 1998; Grotevant, 2020) has served both to demonstrate its complexities and to confirm its advantages overall. However, it has overshadowed and diverted attention from the enduring difficulties for the majority of adopted adults still contending with the restrictions of closed adoption that deny them their own birth certificates and that even restrict them from obtaining the information they seek from the sources of their adoptive placements (Appendix 4). The more recent literature treats closed adoption as a practice of the past (Grotevant & Von Korff, 2011; Grotevant, 2020), but we know from clinical and anecdotal experience, which has not been taken into account in sociological research, that, in fact, its impact continues in the lives of adopted adolescents and adults, regardless of country of birth (Chapter 3). It is the clinical perspective accounting for the life span that informs us that the *results* of closed adoption are far-reaching and endure throughout development for life.

There is no way of knowing the numbers of adopted people from closed adoption who have pursued information and possibly located birth relatives. Therapists do need to be aware that the high demand for infants has resulted for decades in birth mothers being pressured, in various overt and covert ways, to relinquish their babies, without other options being adequately discussed (Madden et al., 2020). In the United States since the 1940s, the promises of "full confidentiality" were silently manipulated to include the child by inference, while the birth mother was coerced to accept these terms by telling her that it was "for the best." This, in turn, has forced searching adopted persons to be in opposition to the law in three-quarters of the states in the United States. Adopted persons have pursued other ways of obtaining information using the internet (Howard, 2012) and through genetic searches. Arrangements for open adoption, now offered through agencies and many public welfare services, have become far more prevalent than closed adoption because we have learned, primarily anecdotally, that open adoption has turned out to be the strong preference of birth mothers. Overall, there have been many variations in the amount of information and contact with birth family that the child has been provided, and in whether the needs and wishes of the child in open adoption have been given priority and professionally mediated. The therapist can still understand that there are many complexities to be considered in the intra-familial experience, in the impact of open adoption on the adopted person's development over time (Siegel, 2012), and in the psychodynamics of adoptive family life that may or may not include members of the birth family, especially as the adopted person grows older.

3. Early/Late Placement

Health-care professionals typically ask when a child was adopted, without understanding that there may be a significant difference between the child's age when arriving at the adoptive home for the first time and the child's age when the legal arrangements were completed. The better wording would be, "How old were you when you joined your adoptive family?" Also, detailed developmental information needs to be obtained whenever possible about the age and development of the child at the time of the final separation from the birth mother, which varies greatly in the lives of adopted children. In many cases, the child will have remained with the biological family for some weeks, months, or years, although it may not be clear whether and to what extent the child may have been directly cared for by the birth mother or other relatives, or whether there was any involvement on the part of the birth father or his family (Chapter 7). Overall, countries differ in their policies for how long the child can or should, or should not, remain in alternative care before adoptive placement, as well as in their procedures for transition to the adoptive home.

Depending on the national and cultural context, there are also great differences in the concept of "early" vs. "late" placement. In Western countries, the general parameters of "early" used to refer to placement by age 1, by which time the child's intelligence could be tested (Appendix 5), (to make sure they were not placing a flawed child) but since the latter part of the twentieth century, with the diminished number of available babies, this has been extended to approximately age 3, when language, memory, and attachment may not yet be fully consolidated in the child's development. These children have typically been placed either from foster care or from international arrangements (Groza & Rosenberg, 2001). In other countries with larger sub-populations of children in care, such as India, placements by age 5 or 6 are considered "early" (Chapter 8). Regardless, for clinical purposes, the therapist's task includes taking a detailed developmental history, carefully noting the areas in which there were evident delays or noted problems physically, medically, socially, in language and cognitive development, and in formation of attachments. As suggested earlier, it is also important for the therapist to recognize that, despite the common assumption that "the earlier the placement, the better," research findings have tended to be inconsistent, and they vary greatly in whether multiple variables were considered in the methodology. There is significant anecdotal material suggesting that there can be serious developmental complexities into adulthood for many who were placed with their adoptive family soon after birth (Appendix 6; Chapter 3). In fact, psychobiological studies maintain that the very young child's *neurophysiological attachment* to the birth mother begins *in utero* (Chapter 6) and, if the child remains with her, continues postnatally into toddlerhood (Hofer, 2005).

4. Domestic/International Placement

There is much in the research literature, particularly since the 1980s, relating to the similarities and differences between children placed for adoption domestically (within their country of birth) and those placed with families in other countries (Bemuz, 2020). The countries allowing international placements have shifted over time, with many variations in both the quality and length of pre-placement care and in the standards and practices in handling the placements. Similarly, there are wide variations *within* individual countries, like the United States, because there is so little consistency in adoption practice from state to state, with no oversight of requirements at the national level, because there is no legally endorsed concept of children's rights (Chapters 1 and 11). Nevertheless, if the latter is to have any priority as a social value on humanitarian grounds, it requires stronger and more explicit advocacy, beginning with the ground roots of social service and law. Most of the serious disadvantages for both the child and the potential adopters appear to apply especially in the case of two "pathways to adoption": the now-dwindling numbers of international adoptions (Chapter 2), often involving delays and misguided practices, such as those requiring psychological testing of the potential parents, along with cumbersome governmental procedures; and within domestic placements, the practices of "private" or "independent" adoptions that provide the child no protection or representation of its own. There is also the inconsistency in the extent and quality of preparation for adoptive parenting and also the problem of limited efforts to provide ongoing help following placement. Perhaps the primary difference between domestic and international adoptions is in the amount of information about the birth parents that is typically limited in transnational placements. The peak of these placements was in 2004 (Selman, 2012), and even though international arrangements have significantly declined over the past two decades, the larger numbers of children placed transnationally are now adolescents and adults, many seeking help from well-attuned clinicians who understand the additional complexities they face. For example, for many, these include the triple disadvantage of minimal available information, significant adversities in caretaking prior to placement, and placement in an adoptive family of a different race and ethnicity (Baden et al., 2013).

5. Same/Different Race and Culture as Adoptive Parents/Family

The first three dyads, and perhaps the fourth regarding factors in adoptive status, have in common the fact that differences between the adopted child and the adoptive parents are not evident to those outside the family. However, this does not apply with regard to transracial or mixed-race adoptions (typical in international placements), because the child's differences in appearance from the adoptive parents, and perhaps siblings, are usually evident visually. This announces the lack of a biological relationship between child and parents, which is followed by a number of reactions, one of them confusion in the adopted child around the time of entering school, when differences become more likely to be noticed, and there may be uneasy reactions in the social environment. If the latter appears to be distant, critical, or disapproving, or especially if it exposes the child to taunts and other forms of hostile behavior, it sets the child up for struggles with self-doubts, low self-esteem, anxiety about her/his accepted place in the world, and hyper-awareness about potential threats. There is no "tribal safety" to protect them. The critical issue for the fifth and sixth dyads relate to the human inclination, probably based on innate survival impulses, to notice similarities and differences and to attribute particular social meanings and levels of value to them. This likely explains the irrational, subconscious aggressive responses from the environment, such as the community, that are based on invidious comparisons and misperceptions of potential threats.

Thus, the therapist's efforts to understand some clients' difficulties will benefit from an overview of transracial adoptions (Baden, 2007; McRoy & Griffin, 2012; Manzi et al., 2014; Marr, 2017). Particularly needed is the therapist's careful review of the similarities and differences noted by the client, the adoptive family, and their larger community, along with the ways these may have played out in the client's life experience (Annamma, 2012; Jackson & Samuels, 2019). Further, regardless of the degree to which the child's appearance may be very different from that of members of the adoptive family, and regardless of the degree to which the family is/was authentically comfortable with differences (Tessler & Gamache, 2012), it is guaranteed to take on a new and perhaps urgent meaning and importance in adolescence and young adulthood when the adopted person's attention is drawn to bodily changes, family expectations, sexuality, choices in love relationships and employment, and perhaps eventually to questions around marriage and having children. Racial and cultural similarities and differences between the adopted child and the parents have been addressed a good deal in the literature (Baden, 2007) but is more limited in addressing these concerns in adolescence and young adulthood (O'Connor et al., 2016).

A French team focusing on internationally placed adopted children noted the differences between the French/European literature and the English-language literature (Hart et al., 2015). They observed that the latter tends to emphasize the importance of maintaining connections with the country and culture of the child's birth, as in "heritage travel" programs. However, they state that the majority position in Europe, and especially France, is that "the emphasis needs to be on belonging to the receiving country and its culture," because promoting connections with the birth culture creates the risk of accentuating the differences between the child and the parents, "differences that should be erased to construct a family" (ibid., p. 2). Depending on additional variables that must be taken into account, such as the child's age and memories, the French viewpoint has great merit, although, in deference to the great importance of timing, cultural differences need to be set aside rather than "erased." Regardless, and most fundamentally, as with so many questions, the developmental readiness and voice of the adopted person need to take priority over the parents concern to "do the right thing".

6. Same/Different Gender/Sexual Identity as Adoptive Parents

With the change in adoptive placement practices in the 1990s to being somewhat more open to placement of young children with same-sexed parents, having begun originally with lesbian parents, research into these families' adjustments, both within the family and vis-à-vis the community, is still relatively recent (Brodzinsky & Pertman, 2012; Goldberg & Smith, 2013; Goldberg & Allen 2013b; Farr et al., 2013; Farr & Vazquez, 2020; Messina & Brodzinsky, 2020; McConnachie et al., 2020). A Canadian attorney notes that "the reforms in the UK and Quebec . . . most marginalize those whose kinship configurations are least like the two-parent nuclear model" (Leckey, 2015, p. 22). The literature on "assisted procreation" for LGBTQ persons who may or may not be in a legalized marriage addresses numerous variations in regulatory details between countries, but also whether and how the acquisition of a child through assisted technology involves legal adoption. There are likely to be increased legal debates as these complicated routes to parenthood are taken (Boucai, 2016). However, to date, the literature tends to focus on parenthood rather than on the impact of these complexities on the child over time. On the other hand, protocols and recommendations are being developed for such matters, as what information about the sources of conception is made available to the adopted "child" at the age of majority, and whether and how actual contact between the child and the "co-procreators" might be regulated (Leibetseder & Griffin, 2019). Themes in the literature include redefining the family, that is, problems with heteronormativity, questions about the need for gender role models, complexities around identity (Messina & Brodzinsky, 2020), and stigma in the community (Kuvalanka et al., 2019; Allen & Goldberg, 2019). Quantitative studies have generally focused on the children in LGBTQ families but have expanded somewhat to addressing the longitudinal impact of these developmental complexities when these children become adults (Brodzinsky & Pertman, 2012; Clarke & Demetriou, 2016). Once again, the clinical usefulness of research findings will depend on what questions are asked, whether they are informed by clinical perspectives, and the meanings derived from the answers given.

There can be variations in the "significance of differences" even within communities with diversity. The problem remains that despite the general expectation that there may be some complexities or difficulties at different times in the LGBTQ family's life, such as in the mutual adjustment between the child and the school community, or when the parents separate or divorce, or litigate custody (Goldberg & Allen, 2013a; Kuvalanka et al., 2019), with very few exceptions, no substantive services for adoptive families have been provided by any segment of the adoption system beyond the initial weeks after placement. Adoption placement sources, along with some adoption medicine programs, are sometimes remiss in their referral practices to resources for ongoing help if they are handled in a perfunctory way (e.g., simply taken from a list) or if the resources are not adequately known or kept updated. Some adoption placement services have transitioned to working within the auspices of family counseling agencies, but study is needed of the level and extent of adoption-specific training, including clinical perspectives, of the practitioners in these settings. Further and most troubling, in the current culture of family therapy, there is no consideration of the adoptive family being a special needs family. In short, regardless of the sexual orientation of the parents, or of any other factors involving the identities and needs of the adoptive parents, on the basis of what has been learned through direct outreach, the adoption system overall has not assisted families in a responsible or professional way with accessing suitable and affordable ongoing services over time, nor has it actively advocated for funding in order to expand their services.

Demonstration of the Complexities in Assessing the Adopted Client's Development

This section alerts the therapist to the *combination of factors*, as organized around the six dyads discussed earlier, that attempt to explain the adopted client's likely multiple vulnerabilities and adjustments that need to be integrated into the clinical formulation. The following hypothetical case examples are composites, all with authentic details derived from adopted patients who, at one time, were in treatment. Consider, for example, someone in a kinship domestic adoption who is raised by an aunt or grandparent, members of the birth family, who represent the full spectrum of health and illness, physically and in personality, culture, and the population at large. The adopted person usually has access to information within the family that includes bodily features, health histories, photographs, talents, personalities, and family stories – along with at least some information about the reason for their needing to grow up with relatives. These become woven into the child's self-image, body image, and personal identity, in their own physical and personality development. Granting the advantage of such ties with the birth family, for better or worse, it still represents the full gamut of the familiar social, health, and mental health problems that the court and the social service workers may tend to minimize because of the expedience of kinship placements.

Still, such a child will have a very different experience and development from an adopted person separated from the birth mother in infancy, in foster care for several months, and then placed through a county child welfare department in a non-kinship domestic closed adoption with heterosexual parents in their early 40s. Such a child's development will be different still from someone placed at the estimated age of 3 through an international adoption arrangement but having remained with the young birth mother and her parents through the first few months of life, then spending a year in a "baby home," where there was no consistency or stimulation in caretaking, minimal record-keeping, and conditions that left the child with a chronic pulmonary disorder. When the child is finally placed with the adoptive parents, the typical background they are given is that "the family was very poor, the birth mother was not well, and no information was given about the birth father." The child is then transported to another country, where no one speaks any words that the child can comprehend. This child's development and internal construction of identity will differ, in turn, from someone placed domestically by the welfare department at 1 year of age, following two abrupt changes in foster care, in an open-adoption arrangement with a same-sex couple of different races from the child. Consider, still, the complexities for the child found online, her/his placement secured by a lawyer representing financially advantaged adults old enough to be grandparents, with significant but concealed health problems, and intending to hire caretakers for both the child and the household.

A therapist might see a high school student presenting, commonly enough, with anxiety about going away to college. Asked about her background, the girl explains that she is adopted, having been placed privately (legal contract) with a late-middle-aged couple when she was "a few months old." The therapist learns that the adoptive father is several years older than the mother and had grown children from his first marriage. This second marriage had become increasingly troubled over the years prior to their adopting her. Having focused for years on her career, the adoptive mother had wanted a last chance to raise a child, and eventually her wishes prevailed over his. Over the next decade, not only did the adoption fail to stabilize their relationship, but it also created more conflict between them as they were forced to face their long-standing difficulties with each other. From the beginning, the "outsourced" social worker had not been adequately skilled in doing the home study, focusing primarily on the couple's concrete assets, high level of education, and superficial accomplishments, but lacking critically important skills in her assessment of their relationship, their personalities, and their reasons for wanting to adopt. The girl is exposed to much intense arguing in the household throughout her childhood, and when the parents finally separate, one of them, seeking to "start over," takes up residence in another part of the country to be in a new job and new relationship. Unlike the usual anxiety many high school students experience about "going away to college" – although when divorce is involved, there is often the burden for the "child" of the parents' arguments over who will pay the college expenses – this girl is already very anxious as she automatically (neuropsychologically) anticipates frightening changes she cannot control. She is vulnerable to anxiety states and sleep difficulties and experiences the betrayal of her parents in the divorce as a second abandonment because they had told her they would "always be there for her." She now needs to prepare for another separation and loss as she is about to leave for an environment that will challenge her cognitive abilities and concentration, her efforts to develop close and trusting friendships in her social relationships, and her ability to remain hopeful for a future life that she has difficulty conceptualizing.

> *The idea of graduating from college was like steeling myself for the time I would come to the edge of a high cliff: beyond the edge, there wasn't anything there, just empty space. I had no idea at all what I would do from there.*

> *How can I figure out where I'm going or what I'm going to do when I can't even figure out where I came from?*

> *I have no way of envisioning my future, so I don't know what I'm doing anything for.*

If the therapist's effort to weigh the multiplicity of these factors in order to understand the adopted person's development is not sufficiently daunting, consider the implications for the complexities and time involved for the adopted person themselves regarding their own internal integrative process from childhood into adolescence and young adulthood. Similarly, if ordinary (non-adoptive) parents are surprised by the capacities, talents, seeming oddities, differences, and limitations of children born to them, consider the shared perplexities and unknowns in the experience of the adoptive family, especially for the adopted person.

Conclusion

This chapter makes the argument that every adopted person is very different from every other in their early development, not only because they bring within them their genetic template for internal assets and vulnerabilities, but also because of differences in the combination of pre-placement factors, and then because of the unique mix of features and circumstances in their adoptive families. Early in the evaluation, it is recommended that the therapist review six demographic dyads regarding the client's adoptive status and the clinical significance of each. Altogether, their combination makes adopted persons an entirely different sub-population from those discussed in the literature on "early childhood adversities." Overall, a clinical approach to treating the adopted client benefits most if the therapist is aware of not only the *external* factors in adoption and law that impact, and sometimes interfere with, development, as in the case of the dyads discussed in this chapter, but also of their potential sequelae *internally* (emotionally) that need consideration (Chapter 11), regardless of whether they meet criteria for a formal diagnosis.

Endnotes

Ainsworth, M.D.S., Blehar, M.C., Waters, E., & Wall, S. (1978). *Patterns of Attachment: A Psychological Study of the Strange Situation Procedures*. Hillsdale: Erlbaum.

Allen, J., Fonagy, P., & Bateman, A. (2008). *Mentalizing in Clinical Practice*. Washington, DC: American Psychiatric Press.

Allen, K.R., & Goldberg, A.E. (2019). Lesbian women disrupting gendered, heteronormative discourses of motherhood, marriage and divorce. *Journal of Lesbian Studies*, 1–13.

Annamma, S. (2012). Gazing into the mirror: Reflections of racial identity transformation in transnational and transracial adoptees. *Journal of Social Distress and the Homeless*, 21 (3–4), 168–220.

Atkinson, A.J. (2020) Adoption competent clinical practice. In G.M. Wrobel, E. Helder, E. Marr (Eds.), *The Routledge Handbook of Adoption*. London & New York: Routledge.

Baden, A. (2007). Identity, psychological adjustment, culture, and race: Issues for transracial adoptees and the cultural-racial identity model. In R.A. Javier, A.L. Baden, F.A. Biafora, & A. Camacho-Gingerich (Eds.), *Handbook of Adoption: Implications for Researchers, Practitioners, and Families*. Thousand Oaks: Sage Publications, pp. 359–378.

Baden, A.L., Gibbons, J.L. Wilson, S.L., & McGinnis, H. (2013). International adoption: Counseling and the adoption triad. *Adoption Quarterly*, 16 (3–4), 218–237.

Baran, A., Pannor, R., & Sorosky, A. (1976). Open adoption. *Social Work*, 21, 97–105.

Bemuz, M.R. (2020). Unique challenges and strengths for families formed through international adoption. In G.M. Wrobel, E. Helder, & E. Marr (Eds.), *The Routledge Handbook of Adoption*. London & New York: Routledge, pp. 107–119.

Berens, A.E., Jensen, S.K.G., & Nelson III, C.A. (2017). Biological embedding of childhood adversity: from physiological mechanisms to clinical implications. *BMC Medicine*, 15 (135), 1–12.

Bergman, N.J. (2019). Historical background to maternal-neonate separation and neonatal care. *Birth Defects Research* (Special Issue – Birth Practices), 111 (15), 1081–1086.

Berry, M., Cavazos-Dylla, D.J., Barth, R.P., & Needell, B. (1998). The role of open adoption in the adjustment of adopted children and their families. *Children & Youth Services Review*, 20, 151–171.

Boucai, M. (2016). Is assisted procreation an LGBT right? *Wisconsin Law Review*, 1065–1125.

Bowlby, J. (1969). *Attachment and Loss*, Vol. 1. New York: Basic Books.

Bowlby, J. (1969, 1973, & 1980). *Attachment and Loss*, Vol. 1, 2, & 3. New York: Basic Books.

Brinich, P.M. (1980). Some potential effects of adoption on self and object representations. *Psychoanalytic Study of the Child*, 35, 107–133.

Brinich, P.M. (1990). Adoption from the inside out: A psychoanalytic perspective. In D. Brodzinsky & M. Schechter (Eds.), *The Psychology of Adoption*. New York & Oxford: Oxford University Press, pp. 42–61.

Brodzinsky, D. (1990). A stress and coping model of adoption adjustment. In D. Brodzinsky, & M. Schechter (Eds.), *The Psychology of Adoption*. New York: Oxford Press, pp. 3–24.

Brodzinsky, D., & Palacios, J. Eds. (2005). *Psychological Issues in Adoption: Research and Practice*. Westport: Praeger.

Brodzinsky, D., & Pertman, A. Eds. (2012). *Adoption by Lesbians and Gay Men: A New Dimension in Family Diversity*. New York: Oxford University Press.

Brodzinsky, D., & Schechter, M. Eds. (1990). *The Psychology of Adoption*. New York & Oxford: Oxford Press.

Brodzinsky, D., Smith, D.W., & Brodzinsky, A. (1998). *Children's Adjustment to Adoption: Developmental and Clinical Issues*. Thousand Oaks: Sage Pub.

Clarke, V., & Demetriou, E. (2016). 'Not a big deal'? exploring the accounts of adult children of lesbian, gay and trans parents. In *Psychology & Sexuality*. London: Taylor & Francis, pp. 1–18.

Cohen, M.M., Tottenham, N., & Casey, B.J. (2013). Translational developmental studies of stress on brain and behavior: Implications for adolescent mental health and illness. In *Neuroscience (Special Edition): Stress and the Adolescent Brain*. Amsterdam: Elsevier, pp. 1–10.

Courtois, C.A., & Ford, J.D. (2013). *Treatment of Complex Trauma: A Sequenced, Relationship-Based Approach*. New York: The Guilford Press.

Csaszar-Nagy, N., & Bokkon, I. (2017). Mother-newborn separation at birth in hospitals: A possible risk for neurodevelopmental disorders? *Neuroscience and Biobehavioral Reviews*, 8 (13), 1–18.

Dalley, T., & Kohon, V. (2008). Deprivation and development: The predicament of an adopted adolescent in the search for identity. In D. Hindle, & G. Shulman (Eds.), *The Emotional Experience of Adoption: A Psychoanalytic Perspective*. London & New York: Routledge, pp. 225–236.

Dekker, M.C., Tieman, W., Vinke, A.G., van der Ende, J., Verhulst, F.C., & Juffer, F. (2016). Mental health problems of Dutch young adult domestic adoptees compared to non-adopted peers and international adoptees. *International Social Work*, 1–17. isw.sagepub.com.

Farr, R.H., & Vazquez, C.P. (2020). Adoptive families headed by LGBTQ parents. In G.M. Wrobel, E. Helder, & E. Marr (Eds), *The Routledge Handbook in Adoption*. London & New York: Routledge, pp. 164–175.

Farr, R.H., Vazquez, C.P., & Patterson, C.J. (2013). LGBTQ Adoptive parents and their children. In A.E. Goldberg, & K.R. Allen (Eds.), *LGBTQ-Parent Families: Innovations in Research and Implications for Practice*. New York: Springer Nature, pp. 45–64. https://doi.org/10.1007/978-3-030-35610-1_3

Fonagy, P., Gergely, G., Jurist, E., & Target, M. (2002). *Affect Regulation, Mentalization, and the Development of the Self*. New York: Other Press.

Goldberg, A.E., & Allen, K.R. (2013a). Same-sex relationships dissolution and LGB stepfamily formation: Perspectives of young adults with LGB parents. *Family Relations*, 62, 529–544.

Goldberg, A.E., & Allen, K.R. (2013b). *LGBTQ-Parent Families: Innovations in Research and Implications for Practice*. New York, NY: Springer.

Goldberg, A.E., & Smith, J.Z. (2013). Predictors of psychological adjustment in early placed adopted children with lesbian, gay, and heterosexual parents. *Journal of Family Psychology*, 27 (3), 431–442.

Grotevant, H.D. (2020). Open adoption. In G.M. Wrobel, E. Helder, & E. Marr (Eds.), *The Routledge Handbook of Adoption*. London & New York: Routledge, pp. 266–277.

Grotevant, H.D., & Von Korff, L. (2011). Adoptive identity. In S. Schwartz, K. Luyckx, & V. Vignoles (Eds.), *Handbook of Identity Theory and Research*. New York: Springer.

Groza, V., & Rosenberg, K.F. (Eds.). (2001). *Clinical and Practice Issues in Adoption: Bridging the Gap Between Adoptees Placed as Infants and as Older Children*. Westport & London: Bergin & Garvey.

Hambrick, E.P., Brawner, T.W., & Perry, B.D. (2019). Timing of early-life stress and the development of brain-related capacities. *Frontiers in Behavioral Neuroscience*, 13 (183), 1–14.

Hambrick, E.P., Brawner, T.W., Perry, B.D., Brandt, K., Hofmeister, C., & Collins, J.O. (2019). Beyond the ACE-score: Examining relationships between timing of developmental adversity, relational health, and developmental outcomes in children. *Archives of Psychiatric Nursing*, 33 (3), 238–247.

Hart, A., & Luckock, B. (2004). *Developing Adoption Support and Therapy: New Approaches for Practice*. London & Philadelphia: Jessica Kingsley.

Hart, A., Skandrani, S., Sibeoni, J., Pontvert, C., Revah-Levy, A., & Moro, M.R. (2015). Cultural identity and internationally adopted children: Qualitative Approach to Parental Representations. *PLOS ONE*, 1–19. https://doi.org/10.1371/journal.pone.0119635

Henry, D. (2012). *The 3-5-7 Model: A Practice Approach for Permanency Work with Children and Youth*. Pennsylvania: Sunbury Press.

Hindle, D., & Shulman, G. (Eds.). (2008). *The Emotional Experience of Adoption: A Psychoanalytic Perspective*. London & New York: Routledge.

Hofer, M. (2005). The psychobiology of early attachment. *Clinical Neuroscience Research*, 4 (5–6), 291–300.

Howard, J.A. (2012). *Untangling the Web: The Internet's Transformational Impact on Adoption*. New York: Donaldson Adoption Institute.

Howard, J.A., & Smith, S.I. (2003). *After Adoption: The Needs of Adopted Youth*. Washington, DC: Child Welfare Leagues of America Press.

Jackson, K.F., & Samuels, G.M. (2019). *Multiracial Cultural Attunement*. Washington, DC: NASW Press.

Johnson, D.E., Eckerle, J., Bresnahan, M., & Kroupina, M. (2020). Adoptees with disabilities or medically involved children: A multidisciplinary approach for preparing parents, assessing the child, and supporting successful family formation. In G.M. Wrobel, E. Helder, & E. Marr (Eds.), *The Routledge Handbook of Adoption*. London & New York: Routledge, pp. 188–201.

Juffer, F., Palacios, J., Le Mare, L., Sonuga-Barke, E.J.S., Tieman, W., Bakermans-Kranenburg, M. J., Vorria, P., van Ijzenjoorn, M.H., & Verhulst, F.C. (2011). Development of adopted children with histories of early adversity. *Monographs of the Society for Research in Child Development*, 31–61.

Julian, M.M. (2020). Post-institutionalized adopted children: Effects of prolonged institutionalization and adoption at an older age. In G. M. Wrobel, E. Helder, & E. Marr, (Eds.), *The Routledge Handbook of Adoption*. London & New York: Routledge, pp. 176–187.

Koh, B., Kim, J.R., & McRoy, R. (2020). Adoption-specific curricula in higher education. In *The Routledge Handbook of Adoption*. London & New York: Routledge, pp. 493–507.

Kreider, R.M., & Lofquist, D. (2014). Adopted children and stepchildren in the U.S.: 2010. *Current Population Reports* (P20–572). Washington, DC: U.S. Census Bureau.

Kuvalanka, K.A., Bellis, C., & Goldberg, A.E. (2019). An exploratory study of custody challenges experienced by affirming mothers of transgender and gender-nonconforming children. *Family Court Review*, 57, 54–71.

Leckey, R. (2015). Identity, law, and the right to a dream? *Dalhousie Law Journal*, 38 (2), 525–547.

Leibetseder, D., & Griffin, G. (2019). States of reproduction: The co-production of queer and trans parenthood in three European countries. *Journal of Gender Studies*, 29 (3), 310–324.

Lipschutz, R., & Bick, J. (2020). The neurobiological embedding of early social deprivation in children exposed to institutional rearing. In G.M. Wrobel, E. Helder, & E. Marr (Eds.), *The Routledge Handbook of Adoption*. London & New York: Routledge, pp. 367–380.

Luyten, P., & Fonagy, P. (2014). Assessing mentalising in attachment contexts. In S. Farnfield, & P. Holmes (Eds.), *The Routledge Handbook of Attachment: Assessment.* London & New York: Routledge, pp. 210–226.

Madden, E.E., Aguiniga, D.M., & Ryan, S. (2020). Birth mothers' options counseling and relinquishment experiences. In Wrobel, Helder, & Marr (Eds.), *The Routledge Handbook of Adoption.* London & New York: Routledge, pp. 219–237.

Mahler, M.S., Pine, F., & Bergman, A. (1975). *The Psychological Birth of the Human Infant: Symbiosis and Individuation.* New York: Basic Books.

Manzi, C., Ferrari, I., Rosnati, R., & Benet-Martinez, V. (2014). Bicultural identity integration of transracial adolescent adoptees: Antecedents and outcomes. *Journal of Cross-Cultural Psychology,* 45. Sage Publications, pp. 888–904.

Marr, E. (2017). U.S. transracial adoption trends in the 21st century. *Adoption Quarterly,* 20 (3), 222–251.

McConnachie, A.L., Ayed, N., Foley, S., Lamb, M.E., Jadva, V., Tasker, F., & Golombok, S. (2020). Adoptive gay father families: A longitudinal study of children's adjustment at early adolescence. *Child Development,* 92 (1), 425–443.

McRoy, R., & Griffin, A. (2012). Transracial adoption policies and practices. *Adoption and Fostering,* 36 (3–4), 38–49. https://doi.org/10.1177/030857591 203600305

Melo, A.I. (2015). Role of sensory, social, and hormonal signals from the mother on the development of offspring. In M.C. Antonelli (Ed.), *Perinatal Programming of Neurodevelopment, Advances in Neurobiology,* 10. New York: Springer Science + Business Media, pp. 219–248.

Merritt, M. (2022). Rediscovering latent trauma: An adopted adult's perspective. *Child Abuse & Neglect,* 130, 1–11.

Messina, R., & Brodzinsky, D. (2020). Children adopted by same-sex couples: Identity-related issues from preschool years to late adolescence. *Journal of Family Psychology,* 34 (5), 509–522.

O'Connor, S.H., Christian, D.R., & Ellerman, M.A. (2016). *Black Anthology: Adult Adoptees Claim Their Space – A Diverse Exploration of the Black Adoptee Journey.* The An-Ya Project. Middletown, DE: Self-published.

Palacios, J., & Brodzinsky, D. (2010). Adoption Research: Trends, topics, outcomes. *International Journal of Behavioral Development,* 34, 270–284.

Perry, B.D. (2019). The neurosequential model: A developmentally-sensitive, neuroscience informed approach to clinical problem solving. In J. Mitchel, J. Tucci, & E. Tronick (Eds.), *The Handbook of Therapeutic Child Care: Evidence-informed Approaches to Working with Traumatized Children in Foster, Relative and Adoptive Care.* London: Jessica Kingsley.

Perry, B.D., & Winfrey, O. (2021). *'What Happened to You?": Conversations on Trauma, Resilience, and Healing.* New York: Flatiron Books

Priel, B., Kantor, B., & Besser, R. (2012). Two maternal representations: A study of Israeli adopted children. *Psychoanalytic Psychology,* 17 (1), 128–145.

Reinoso, M., Juffer, F., & Tieman, W. (2012). Children's and parents' thoughts and feelings about adoption, birth culture identity, and discrimination in families with internationally adopted children. *Child and Family Social Work,* 18, 264–274.

Roszia, S., & Maxon, A.D. (2019). *Core Issues in Adoption and Permanency: A Comprehensive Guide to Promoting Understanding and Healing in Adoption, Foster Care, Kinship Families, and Third Party Reproduction.* London: Jessica Kingsley Pub.

Rutter, M., & the English & Romanian Adoptees Team (1998). Developmental catch-up and deficit following adoption after severe global early privation. *Journal of Child Psychology and Psychiatry,* 39 (4), 465–476.

Schore, A.N. (2001). The effects of secure attachment relationships on right brain development, affect regulation, and infant mental health. *Infant Mental Health Journal,* 22, 7–66.

Schore, A.N. (2013). Relational trauma, brain development, and dissociation. In J.D. Ford, & C.A. Courtois (Eds.), *Treating complex traumatic stress disorders in children and adolescents. Scientific Foundations in Therapeutic Models.* New York: The Guilford Press, pp. 3–23.

Schore, A.N. (2015). *Affect Regulation and the Origin of the Self*. London & New York: Routledge.

Selman, P. (2012) The rise and fall of intercountry adoption in the 21st century: Global trends from 2000 to 2010. In J.L. Gibbons, & K.S. Rotabi (Eds.), *Intercountry Adoption: Policies, Practices, and Outcomes*. Surrey: Ashgate, pp. 7–28.

Siegel, D.H. (2012). Growing up in open adoption: Young adults' perspectives. *Families in Society: The Journal of Contemporary Human Services*, 93 (2), 133–140.

Steele, H., & Steele, M. (2018). *Handbook of Attachment-Based Interventions*. New York & London: The Guilford Press.

Szalavitz, M., & Perry, B.D. (2010). *Born for Love: Why Empathy Is Essential – and Endangered*. New York: HarperCollins Publishers.

Tessler, R., & Gamache, G. (2012). Ethnic exploration and consciousness of difference: Chinese adoptees in early adolescence. *Adoption Quarterly*, 15, 265–287.

Van der Kolk, B. (2005). Developmental trauma disorder: A new rational diagnosis for children with complex trauma histories. *Psychiatric Annals*, 35(5), 401–408.

Van der Kolk, B. (2015). *The body keeps the score: Brain, Mind, & Body in the Healing of Trauma*. New York: Penguin Books.

Van der Vegt, E.J.M., Tieman, W., van der Ende, J., Ferdinand, R.F., Verhulst, F.C., & Tiemeier, H. (2009). Impact of early childhood adversities on adult psychiatric disorders: A study of international adoptees. *Social Psychiatry and Psychiatric Epidemiology*, 44, 724–731.

Van Ijzendoorn, M.H., & Juffer, F. (2006). Adoption as intervention: Meta-analytic evidence for massive catchup and plasticity in physical, socio-emotional, and cognitive development. *Journal of Child Psychology and Psychiatry*, 47 (12), 1225–1245.

Ventura-Junca, R., & Herrera, L.M. (2012). Epigenetic alterations related to early-life stressful events. *Acta Neuropsychiatrica*, 24 (5), 255–265. https://doi.org/10.1111/j.1601-5215.2012.00683.x

Waterman, J., Langley, A.K., Miranda, J., & Riley, D.B. (2018). *Adoption-Specific Therapy: A Guide to Helping Adopted Children and Their Families Thrive*. Washington, DC: American Psychological Association.

Welsh, J.A., Viana, A.G., Petrill, S.A., & Mathias, M.D. (2007). Interventions for internationally adopted children and families: A review of the literature. *Child and Adolescent Social Work Journal*, 24 (3), 285–311.

Winnecott, D.W. (1971). Adopted children in adolescence. In R. Tod (Ed.), *Social Work in Adoption* (Collected Papers). London: Longman, pp. 135–143.

Wrobel, G.M., Helder, E., & Marr, E. (2020) *The Routledge Handbook in Adoption*. London & New York: Routledge.

Zilberstein, K. (2011). Multiple attachment representations in clinical practice: Case study of a six-year-old maltreated child. *Psychoanalytic Social Work*, 18, 23–38.

APPENDIX

1. The term "mentalizing" or "mentalization" refers to a mostly preconscious capacity to imagine, perceive, and interpret the meanings of behavior in others and in oneself with regard to needs, desires, feelings, beliefs, goals and intentions, purposes, and reasons. This capacity is vital for self-organization, affect regulation, and secure attachment (Allen et al., 2008; Fonagy et al., 2002). This presents a problem for the many adopted people who, for good reason, would be recognized as having insecure or anxious attachments. From the beginning, the capacity for its development is said to depend on early attachments to a caretaker or caretakers who are able to engage in a two-way process of mirroring affective states (Luyten & Fonagy, 2014). There are no known studies of mentalization capacities in adopted individuals, particularly those whose earliest months and years involved care that was perfunctory and lacked consistent "emotional attunement." But there is reason to believe, based on extensive anecdotal material from adopted adults, that there are exceptions: we know of cases of mentalization capacities still being possible, perhaps an innate talent, regardless of early prenatal and postnatal experiences that failed to engage the child in a way that helped secure attachment.
2. The concept of "adoption competence" as developed for trainings for the social service field has its own criteria for the parameters of necessary skills for adoption professionals, although clinicians have raised concerns about its implicitly judgmental tone. Regardless, the knowledge base and skill sets needed by psychotherapists, particularly those in the traditional mental health disciplines with psychodynamic training, are more diverse and complex and require more years of training. In adoption, there are many different areas of skill sets that are determined by the setting, for which reason the preferable (to the author) concept of "adoption knowledgeable" still requires a subtext specifying the areas of the practitioner's range and level of skills. "Expertise" is always relative and limited to specific areas.

3. Regarding the qualifications of therapists, given what we know about the adopted person's great sensitivity to externally imposed change and loss, about the importance of continuity in important relationships, and about their need and entitlement to have highly skilled psychotherapists, the question should be raised as to how the assignment of adopted clients as training cases (another "placement") can be justified on ethical grounds, regardless of the supervision. When adopted young adults have become more aware of certain details in their early lives, many have expressed to their therapists resentment about "being used to meet someone else's needs." This is indeed the situation when the adopted client becomes a training case, particularly if the treatment is primarily supportive and time-limited, and also if the trainee has limited wisdom from life experience.
4. Within the relatively few private adoption agencies still operating, along with the increasing majority of adoptions handled by welfare services, their responses to the adult adopted person returning for information are, on the basis of many anecdotal accounts, mechanical and perfunctory at best, replicating for many their earliest experiences. These typically involve lengthy delays and, at times, a begrudging attitude, beyond which there is no service because they do not consider the adopted person's ongoing needs to be any part of their mission, which they view as protecting both sets of parents. Instead, placement sources tend simply to defer to the law in the hope that it will protect them (the sealed adoption record pertains only to original birth certificates, not to information in agency records). At best, they may suggest some resources where the adopted person might find further help. Such an attitude of indifference to their needs leaves the adopted person feeling profoundly betrayed.
5. It is one of the dark secrets in the history of American adoptions and serves as evidence of the true priority of the adoption field that has not necessarily changed over the decades that in the 1930s and 1940s, it was standard practice to keep babies in foster care or group homes for a full year before being released for adoptive placement. The reason was to ensure that the adoptive parents would receive a baby that had no significant health or developmental problems. Also, in those days, the child's intelligence was of utmost importance, and it was believed this could not be tested before the age of 1. The placement services also wanted to ensure that the baby would have no difficulty making attachments to the adoptive parents, for which reason young babies were shifted through several foster homes for a full year before being placed, that is, so that they could "save" their attachment capacities for the parents who would eventually adopt them.
6. From a private communication, a professional social worker and her husband adopted an infant within days of birth, having found the pregnant birth mother online. A lawyer within the same highly educated suburban community had a specialty of handling the legal arrangements for prospective adoptive parents. In time, through the lawyer, this gave the social worker access to 11 other families for whom she organized and led a support group for over two decades. All the

Life Begins Before Adoption

children had come into the adoptive homes within the first month or two after birth, having also been found online. During the time that her adopted child was growing up, the mother decided to develop a specialty in working with adoptive families and took additional training through one of the well-known adoption training programs for the social service field.

As an overall observation, our children's development throughout their first year seemed entirely typical of babies through that time. However, variations on the norm became gradually evident in the second and third years, particularly in learning and language skills, but also in various forms of difficult behaviors, such as tantrums, withdrawal, hyperactivity, and difficulty joining in age-appropriate group activities. However, the families' pediatricians continued to offer reassurances that the problems of concern to the parents would work themselves out. However, into the latency and early-adolescent years, in many children the difficult behaviors not only increased but also expanded in range, such as crises with volatility, aggression, suicidal thinking, and early drug use. These led to neuropsychological testing and, for most of the children, diagnoses of ADHD, with many assorted trials of medication intended to "fix" the behavioral problems. But the families were given little more in the way of help, even from some of the top-notch university-based outpatient children's programs in the metropolitan area. When we asked whether and how our children's adoptions may be a factor, we were met with silence.

Over time, of the 17 adopted children in these families, 14 had significant learning problems, and half needed help with substance abuse problems, ten — some in their middle school years — felt the need to know about their birth families and later searched for them. Their struggles did not subside once they became young adults: one-third graduated from college, although often with bumps along the way, while others had extensive difficulty, going from one school to another, unable to find consistent work while living back and forth between home and apartments with friends. For every family, some level of mental health care needed to be accessed for each child at various ages, for different needs, throughout adolescence and young adulthood. When families seek mental health care, they encounter society's "conspiracy of silence" from therapists everywhere. An adoption-specialized *clinical* training venue needs to be prioritized for mainstream mental health.

(personal communication from the author of the report)

Note from DB: The previous account may or may not be typical of children placed soon after birth: we cannot know because outcomes, especially of private/independent adoptions, have never been studied. Research involving "early placement," such as in all cases of the families described in the report, still has inadequate details of many important variables, such as age and developmental profile, within the particular context being discussed. For example, in her report, the social worker did not provide any information about the birth mothers' health or mental health during their pregnancies (e.g., health histories, obstetrical care, medications, possible drug use) or anything about the biological family's medical or psychiatric history that may have been known.

5

THE ADOPTIVE FAMILY NARRATIVE AND ITS EFFECTS ON THE ADOPTED PERSON'S DEVELOPMENT

Steven L. Nickman, MD

Introduction

Psychotherapy and satisfactory family life have in common the sharing of stories in a safe setting. The therapist elicits the client's story, does her/his best to understand it, and tries to clarify and make sense of the different parts with the client. Having a personal story is like wearing clothes suitable for the occasion; it is being able to locate yourself in the long succession of previous generations/family history/cultural background. Adoptees, particularly in non-kinship adoption, often feel they have an incomplete story. Many do not have a sense of authentic belonging in a family, community, ethnicity, or nation. Some adoptees report experiencing an "as if" position; their lives are straddled within the adoptive family they know and a birth family they do not know at all or do not know well. Regardless of whether adoptees enter treatment, depending on a number of factors, some adopted people feel they had not really been born or were not truly connected to the human race. A lack of empathic and open dialogue in the adoptive family has often contributed to such convictions.

As the adopted person matures, the adoptive family narrative becomes the nucleus of the person's adoption story. It includes the words, language, and attitudes conveyed in family conversations during childhood, the feelings aroused at those times, and the ways in which the conversations have been remembered. The adoption story comes to include fantasies based on what the adoptee was told and feelings that evolve about what is and is not known. In adulthood, it becomes the adoption-related component of an individual's self-concept and self-presentation in social situations. Thus, the adoption story consists of:

1. What was told to the adoptee in early childhood and/or later.
2. How this was understood and became part of the adoptee's own self-narrative.
3. How the maturing adopted person came to talk about his or her own adoption with others.
4. How adoption affected the adoptee's broader interactions with the world in adolescence and adult life.

Because of its importance for clinical work, this chapter will first address general considerations about when and how someone learns about being adopted, how they understood what they have been told, and the effects of the disclosure of adoptive status as they understand it at different stages of development. The discussion will be predicated on the idea that there are many kinds of loss in being adopted (Nickman, 1985). One type relates to overt losses; this includes separations, disrupted placements, and loss of familiar surroundings. A second type relates to covert losses; these relate to the *inner responses* to external separations (Nickman, 1996). The third type refers to status losses; these are the experiences of social stigma, even in subtle forms, related to some aspect of adoption. The importance society attributes to blood ties and genetics may decrease social status because they are adopted, increasing feelings of loss or inadequacy (Leon, 2002; Barroso & Barbosa-Ducharne, 2019). The experiences of loss depend on the adoptee's particular life context, the meanings attributed to his or her losses, his or her adoption and pre-adoption life, as well as his or her cognitive and developmental stage (Smith & Brodzinsky, 1994, 2002)

General Considerations

There are several general issues when working with adopted people in adolescence and early adulthood. The first has to do with issues of bias against adoption, that is, the view of it being "second best" as a way of forming family life. The second is about the changing nature of adoption policy and practice, especially over the past five decades. It is important for the therapist to take them into account because the adopted patient's particular circumstances are an integral part of their experience and development.

Prejudice and bias exist in many cultures and countries against adoption. In non-kinship adoption, adoptees' connection with their adoptive parents is non-biologic and the genetic discontinuity implies that something went wrong (Brinich, 1980; Wegar, 2000; Wieder, 2001; Roy, 2020). Adopted people may absorb this cultural attitude, and some take it a step further, assuming that something went wrong with them. In a global context, this bias persists in biological family opposition to adoptees' inheriting property, closed or missing birth records, social stigma that is generally unacknowledged, and with an array of losses (Barroso & Barbosa-Ducharne, 2019). Some adoptive families encounter a lack of support from their own parents and negative attitudes about adopting an unrelated child. There have been media accounts about adult adopted people placed internationally that were deported or were at risk of being deported to a country they did not know and a language they did not speak (Kim, 2021). Microaggressions are examples of adoption bias; this includes attitudes, judgments, prejudice, and racism that can be subtle, overt, or hostile in everyday interactions (Baden, 2016). They are innocent, unintentional, ignorant, or blatant. Adoptees will often not tell their parents about these experiences (Reinoso et al., 2013).

Adoption policy and practice have undergone major changes throughout the twentieth century and into the twenty-first. Starting in the 1950s, there was an increase in both intercountry adoption and transracial adoptions (Baden, 2007; Biafora & Esposito, 2007). Beginning in the 1980s, a substantial proportion of adoptees was placed with their families when they were older, often with a history of foster care, or from other countries with a history of institutionalization before adoption (Zamostny et al., 2003; Selman, 2009; Wiley, 2017). Their stories contain layers of narratives involving the birth mother and relinquishment, the "ghost" of the birth father, about whom there is typically little or no information (Chapter 7), changes in caretakers, trauma and its sequelae, and additional kinds of losses beyond those experienced by adoptees who were placed early in life as infants.

As a result of these issues, mental health providers need to be alerted to missing parts of an adopted person's history. In addition, details may have great importance during adolescence. The "medical passport" has been needed to ensure continuity of pediatric care for children who go from one caretaker to another when their foster placement changes. Some adolescents adopted at a young age from other countries have surgical scars from procedures, the nature of which is unknown and undocumented in the records provided to adoptive parents. Less well recognized is the importance of a full assessment of psychosocial history and of details of the child's pre-placement development. Adopted people who require mental health services may lack information and/or memory about periods of their childhood prior to adoptive placement. As a guide to mental health practice, the following are important to note:

1. When early information is available, either in written records or directly from the adoptee or adoptive parents, a therapist must understand the importance of knowing this information when the initial history is taken. To view the early history as irrelevant or too painful to talk about, or to be concerned about upsetting the patient, may represent the therapist's bias or subconscious anxiety related to the material. This is not likely to correspond with the adoptee's feelings that are already there, or those of the family. In fact, a common disappointment and complaint of adopted young adults is that they had to see a number of therapists when they were younger and that the therapists "never brought the subject up." But early experiences have lifelong consequences, for which reason best practices require the therapist to take them into account. As an example, when an adopted person as a child had interrupted or impersonal care, such as found in institutional settings, the implications of these experiences are not well

understood by the adoptive parents. A lack of understanding affects parental expectations that may have been problematic for both the adopted person and the adoptive family. Similarly, a lack of understanding also affects both the therapy and the therapist's expectations regarding the treatment goals.

2. There is no reason to assume *a priori* that the presenting problem has resulted from interactions within the adoptive family. In fact, difficulties may have arisen from early trauma or pathological interactions before adoption, from adoptive family dynamics, or from interactions between pre-adoptive and post-adoptive experiences (Grotevant & McDermott, 2014). When parents know the early history and its implications, they have some knowledge about the damage their child likely sustained before joining their family. However, often the professionals blame them for the resulting emotional and behavioral problem. Or when the parents or the adoptee try to explain the complexities of the early history, the therapist may wave it aside and communicate that they do not feel it is necessary. This is an affront to the adopted patient for whom the primary agenda for treatment is to be understood.

3. As in the case of other patients who have very complicated earlier lives or circumstances, in evaluating and treating an adopted client/patient, the clinician must be prepared to devote the time required in order to explore the topics and details as fully as possible in order to reach a suitable differential diagnosis and consider a treatment plan. If the clinician or the setting cannot allow for what is likely to take additional time for the service, and depending on the mutual goals for treatment, the therapist must give careful thought to discussing this with the patient and reviewing options for referral to a resource that would better meet the patient's needs. Clinical specialists believe this is the therapist's obligation, including those in private practice.

Apart from therapists' not considering historical information, adoptees or adoptive parents may omit or minimize background information. When clinicians do not ask about the full time span of an adoptee's life, they may be colluding in disregarding history that is essential for effective treatment. From the standpoint of best clinical practice, neglecting or avoiding any information is an error of omission. When a blank space emerges in the course of inquiry – as happens with an adopted person – it is significant; it points to a missing piece of knowledge that may be associated with feelings of loss or a gap in memory related to repression, or the suspicion that the information may be "bad." The best metaphor may be missing an important body part. Any of these presents the opportunity for therapeutic exploration.

Adoptees' interactions with peers and adults over time about their adoption, and the societal attitudes about adoption, are important contributors to their experience. This includes their communities and the broader culture presented in films, television, fiction, and social media. As adoptees move from the family circle into broader social contexts, they become more aware that being adopted is a non-normative or abnormal life circumstance; this may affect self-perception, self-esteem, and self-confidence.

Mental health professionals working with adoptees need to assess adoption discussions within the adoptive family – whether they were brief and unsatisfying or empathic and ongoing. They also need to consider how adoption has been experienced throughout an adopted person's life, including both inner experiences (a sense of loss, unanswered questions, preoccupations, frustrations) and reactions of important others to the adoption. Of special importance for adoptees is the *autobiographical capacity* – the ability to tell their own story coherently and in sequence. Such ability has consequences throughout the life cycle. The adoption story is an opportunity for adoptive families to discuss the circumstances of the adoption in a way that emphasizes the adults' care and concern. If the family engages in open communication about the adoption, the adoptee's questions about the adoption facts can be answered and the parents can find out whether he/she wishes to learn more (Wydra et al., 2012; Horstman et al., 2016). When parents are able to permit inquiry and respond non-defensively to the expression of feelings an adopted person experiences, they are more likely to promote healthy personality development, high self-esteem, creativity, and mature social interactions (Hauser et al., 1991; Ranieri et al., 2021). It is an important part of assessment to review these details of family communication patterns. The following is a guide to questions the therapist can ask:

- Would you be comfortable if I could ask you some questions about your adoption?
- What do you remember about when and how your parents let you know that they adopted you? How old were you at that time? How did they try to explain it, and what did they actually tell you? What words did they use? Do you remember how you reacted or what it meant to you at that time?
- To what extent was there a comfortable atmosphere that encouraged you to ask any questions you may have had or express feelings about being adopted over time? Were your questions answered? Did your parents bring up the subject occasionally? Frequently? Or never?
- How did conversations about adoption within the family influence the way you thought of yourself or who you are and how you felt about yourself?
- Have you known other people who were adopted?
- Do you know whether your parents had any preparation either for what would be involved in becoming adoptive parents or for how and when to begin telling you of your adoption?
- Did your being adopted ever come up in your friendships or in school? Do you remember how it may have come up and how you felt about it?
- Did your parents mention your biological parents? What did they say about them? Did they say anything about the reason your birth parents could not raise you themselves?

- If age-appropriate, has/did your being adopted ever come up in your dating life?
- Is there anything about being adopted that is on your mind now?

At the same time, open communication does not mean telling everything, or most things, all at once. In some cases, parents may say too much too soon, likely out of anxiety and a wish to "get it over with." Rather, "the telling" or disclosure needs to be a process over time, guided by the child's developmental capacities and by the child's questions.

The Particulars of How and When Adoption Was Disclosed and Its Impact

A common practice in adoption social work over the decades has been the encouragement that adoptive parents tell about the adoption "early and often" (MacIntyre, 1990). This was intended to make the process seem as normal and familiar as possible as well as protect from sudden disillusionment or revelations from others (Brinich, 1980). However, disclosure "from the beginning" (prior to about age 3) was not based on any understanding of early childhood development, particularly in the case of adopted children, and even more so if they experienced severe early trauma. The practice of "early telling" was challenged by some child psychiatrists (Wieder, 1977, 1978) on the grounds that adoption disclosure contributed to a splitting in the child's mind between good parent and bad or abandoning parent and, subsequently, good and bad self. This perspective was based on psychoanalytic case reports and suggested that:

1. Introducing knowledge of adoption before the latency period (before age 6 to 7), or especially in the pre-school years, before the child has developed relationships outside the immediate family, would result in threats to self-esteem because the sense of abandonment by the birth parents was felt concretely and took a prominent place in their evolving sense of themselves.
2. Children could become deeply confused by having to live with shifting fantasies about their birth parents, while the priority in the early years should be consolidating their attachment to their adoptive parents. Introducing the fact that there is "another set of parents" can interfere with this process within the child. A best practice within the adoption community developed that secrecy could not be defended and secrecy or denial about adoption had long-lasting negative effects.

But this does not actually contradict the arguments about basing the initial disclosure on the child's developmental readiness, as discussed in Wieder (2001). A study by counseling psychologists concluded that any disclosure past the age of 3 fell into the category of "late disclosure" (Baden et al., 2019), but this is not the clinical perspective based on what is being learned about the very fragile first three years of life, especially if the child experienced early trauma. Inquiry about all the previous text is an important part of the extended evaluation of the adopted client, but it is also an issue that may warrant the parents seeing an adoption-specialized consultant, in collaboration with the child/adolescent's therapist, to discuss their own family situation.

Since the adopted client sets the agenda as therapy begins, the psychodynamically informed clinician waits to hear whether, and in what context, being adopted comes up. It is sometimes proposed that adoptive status be a standard intake question, but this may seem strange and out of context, but it is also unnecessary, because there are other ways to "invite" the topic and to "listen for it." One of the best ways is to ask the patient who they resemble in their family. Another is to ask, perhaps in the context of taking a medical history, if there is any information about their birth or about the early part of their life that they may have questions about. A clinician will want to understand the role of the person who disclosed the adoption. If it is a two-parent family, did each parent participate equally in deciding to adopt and in the adoption disclosure? Were there ongoing conversations about adoption over time? Was it a process that both parents participated in, or was it primarily one parent who discussed adoption, especially over time? For the adopted individual, rarely is there a single conversation about adoption, although one interaction may stand out in memory as a critical incident.

In adoption, the idea of physical resemblance serves as a metaphor for whether and how the adoptee feels a connection and bond with the adoptive family. With suitable context and timing, it can be important to inquire about physical attributes or parts of the body: Does the client like certain attributes or dislike specific features or traits. What is it about these traits that make them proud or unhappy? Was there post-infancy circumcision of young boys after joining their adoptive families to resemble the circumcised father?

The therapist needs to be aware that if an adoptee was placed in early infancy, a wealth of sensory memories already exists, and receptive, preverbal, and expressive language may have developed. This is somewhat different from disclosure with older child adoptees, who likely have memories, although they may be fragmented and vague. Even when there have been contacts with the birth family or adoption workers after placement, adoptive parents cannot assume the adoptee understands the role of different adults, the circumstances leading to adoption, or memories they have pre-adoption. Empathic disclosure and ongoing dialogue are essential in the family, along with re-working of events as cognitive development advances and opportunities to revisit affectively past times of sorrow and confusion about the adoption (Brodzinsky et al., 1984; Brodzinsky, 2006; Colaner & Soliz, 2017). However, the therapist cannot assume that the disclosure of adoptive status, or the communications over time, met these conditions.

One tool that has helped in this process is an adoption lifebook which the parents may have developed (Backhaus, 1984). This records an adopted person's life using words, photos, graphics, artwork, videos, and memorabilia. They can contain early photographs and mementoes of the child, first family information, previous homes, and previous caretakers. Especially in the case of an older child, they may have been compiled by adoption placement workers as a resource. The lifebook, and the stories associated with it, may be helpful if the therapist invites an adolescent, or even a young adult, to share in therapy. If the adopted person does not have an adoption lifebook, part of initial therapeutic work, especially with a young adolescent, may focus on developing one.

Overall, adoption disclosure should have been individually paced and based on the adoptee's cognitive and developmental abilities (Brodzinsky, 2011). It would have taken into consideration times of stress or change in family life, and the therapist will want to note the adoptive parents' sensitivity and skills in handling any complications. Consultation with a qualified adoption-informed professional is a good practice, prior to and as part of the adoption telling, and of the retelling process over time. On the other hand, sometimes the disclosure occurs in adolescence, young adulthood, or later in life (Chapter 3), which, depending on when this occurred, may actually become a psychological emergency for the adoptee that the therapist must immediately recognize and be prepared to attend to. The late disclosure or discovery of adoption creates an array of emotional difficulties and psychological distress (Sherr et al., 2018; Baden et al., 2019), and the therapist should not underestimate the impact on the adopted client.

There may be periods of time when the adoptee is not interested, but during adolescence and early adulthood, there is often a renewed interest in the birth/first family. When adoptive parents are aware of circumstances that might be considered shameful, stigmatizing, or disturbing, truth-telling becomes more complex, and it takes great skill to do this. The most difficult information has to do with either rape or incest, but hopefully, the parents will consult an adoption specialist, to consider whether, how, and when to tell some parts of the history and to manage the adoptee's reaction to the information, particularly when questions may come up in adolescence. The adoptive parents are the custodians of the adoptee's history and are required to preserve and pass on whatever they know as important building blocks for the construction of self-identity. These include the parents' reasons for adopting, which might include infertility, genetically transmitted illness, or other reasons. Eventually, it includes what is known about the adoptee's first family and culture of origin and perhaps, most importantly, the birth parents' own interests, life histories, and enthusiasms, if they can be known, that the adoptee will use as a framework for identification, differentiation, and integration of their full family history. But therapists need also to consider the possibility that the adoptee's parents were inadequately prepared by the placement source, a very common complaint from adoptive parents, and that they may not have some of this information.

A Case of Late Disclosure

Mrs. S, the mother of a 16-year-old girl, had not found a way to tell her daughter about her adoption until the week before the two of them presented for a clinic visit. This was a family that I saw only twice, so I had little background or context and no follow-up. The mother and daughter were seen separately and together. Mrs. S was angry and dismissive toward her daughter because she had been difficult to raise. The two of them had a bitter argument, but things had calmed down somewhat and they were watching television together. By chance, the program had an adoption theme. The teenager turned to her mother and asked, "I'm not adopted by any chance, am I?" Her mother said, "Well, actually, you are. We didn't know how to tell you." The girl cursed and stormed out of the house. She returned later in the evening, but little had been said during the intervening days.

This example underscores the risk of parents' not being in empathic connection with their daughter or son when discussing adoption. It also raises the question of timing. The fact that the mother had not been able to discuss adoption with her daughter suggests that she felt it was so potentially harmful that it had to be avoided, yet she knew it needed to be disclosed at some point. It was only at a moment of angry disconnection that the negative aspect of her ambivalence took charge (Bonovitz, 2006; Brinich, 1980). While young adoptees inevitably experience loss as a result of learning about their adoptions, they are usually fairly resilient; when parents cannot believe in that resilience, there may be reasons that belong to their own past histories of loss, injury, or betrayal (Nickman, 1999).

Adolescence

The prominence of sexuality in teenagers accompanies their rapid physical maturation and cognitive development. Group membership becomes crucial as they continue to define themselves as individuals with identities that do not depend on their roles in their families. Their maturing cognition and social perception allow them to see things from different points of view. They have their own culture based largely in social media. Adolescents have acquired some understanding of procreation, pregnancy, childbirth, adoption, and what is involved in being a parent. Adopted adolescents' earlier fantasies about their birth parents may move toward active desires to learn more about the birth parents or to seek them out, to substitute fantasy with reality (McRoy et al., 1988). They feel more acutely these questions:

- Can I understand what their experiences must have been like?
- Are they still alive and in good health?
- What do they each look like? Do I resemble them? Do I have siblings?
- If I don't look for them now, will they still be there later on?
- Does my birth mother think about me on my birthday?
- Does she ever wonder how I'm doing?

Often, questions are about the birth mother, but some adopted adolescent boys also have the same questions about their birth fathers (Henderson, 2007) (Chapter 7).

It has been observed that in some cases, the adoptee is so preoccupied with the birth mother that the birth father remains in the background or even "out of mind" (Chapter 7). Although this may also relate to the adoptive parents having no information about him, this is likely because the need for connection with the birth mother can be so overwhelming that the adoptee, as it were, cannot get past it at that time. But this does not mean it is not important for many adoptees.

On the other hand, since open adoptions have become more common, additional information about birth parents may be available. Contact with birth relatives, directly or indirectly, in open adoption, often yields more frequent adoption-related family conversations (Von Korff & Grotevant, 2011). Adoptive parents sometimes assume that, if the adoptee is not talking about their adoption, they are not interested. This is not an accurate assumption; it means that they are not talking to the adoptive parents about their questions or concerns. Lodz (2014) identifies the family obligation as not interfering with the adolescent's questions about the birth parents. According to Lotz (2014), adoptive parents need to actively help the adoptee further the search for answers to questions about the birth family. But therapists need also to be alert to situations in which it is more the parents than the adopted daughter/son who want to "help them" with the search, and the therapist may need to consider intervening in this. It should be noted that the sense of loss and the search for the birth family in the development of identity become more urgent with the anxieties of leaving home for college or for the experience of working and living with a friend (Dalley & Kohon, 2008). Three cases illustrate different points about adolescent development:

> Phil had been adopted through a religious agency at 2 months of age. I saw him in weekly therapy for two years beginning when he was 13 1/2. His parents divorced when he was 3, and he lived with his mother, an adopted sister, and another sister who was born to the parents. His mother sought therapy for him because "[she was] afraid his adolescence [was] getting out of control." She suspected he had begun to drink, and in his social studies class, he had expressed admiration for Hitler's personality. The family was Jewish. His adoptive father was a businessperson, and Phil saw him only on alternate weekends. His father took him to lunch at expensive restaurants, and their time together was limited to such special occasions. Phil was good at sports, enjoyed being in motion, but performed poorly in school. He spent much of his time daydreaming. In a therapy session, he said, "If I knew what my birth parents did, what they're good at, it would help. Like, I think I heard somewhere he was a professional boxer. If I knew that for sure, I would be able to aim at that. I would know it was something I could do." His adoptive father remained relatively unavailable as a role model, but also emotionally, because their temperaments were so different.
>
> Seventeen years after his therapy ended, when Phil was 32, I invited him to tell me how things had gone for him, explaining that I had worked with a number of adoptees and was beginning to write about their experiences to

help other therapists learn about adoption. He was quite willing. He looked around my office and commented that it felt like a déjà vu experience. After high school, he had taken some college courses but was not motivated. Discouraged after a failed relationship, he left college and was now working in a computer software company as a low-level manager. He said, "Motivation is a problem for me. That's one of my problems with adoption. I'm too complacent. Let the world do with me what it will. Something was done without my consent, decisions other people made. So it's okay for me to make the best of what I've got." He was living with a male roommate, feeling bored with his bachelor life. He had been close to marriage twice and thought he would make a good father. He thought his parents' divorce had had a greater effect on him than his adoption. His father had remained self-centered, and his mother had died several years before. After she died, he thought, "I don't know anyone I'm related to by blood." He felt orphaned once again. His mother had known the name of the lawyer who arranged the adoption, "but that knowledge died with her." He didn't want to ask his father, because his father might hold it against him. He would have liked to have information about his birth mother or a photograph. He said, "One reason I might follow up on this someday is out of concern for her. She's got to wonder what happened to that baby she had. I'd want to say, 'I appreciate your not aborting me, and I think I'm a pretty good kid.'"

Matt, age 12, had been adopted in infancy by a professional family living in a high-income suburb. He was bright and popular, but overly aggressive and pushed limits. The family went skiing, but Matt spent much time with another family at the same resort. As one long weekend came to a close, the other family came to say goodbye, and they were overheard to say to Matt, "Have a good trip back to Dorchester," naming a blue-collar neighborhood of the city. Matt's parents looked at him, and he shrugged. It was clear that he had told the other family he lived in Dorchester, acting out his fantasy that he belonged to a blue-collar family. He preferred his own narrative. When his misrepresentation was exposed, his parents chose not to pursue it because they knew he would feel they were blaming him.

Brian, age 14, had been adopted at 6 weeks of age. He wrote a story in which he identified himself with the protagonist, a king who assembles a large army to conquer evil spirits and ogres, helped by a wizard. Asked about the meaning of evil in the story, he said, "If you can see it from an adopted kid's point of view, you're trying to find your parents. Evil is what keeps you from finding them. Once the battle is over, you settle down and live a quiet life."

These three boys presented for treatment in early adolescence and made use of fantasy in different ways. All had been adopted in infancy and had grown up in different circumstances. Phil's parents divorced when he was in pre-school; he was close to his mother, but his father was somewhat unavailable. Matt's extended family was intact, but his only connection was with his mother, while he maintained a psychological distance from everyone else. He had begun to show evidence of a private, unshared self that manifested by aggression and distortion of the truth. Brian was sent to a boarding school on the East Coast, far from his adoptive family's home in California, and felt rejected not only by his birth family but also by his adoptive family. Each boy's fantasy reflected an aspect of the ongoing situation. For Phil, fantasy brought him closer to the inner image of himself that he wanted to become (regarding ego ideal). For Matt, fantasy served his need to establish distance from his adoptive parents. Brian constructed a story that put him in charge, changed passive to active, and undid (freed him from) his sense of abandonment.

Many adoptees confront a developmental challenge that is peculiar to them and is not shared by their non-adopted peers as they transition to adulthood. They must grapple with the question of whether or not they want to seek information about or actual contact with first parents whom they have constructed in fantasy but who they know exist in the real world. There is a point in mid-to late adolescence that corresponds with cognitive development. It has become significantly harder to keep the birth parents, and the part of one's history that corresponds to them, contained within fantasy. Therapists of adolescent and young adult adoptees commonly witness this transition. They have the opportunity to help the adopted person understand that the dilemma and mix of emotions is a normative one, that feeling guilt toward the adoptive parents is common, that thinking about doing something is not the same as doing it, and that the prospect of embarking on this decision is both exciting and frightening.

Early Adulthood

Reflective thinking about adoption starts in adolescence and continues into adulthood (Wrobel & Grotevant, 2019). Young adult adoptees may attribute little importance to adoption or may see it as the central experience of their lives. About one-third actively engage in search for the first family (Tieman et al., 2008). With the rise of social media and technology, many barriers have been reduced for those who engage in search (Shier, 2021), while others remain in place (Schechter & Bertocci, 1990).

In the last part of the twentieth century, a great deal of research focused on the long-term physical, cognitive, and psychosocial development of young adults adopted from traumatic or extreme deprivation early in life. Extended early deprivation (more than six months) results in long-term deleterious effects that last into adulthood even after years of nurturance in a higher-resource adoptive family (Sonuga-Barke et al., 2017). Early childhood deprivation alters brain structure into adulthood (Mackes et al., 2020). This means that the clinical issues for this subgroup of adoptees is more complex, especially when the adoption was transracial, international, and/or transcultural. Even those that are resilient after early adversity may have mental health issues such as depression that may resurface and become an extension of depression and trauma in early childhood (Dekker et al., 2017), but sometimes the mental health issues have late onset. Older age at adoption increases the complexity of issues that adult adoptees encounter (Côté & Lalumière, 2020) and, in turn, complexities for diagnosis and treatment.

Implications for Treatment

The adoptive family's shared dialogue about adoption is a framework for discussing therapeutic approaches to adoptees' difficulties. The "adoption story" can be viewed as *dynamic* in the sense that it evolves gradually from what a child is told by adults into the ways in which that adult adoptee comes to understand the past and its influence on his/her development. Topics that often arise in psychotherapy are knowledge (or lack of it) of origins, whether and how more knowledge can be obtained, and how this may be related to the way the initial adoption disclosure was experienced. With the increased freedom of adolescence and young adulthood, adoptees may need help in deciding whether, at a given moment in time, they want to pursue information, which may be sufficient at the time, or actual contact with the birth family. A common dilemma has to do with the unknown, which often involves fantasizing but also deciding whether they are ready for additional information. A dilemma when birth parents are known is how the adoptee can be part of both an adoptive and a birth family. With adult adoptees from other countries, they may or may not have access to information through multimedia or through the recent development of online groups of adoptees from their country. The information they learn may not be consistent with the information they were originally told. Many adult adoptees need to be able to process conflicting and disturbing information. Ambiguous loss is a prevailing clinical theme in working with adoptees.

Summary and Conclusion

The adoptive family's shared dialogue about adoption is used as a framework for discussing therapeutic approaches with adopted youth and young adults. At the outset of treatment, the therapist notes whether the topic of adoption is first mentioned by the client and the context in which it comes up. The therapist then explores with them how they have experienced their adoption and how it has interacted with other themes in their development and current lives. Treatment of adopted patients is most effective when therapists view adoptive status as an important, enduring life circumstance that affects self-regard, relationships, an internal sense of security (ability to trust, closeness in relationships), creativity, and even potential occupational success. Important variables that serve as a foundation are the details of their birth and of their pre-placement experiences, age and development at placement with the adoptive parents, and shifts in relationships within the adoptive family as the adopted person matures into adulthood. Therapists are likely to hear themes of loss and deprivation (neediness), anger, guilt about feeling angry, anger about "being made to feel guilty," conflicts of loyalty, and inhibitions around autonomous decision-making. Although we may sometimes hear some of these expressions from non-adopted adolescents, adopted young adults may be more likely to struggle with feeling infantilized because society has made decisions for them that were never made for their peers, with potentially profound lifelong results that, for those in closed adoptions, began with denying them access to their birth records.

A broader dilemma for them is whether and how to deal with the unknown and the powers over them. They say they tend to worry about everyone else's feelings and needs while not sensing that they receive the same in return. In their encounters with "the system" (agencies, welfare departments, placement organizations), they readily sense the degree to which they are still regarded as a threat to the "status quo." Thus, transference and countertransference problems may arise around issues of forbidden vs. permitted knowledge, idealization or denigration of the therapist, depending on what the therapist may represent internally from time to time, with counter-balancing shifts in feelings about the adoptive parents, and rescue fantasies, although at times the therapist may be confused about who needs rescuing from what.

The foregoing complexities warrant a good deal more examination and discourse as the psychology and treatment of adopted individuals become better understood.

Endnotes

Backhaus, K.A. (1984). Life books: Tools for working with children in placement. *Social Work,* 29, 551–554. www.jstor.org.stable/23713798

Baden, A. (2007). Identity, psychological adjustment, culture, and race: Issues for transracial adoptees and the cultural-racial identity model. In R. Javier, A. Baden, & F. Biafora (Eds.), *Handbook of Adoption: Implications for Researchers, Practitioners, and Families* (pp. 359–378). Sage Publications, Inc. www.doi.org/10.4135/9781412976633.n23

Baden, A.L., Mazza, J.R., Kitchen, A., Harrington, E., & White E. (2016). Mental health issues. In R. Fong, & R. McRoy (Eds.), *Transracial and INTERCOUNTRY Adoption* (pp. 193–236). New York: Columbia University.

Baden, A.L., Shadel, D., Bates, T.A. et al. (2019). Delaying adoption disclosure: A survey of late discovery adoptees. *Journal of Family Issues,* 40 (9) (Sage Pub). https://doi.org/10.1177/0192513x19829503

Barroso, R., & Barbosa-Ducharne, M. (2019). Adoption-related feelings, loss, and curiosity about origins in adopted adolescents. *Clinical Child Psychology and Psychiatry,* 24 (4), 876–891. https://doi.org/10.1177/1359104519858117

Biafora, F.A., & Esposito, D. (2007). Adoption data and statistical trends. In R.A. Javier, A.L. Baden, F.A. Biafora, & A. Camacho-Gingerich (Eds.), *Handbook of Adoption: Implications for Researchers, Practitioners, and Families* (pp. 32–43). Thousand Oaks, London, & New Delhi: Sage Publication.

Bonovitz, C. (2006). Unconscious communication and the transmission of loss. In K. Hushion, S. Sherman, & D. Siskind (Eds.), *Understanding Adoption* (pp. 11–33). Lanham, MD: Rowman & Littlefield.

Brinich, P.M. (1980). Some potential effects of adoption on self and object representations. *The Psychoanalytic Study of the Child,* 35, 107–133.

Brodzinsky, D. (2011). Children's understanding of adoption: Developmental and clinical implications. *Professional Psychology: Research and Practice,* 42, 200–207.

Brodzinsky, D.M. (2006). Family structural openness and communication openness as predictors in the adjustment of adopted children. *Adoption Quarterly,* 9 (4), 1–18.

Brodzinsky, D.M., Singer, L.M., & Braff, A.M. (1984). Children's understanding of adoption. *Child Development,* 55 (3), 869–878. https://doi.org/10.2307/1130138

Colaner, C.W., & Soliz, J. (2017). A communication-based approach to adoptive identity: Theoretical and empirical support. *Communication Research. Sage Journals,* 44 (5), 611–637.

Côté, K., & Lalumière, M.L. (2020). Psychological adjustment of domestic adult adoptees. *Journal of Adult Development,* 27, 118–134.

Dalley, T., & Kohon, V. (2008). Deprivation and development: The predicament of an adopted adolescent in the search for identity. In D. Hindle & G. Shulman (Eds.), *The Emotional Experience of Adoption: A Psychoanalytic Perspective.* London & New York: Routledge. 225–236.

Dekker, S.L., Tieman, W., & Vinke, A.G. (2017). Mental health problems of Dutch young adult domestic adoptees compared to non-adopted peers and international adoptees. *International Social Work,* 60 (5), 1201–1217.

Grotevant, H.D., & McDermott, J.M. (2014). Adoption: Biological and social processes linked to adaptation. *Annual Review of Psychology,* 65, 235–265.

Hauser, S.T., Powers, S.I., & Noam, G.G. (1991). *Adolescents and their Families: Paths of Ego Development.* New York: Simon and Schuster.

Henderson, D. (2007). Why has the mental health community been silent on adoption issues? In R. Javier, A. Baden, & F. Biafora (Eds.), *Handbook of Adoption: Implications for Researchers, Practitioners, and Families* (pp. 403–417). SAGE Publications, Inc. www.doi.org/10.4135/9781412976633.n25

Horstman, H.K., Colaner, C.W., & Rittenour, C.E. (2016). Contributing factors of adult adoptees' identity work and self-esteem: Family communication patterns and adoption-specific communication. *Journal of Family Communication,* 16 (3), 263–276. https://doi.org/10.1080/15267431.2016.1181069

Kim, E.T. (2021, September 23). Adoptees have the same right to citizenship as biological children. *The New York Times.* www.nytimes.com/2021/09/23/opinion/adoption-immigration-korea.html

Leon, I.G. (2002). Adoption losses: Naturally occurring or socially constructed? *Child Development,* 73 (2), 652–663. https://doi.org/10.1111/1467-8624.00429

Lotz, M. (2014). Adoptee vulnerability and post-adoptive parental obligation. In F. Baylis, & C. McLeod (Eds.), *Family-Making: Contemporary Ethical Challenges* (p. 198). Oxford: Oxford University Press.

MacIntyre, J.C. (1990). Resolved: Children should be told of their adoption before they ask. *Journal of the American Academy of Child and Adolescent Psychiatry,* 29 (5), 828–829.

Mackes, N.K., Golm, D., Sarkar, S., Kumsta, R., Rutter, M., Fairchild, G., Mehta, M.A., Sonuga-Barke, E.J.S., & ERA Young Adult Follow-up Team. (2020). Early childhood deprivation is associated with alterations in adult brain structure despite subsequent environmental enrichment. *PNAS Proceedings of the National Academy of Sciences of the United States,* 117 (1), 641–649.

McRoy, R.G., Grotevant, H.D., & Zurcher, L.A. (1988). *Emotional Disturbance in Adopted Adolescents: Origins and Development.* Westport: Praeger.

Nickman, S.L. (1985). Losses in adoption: The need for dialogue. *The Psychoanalytic Study of the Child,* 40, 365–398.

Nickman, S.L. (1996). Retroactive loss in adopted persons. In D. Klass, P. R. Silverman, & S. Nickman (Eds.), *Continuing Bonds: New Understandings of Grief* (pp. 257–272). London: Taylor & Francis.

Nickman, S.L. (1999). Affect tolerance and adoptive parenting. *Issues in Psychoanalytic Psychology,* 21, 63–76.

Ranieri, S., Ferrari, L., Danioni, F.V., Canzi, E., Barni, P., Rosnati, R., & Rodriguez, M.R. (2021). Adoptees facing adolescence: What accounts for their psychological well-being? *Journal of Adolescence: Special Issue on Resilience in Adolescence*, 89 (1), 10–17.

Reinoso, M., Juffer, F., & Tieman, W. (2013). Children's and parents' thoughts and feelings about adoption, birth culture identity and discrimination in families with internationally adopted children. *Child & Family Social Work*, 18 (3), 264–274. https://doi.org/10.1111/j.1365-2206.2012.00841.x

Roy, A. (2020). *A for Adoption: An Exploration of the Adoption Experience for Families and Professionals*. London: Routledge.

Schechter, M., & Bertocci, D. (1990). The meaning of the search. In D. Brodzinsky & M. Schechter (Eds.), *The Psychology of Adoption* (pp. 62–90). Oxford: Oxford University Press.

Selman, P. (2009). The rise and fall of intercountry adoption in the 21st century. *International Social Work*, 52 (5), 575–594. https://doi.org/10.1177/0020872809337681

Sherr, L., Roberts, K.J., & Croome, N. (2018). Disclosure and identity experiences of adults abandoned as babies: A qualitative study. *Cogent Psychology*, 5 (1), 1–12.

Shier, A.M. (2021). Negotiating reunion in intercountry adoption using social media and technology. *The British Journal of Social Work*, 51 (2), 408–426.

Smith, D.W., & Brodzinsky, D.M. (1994). Stress and coping in adopted children: A developmental study. *Journal of Clinical Child Psychology*, 23 (1), 91–99. https://doi.org/10.1207/s15374424jccp2301_11

Smith, D.W., & Brodzinsky, D.M. (2002). Coping with birthparent loss in adopted children. *Journal of Child Psychology and Psychiatry*, 43 (2), 213–223. https://doi.org/10.1111/1469-7610.00014

Sonuga-Barke, E.J.S., Kennedy, M., Kumsta, R., Knights, N., Golm, D., Rutter, M., Maughan, B., Schlotz, W., Kreppner, J. (2017). Child-to-child neurodevelopmental and mental health trajectories after early life deprivation: The young adult follow-up of the longitudinal English and Romanian Adoptees. *The Lancet*, 389 (10078), 15–21.

Tieman, W., van der Ende, J., & Verhulst, F.C. (2008). Young adult international adoptees' search for birth parents. *Journal of Family Psychology*, 22 (5), 678–687.

Von Korff, L., & Grotevant, H.D. (2011). Contact in adoption and adoptive identity formation: The mediating role of family conversation. *Journal of Family Psychology*, 25 (3), 393–401.

Wegar, K. (2000). Adoption, family ideology, and social stigma: Bias in community attitudes, adoption research, and practice. *Family Relations*, 49 (4), 363–369. https://doi.org/10.1111/j.1741-3729.2000.00363.x

Wieder, H. (1977). On being told of adoption. *The Psychoanalytic Quarterly*, 46 (1), 1–22.

Wieder, H. (1978). On when and whether to disclose about adoption. *Journal of the American Psychoanalytic Association*, 26 (4), 793–811.

Wieder, H. (2001). *Handbook on Adoption: A Psychoanalytic View*. Bloomington: iUniverse.

Wiley, O'L M. (2017). Adoption research, practice, and societal trends: Ten years of progress. *American Psychologist*, 72 (9), 985–995. http://dx.doi.org/10.1037/amp0000218

Wrobel, G.M., & Grotevant, H. D. (2019). Minding the (information) gap: What do emerging adult adoptees want to know about their birth parents? *Adoption Quarterly*, 22 (1), 29–52.

Wydra, M., O'Brien, K.M., & Merson, E.S. (2012). In their own words: Adopted persons' experiences of adoption disclosure and discussion in their families. *Journal of Family Social Work*, 15 (1), 62–77. https://doi.org/10.1080/10522158.2012.642616

Zamostny, K.P., O'Brien, K.M., Baden, A.L., & Wiley, M.O. (2003). The practice of adoption: History, trends, and social context. *The Counseling Psychologist*, 31 (6), 651–678. https://doi.org/10.1177/0011000003258061

APPENDIX

A *medical passport* is an electronic, portable record of the child's medical and family health histories (see https://cbexpress.acf.hhs.gov/index.cfm?event=website.viewArticles&issueid=118&sectionid=5&articleid=2941).

6

UNDERSTANDING THE INNER WORLD OF THE ADOPTED PERSON

A Psychoanalytic Conception of the Psychology of Adoption

Christopher F. Deeg, PhD

The adopted person's life simultaneously contains and masks an inherent contradiction. As they live as the daughter or son of an adoptive parent, their initial connection to the other, the birth parent, is hidden and implicitly denied by both the legal machinery of adoption and by the social/psychological attempts to suppress this anxiety-inducing fact, namely, biological and psychological relatedness to the lost birth parent. Until very recently, the adopted person's "birth certificate" was a fictional creation which listed the adoptive parents as though they were the biological wellspring for the latter's existence. For reasons which I have previously written about (Deeg, 1989, 1990, 1991, 2002) and will describe here, the adopted person often feels conflicted about his or her intense relatedness to the birth parent, typically the birth mother. The connection of the adopted person to the birth parent is experienced in different ways ranging from disguised expressions of denial or nonchalant, superficial "interest" to lifelong searing conflicts surrounding identity and the ability to forge relationships with others.

In previous works (see preceding text), I have attempted to provide a psychological framework for the adopted person's connection to the birth parent. From a psychoanalytic viewpoint, the theory of object relations provides a viable working schema from which to understand this phenomenon. In general, object relations theory attempts to explain human psychological development in terms of internalized relations to others. This internalized relation consists of a self-representation connected to an object representation (an image of another person). The connection consists of a drive derivative or affect that varies according to how psychologically developed and complex the emotion is, ranging from unmitigated split off rage, anger, pure idealizing love to mixtures of love and hate which are described as ambivalent connections or cathexes. Similarly, both the self and object representations themselves are considered along a spectrum of developmental complexity from all-good and all-bad split representations to mature representations which are capable of integrating both loving and hating feelings and are therefore capable of ambivalence – a hallmark of psychological maturity and higher functioning. The framework that I have proposed is dependent on the works of writers such as Jacobson (1964), Mahler (1968), and Kernberg (1976).

In my first paper on this topic, *On the Adoptee's Cathexes of the Lost Object* (Deeg, 1989), I concluded my review of the clinical literature with the proposal that the most salient and important feature of the adopted persons' psychology was their internalized relationship to the birth parent, particularly the mother. That the adopted persons' connection to the birth parent is central in understanding the latter's specific psychology is either implied or directly indicated by literature that either analyzes the institution of adoption itself or the societal attitudes toward adoption, or by a clinical examination of the adopted person (Schechter, 1960; Goodacre, 1966; Tizard, 1977). For example, Friegelman and Silverman (1986) suggested that negative or anxious societal attitudes toward the concept of adoption found expression in the genesis of policies that endeavored to sever the link between adoptive person and birth parent. The connection of birth parent to adopted person could thus be extinguished or at least contained by assuring the anonymity of the birth mother. The instinctual bond between birth mother and adopted person is directly implied by the existence of these policies. Similarly, the feared intensity of the bond is expressed by the intent of the policies to permanently separate and dissolve the connection.

Earlier clinical authors (Barnes, 1953; Berman & Bufferd, 1986; Hodges, 1984), as well as more recent contributions (Grotevant & Korff, 2011; Lifton, 2010), support the idea that the adopted person often experiences a desire for reparation and reunion with the birth mother. Hodges cites the questions, "Who were my first parents?" and "Why did they give me up?" as central in relevance and importance in clinical work with the adopted person. Schechter (1960) described the perceived rejection of the infant by the original parents as a "severe narcissistic injury" which finds later expression in character development or symptomatology. Other authors focused on the reluctance of the adopted parents to openly acknowledge the existence of the biological parents (Goodacre (1966), Tizard (1977). Eiduson and Livermore (1952) pointed to the underlying issue of biological origin as fueling the adopted child's enraged accusation, "You're not my real mother!" Barroso and Barbosa-Ducharne (2019) studied the effects of adoption-related losses and related feelings on subsequent interest in the birth parents.

As I have previously written, I now continue to propose that a direct examination of the specific object relation of adopted self to birth parent underlies the main thrust of the literature and is at the root of the clinical manifestation of typical adoption-related issues of identity, feelings of abandonment and loss, difficulty connecting to others, feelings of insecurity, etc. After 31 years of continued work with adopted individuals, I believe this formulation stands and continues to be the often-neglected or tacit theme which underlies much of the clinical literature on adoption as well as the psychological development of the adopted person. This object relation is the unconscious trace which, from my view, links adopted persons to each other and unites the various clinical manifestations of adopted persons to a common dynamic.

From an object relations perspective, this dynamic consists of an internalized representation of birth parent, usually the mother, in affective connection or cathexis to an internalized representation of self which is typically a conglomeration in various manifestations of all colorings of the adopted self, for example, abandoned self, all-bad unlovable self, or all-good but victimized self, damaged self. The themes correspond to any number of idiosyncratic case factors but typically are an amalgamation of elements of the original surrender and displaced or projected features of significant others, most notably the adoptive parents.

The obverse is similar in terms of diversity and the imprint of specific psychological history. The representation of the birth parent can be encoded as a lost but loving mother, a missing and dangerous mother who may return to claim the adopted person, a hateful mother who has abandoned the adopted self, a magical savior who, upon reunion with the adoptee, will repair and supplant all previous emotional loss and damage.

While the specific content, affective coloring, and developmental level of the object relation of adopted self to birth parent must be discovered in each individual case, several considerations lend themselves to a model which underlies all cases and provides a general understanding of the dynamics of the adopted person: (1) the adopted person's unique circumstance of experiencing the existence of two sets of parents, the original pair absent yet indelible, that is, the lost object; (2) that a direct examination of the internalized relation of adopted person to biological parent is requisite to a complete understanding of the adopted person; (3) that the relative success of the adopted person in adapting to the full range of their experience is commensurate with the quality and maturational level of this object relation.

Before discussing the specific manifestation of the internalized relation of adopted self to birth parent in the development of the adopted person, it is important to attempt to account for the very existence of the object relation particularly in cases where the adopted child had no external contact with the birth mother.

The Origin of the Lost Object: Accounting for the Existence of the Internalized Representation of the Birth Parent

A central tenet of object relations theory is that the inner psychological world is constructed as a representation of external relationships with others. Once an object representation is constructed, it begins to shape the individual's ongoing experience of the interpersonal world. The object and self-representation are therefore in a reciprocal causative relationship with the experience of the outer world.

The adoptive person in treatment, in their relationships with others, and through their external expressions, including in literature and art (Glenn, 1974; Blum, 1969; Bartram, 2003), evidences an emotional connection to the birth parent. Both clinically and theoretically, it is therefore important to account for the origin of an internal object relation in cases (the vast majority of adoption cases) where there has been *no* external contact with the object, the birth mother. What is the content of the representation, where does the content of the representation come from, and what is the mechanism of internalization?

Before discussing the more obvious and empirically verifiable idea that the birth parent representation is essentially an internalization of characteristics of the adoptive parents or other caregivers, it is worthwhile to consider research which suggests a prenatal, embryonic patterning and pre-psychological transmission between mother and fetus (Moon, 2000, 2013; Kisilevsky, 2003; Moon, 2013; Stern, 1985; DeCasper and Fifer, 1980). In essence, these studies suggest that the fetus is able to recognize the heartbeat and voice of the mother, as evidenced by various pre- and postnatal physiological measures. I have previously suggested that the experience of nine months of gestation cultivates a primitive cathexis which gives rise to a primal attachment.

Constructing a theoretical framework for the concept of primal, prenatal attachment is fraught with heuristic peril. Obviously, the fetus cannot be conceptualized in a formal psychological manner; self and object, to any extent that they can be conceptualized at all, are not formed or separated. Discussions of prenatal prepsychological representations of the mother must be tentative and subject to easy modification and discard. I have suggested that a primordial inchoate patterning of the representation based on early somatic auditory and physiological transmissions may occur during this period. Given the preponderance of clinical evidence that, in most cases, the adopted person defends against a primal and all-bad representation of the mother which generally forms the deepest layer of the birth parent representation (Neil, 2012; Derdeyn and Graves, 1998), combined with the idea that the fetus has established a connection with the birth mother before postnatal contact, it follows that disruption of this bond *would* register as a loss. Early loss or trauma is met not by the relatively sophisticated ability to mourn the loss of a loved and hated other but instead by aggressive cathexis, that is, unmitigated aggression or rage. This would explain why, for the adopted person, the image of mother as hating and hateful, the bad object, constitutes the bedrock and most defended against aspect of the representation.

Nonanalytic psychotherapists and others with tacit motivations, such as groups interested in safeguarding the interests of adoptive parents, sometimes ask, "Why should the surrender of the infant by the birth mother necessarily be considered a trauma, loss, or primal wound?" I suggest that the ultimate consequence of the "dialogue" or in utero transmissions between fetus and birth mother is to establish the birth mother as the caregiver, who enjoys a biologically fine-tuned position in later ministering original and early maternal functions. The birth mother alone may therefore be in a physiologically fine-tuned position to provide the newborn with the nurturing, drive-neutralizing, auxiliary ego function necessary for their survival and growth, by virtue of the pre-patterned "eurythmy" (Deeg, 1989) of the neonate's responses to the mother's vocal and physiological sounds and overall biological presence. Returning to the studies noted earlier, the birth mother's presence is recognized by the fetus; conversely, her absence is also recognized and recorded.

The separation of infant and birth mother registers as a rupture of this eurythmy and pre-psychological "dialogue." Even in cases where the adopted infant's early symbiotic needs are met by a caregiver or adoptive parent, the loss of the birth mother's unique presence is encoded in the nascent psyche of the adopted child. The concept of trauma (Fenichel, 1945) denotes an experience or event which overwhelms the ego's capacity for discharge of stimulation. The individual is thus unable to lower levels of excitation and is traumatized. Trauma as applied to the initial weeks of life can be conceived as an experience that overwhelms the discharge capacities of the early ego, resulting in the aggressive infiltration of inchoate self/object representations. The "trauma" of abandonment, the primal loss, encompasses both the emotional "experience" of the overtaking of the early ego by internal and external stimulations which cannot be adequately discharged and the encoding of this experience as a primitive original object relation.

From an object-relational perspective, depressive response occurs later than unmitigated aggression and is more complex since it implies a fusion of aggression and libido and therefore the capacity to experience ambivalence toward the same object in the form of mourning. The primal or bedrock affective quality of the adopted child's response to the severing of the bond with the birth mother would therefore be aggression or rage, which would color the initial object relation as an all-bad mother rejecting, hating, or attempting to destroy the infant. As noted earlier, clinical work with adopted persons of varying diagnoses suggests that the internalization of birth mother as all bad is generally the most disruptive and deeply defended object representation. The discharge of primitive unneutralized aggression toward an inchoate, partially formed object that is not differentiated from an equally primary self exceeds the capacities of the early ego and constitutes a trauma. While subsequent adequate maternal ministrations from caretakers or adoptive parents can ameliorate this experience, the adopted person nonetheless has enshrined the loss and established an object relation which will continue to be projected and re-internalized throughout life, thus creating a pattern or dynamic of interpersonal relations, identity, and defense, albeit often silently or unconsciously.

The expression of this dynamic is varied; however, two fantasies are often expressed in treatment as the all-bad birth mother representation is mobilized: mother abandoned me because she is all bad, devalued, damaged, or evil, or because I am all bad. The primary defensive mode governing this fantasy is splitting, which is observed in adopted person's treatments where there is often a misdiagnosis of borderline personality (Deeg, 2002) due to the manifestation of the split abandoned self/lost object representation. Ultimately, the split object representation evolves and a depressive position can emerge in which an all-good, idealized, perfect mother was lost and, if reunited with the adopted person, would perfect and make whole the latter's personality and life.

A college-bound female adopted patient came to treatment with the information that she was left on the doorstep of a courthouse in her native country rather than being formally surrendered to an orphanage. Originally, her sessions explored and elaborated fantasies in which her birth mother was imagined to be a beautiful but tragic figure caught between her mournful love of the as-yet unborn patient and a variety of circumstances which made the severing of their relationship a sorrowful necessity. The patient, through verbalizing fantasies of her birth mother, described her bright floral native dresses and long flowing dark hair (a projection of her own features and wardrobe propensities). The mother in these fantasies suffered terribly as she slowly and painfully accepted the imminent loss of her baby and tearfully stoked the patient's cheek as she gently lowered her during the night, to the closed door of the courthouse.

During this phase, the patient mourned the loss of her birth mother and discussed her plan to try her best to find her and lovingly reunite with her. The patient's external life remained lively and social at this time, and she flirted with several boys and expressed her sexual fantasies regarding them in explicit terms. Eventually, the patient hesitantly expressed the possibility that her mother had abandoned her rather than keeping her or pursuing a more traditional route of surrender to an orphanage because of indifference or narcissistic self-absorption. The patient's feelings toward her own sexuality underwent a dramatic evolution in which she began to describe disgust at the very idea of intercourse and oral sex. In essence, she swore off becoming sexually involved with anyone and reported that she felt "dead inside" when she thought about the abandoning mother.

Unneutralized aggression directed toward a self/object forerunner threatens to harm the inchoate self because of the lack of separation and differentiation. The aggression must be defended against and can safely be explored in the therapy only after a prerequisite tolerance for fantasy and a general feeling of safety can be established. For both neurotic and borderline adopted patients, splitting of the birth mother representation is utilized. For the higher-functioning neurotic patient, the "bad mother" introject is generally kept from consciousness by a secondary repression, while for the borderline patient, the idealized and devalued version of the birth mother are expressed consecutively without any attempt to integrate them.

Defensive Functions of the Birth Mother Representation and the Addition of Further Content

Clinical work with adopted people readily reveals that the image of the birth parent, typically the mother, is multivariate and embedded within object-relational narratives that are far more detailed than what could arise simply from an internalization of a primitive object forerunner which has derived from a prenatal eurythmy or transmission. Shades and variations of the relationship with the adoptive parents or caretakers are not difficult to discern within the explored fantasies of the birth parent. This leads to a consideration of the process of the internalization of the images of the adoptive parents and their consolidation and embedding within the birth parent image, which is complex and involves variables such as the developmental level of both self and object representations and the underlying motive, drive, or impetus for the internalization. While internalizations can be adaptive when self and object boundaries are well-established and when the identity-enhancing internalization is therefore partial rather than global, more often in treatment, the impetus for the internalization is defensive or part of a compromise formation. In the latter case, aspects of a cathected (including all points on the spectrum of love to hate) object are internalized when the external object is removed so that the experience of object loss is avoided. In other words, while I cannot have you near me, I will now preserve a portion of my experience of being with you by internalizing *some* of your characteristics. In addition to preserving some portion of the attachment to the object, internalizations can be embedded in a number of defensive constellations. The internalization of the biological parent representation therefore serves the adopted person defensively by attempting to maintain psychic equilibrium either by warding off objectionable impulses, affects, or cognitions or by attempting to substitute for absent structure-building, nurturing interactions that an external object would have provided.

In a previous paper (Deeg, 1990), I described six defensive functions of the biological parent representation which emphasized how the representation is used to provide missing gratifications or to achieve psychological compromise formations. Before commenting on some of these functions, I would currently emphasize that after 30 years of further clinical experience, it is my perspective that the adopted person is wont to color their representation of their birth parent with content and that any addition at almost any cost is worth the bargain. One of the primary motivations for the adopted person is to undo or correct the experience of intense connectedness to a nebulous and unknowable other. When defenses are resolved and the path is clear, the adopted person in treatment comes to express the pain that is associated with this difficult and possibly damaging object relation.

The adopted person is in the unique and unenviable position of experiencing waves of affect, sometimes raw and unmitigated by the cognitive ego, toward a nebulous and absent partner. The biological parent representation acquires content as the nucleus of various defensive constellations which serve to attenuate, manage, or fend off these disruptive emotions. Among these are the following possibilities: the birth parent representation as a container for disavowed negative aspects of the adopted parent, as a primitive self-esteem or narcissistic regulator, as a fantasy source of various libidinal gratification, as a defense against conscious rage or dangerous aggressive impulses toward the adoptive parents, as a defense against "dangerous" sexual impulses toward the adoptive parents, as a defense against strong and unyielding symbiotic wishes toward the adoptive parents, and as a means of defense within the dynamics of masochism (Deeg, 1990).

Projecting or displacing negative aspects of the adoptive parent into the representation of the birth parent is a common mechanism. In the non-adopted population, it is akin to the role played by the "family romance" (Freud, 1909, 1933), where a disruptive massive devaluation of the parents is avoided by the cathexes of fantasized ideal set of parents who embody aspects of the actual parents. Here, for the adoptive person, the adoptive parent is perceived as overly symbiotic, seductive, sadistic, negligent, etc., and these characteristics are attributed to the representation of the birth parent, thus protecting the relationship (internal and external) with the adoptive parent.

A young male adult patient began to describe the image he retained of his birth mother with increasing frequency as he began to prepare for an attempted search for her. He imagined that his birth mother was a beautiful, effervescent seductress who had tricked his birth father into bed and, once captivating him, enslaved him through sexual domination. The patient's adoptive mother was described as obese, repulsive, and fierce when she was enraged. Further exploration revealed that the adoptive mother in the patient's youth had been openly devaluing of the adoptive father and had turned her sensuality to the patient, asking him to massage her back and to adjust her garters. The description of her as fat and repulsive was a reaction formation to his longing for her. The image of the birth mother as a beautiful and dangerous femme fatale fortified this defense. As he derided the birth mother in treatment, the patient reported feeling energized and awake. His interest in her contained his sexual attachment to both mothers and, when interpreted, initiated a period of increased sexual activity for him.

Similarly, the birth parent representation can be cathected when the adoptive parent is overly gratifying or enveloping in a pre-oedipal manner, that is, when the adopted person needs to separate and individuate. For example, if the adoptive parent becomes anxious when the child pushes away and asserts a need for independence, the parent may fortify their attempts to envelop the child and block the child's paths away from the parent. The biological parent can then be imagined to be a steady but lenient approver of these explorations, or a negligent, uninterested onlooker from whom escape is relatively easy. Once again, the relationship with the adoptive parent (both internal and external) is protected; the representation of the birth parent acquires content as a narrative describing the internal object relation is elaborated.

The biological parent representation can also be mobilized when the adoptive parent maintains an appropriate or overly severe oedipal boundary. Since the birth parent representation is not exposed to actual ongoing contact with an external person, it retains its fluid and plastic state and can therefore become a fantasized source of gratification.

When the adoptive mother of a young adult male adopted patient expressed disapproval or disappointment with his career aspirations, he angrily denounced her middle-class values and lack of creative interest and achievement. He fantasized that his birth mother, although irresponsible and selfish, was a youthful, artistic woman who had the courage to live a free, bohemian lifestyle. He imagined that few men would be able to resist her charms, and his previous disgust at her indiscretions became supplanted by a view of her as witty and seductive. He was resistant to discussing how his feelings about her had changed in a few sessions and was upset by the idea that this change signaled a shift in his feelings and fantasies that deserved exploration.

A frequent presenting issue in the treatment of the adopted child or adolescent is uncontained anger at the adoptive parent forged within the mold and narrative of adoptive dynamics. The adopted parent often reports that the child openly states that the birth parent would have made a better parent, often in providing a missing or limited gratification. Even when the biological parent is not overtly idealized, when the child screams, "You're not my mother" or "Why should I love you?" there is generally an accompanying idealization of the birth parent representation. In some cases, the birth parent representation is cathected and labeled the "real" parent without being idealized, in contrast to the devaluation of the adoptive parent. The relationship with the adoptive parent is protected by a de-emphasis and disavowal of anger by the thought, "My anger toward my adoptive parents is not important because they are not my real parents. I can tolerate it and keep it from contaminating my loving feelings for them." The aggressive affect is not repressed, and the dynamic as a whole operates as a form of splitting even in adopted people whose personality structure more typically relies on repression and other "higher-order" defense mechanisms. The anger toward the adoptive parent takes on an "as-if" quality, which can infect the overall relationship and substantially weaken or derail it.

For many adopted persons, the lifelong experience of being adopted and the effects of the inner object relation of abandoned adopted self to lost birth parent creates a perduring challenge to self-esteem regulation. The classical formulation of self-esteem involves the gradual internalization of a nurturing and sustaining object which ultimately becomes the portion of the superego known as the ego ideal. The internal object then provides the individual with feelings of warmth and well-being that are derivatives of this earlier oral gratification (Fenichel, 1945). Kohut (1966, 1971) emphasized that the internalized object which supplies the ego with narcissistic supplies (self-esteem) is both admired and admiring.

The birth parent representation can be mobilized as a source of narcissistic gratification. The birth parent is fantasized to be a lost object who nonetheless loves and approves of the adopted person (often in contrast to the adoptive parent). The birth parent as a source of narcissistic supplies can also be camouflaged as a magical fantasy figure, such as a witch, ghost, or in a case of a borderline adolescent I have previously described (Deeg, 1990), a powerful but benevolent religious figure such as Satan. In all these cases, the underlying dynamic remains the same: the cathexis of the birth parent representation provides the adopted person with narcissistic supplies in the form of feelings of adequacy, approval, and in more regressed personality organizations, warmth, fullness, and satiety.

Although the cathexis of the adopted self representation as abandoned because of badness, defect, or worthlessness is quite painful, when the capacity for an even more disintegrating or annihilating form of guilt threatens the personality, the adopted person may utilize a masochistic defense to avoid these latter feelings. The adopted person mobilizes the object relation of worthless self to abandoning mother as an unconscious means of avoiding the searing guilt that would be experienced for a mistreatment or offense against another person, and frequently as a means of preventing the wronged person from abandoning the adopted person. This is more complex than the conscious rationalization that the adopted patient first offers as a result of this defense: "I hurt you because I am adopted and can't help doing this." The masochistic defense is predicated upon an unconscious mobilization of the birth parent representation and adopted self representation. The individual is not aware, or not fully aware, of the defensive reference to the object relation. Were it to be consciously articulated, the adopted person is saying, "I hurt you because you represent my sadistic birth mother, upon whom I am now exacting revenge. Please do not hurt me in response, because I have already been abandoned and damaged and must now hurt others."

A female adopted patient routinely betrayed close friends by sharing information about them that she had been entrusted with. In session, she said, "Isn't this what adoptees do? We can't keep our friends." Although she was able to offer this facile explanation of her behavior which was superficially linked to her adoptive psychology, further exploration of her fantasies of being abandoned by her mother because she was the tainted offspring of a rape brought into focus her depression about this fantasy and ultimately made her masochistic defense less available. Her defensive excuse that she was adopted and couldn't help being unreliable had previously enabled her to avoid the deeper, more disturbing fantasy that others would ultimately perceive her true inner badness and the dissolute nature which had been "stamped" into her being as a magical consequence and permanent connection to the circumstances of her conception. She began to perceive the conflicts and outcomes of her relationships as more self-directed and was enabled to explore her motivations for the impediments she created in her friendships.

The Adopted Person's Search for Identity

Clinical work with adopted people reveals the high frequency with which a struggle surrounding the issue of identity dominates the picture. Adopted persons often present a spectrum of identity diffusion ranging from a vague sense of "not knowing who they really are" to global difficulties maintaining a sense of separateness and independence from others which challenges and often destroys their capacity for intimacy and connection.

The issue of identity formation considered psychoanalytically or metapsychologically is complex but ultimately focuses on the status of internalized representations of self and others. The central idea that identity evolves from a state of merged unity with the representation of the mother is discussed by various writers with differing emphases (Jacobson, 1964; Mahler, 1965, 1968; Mahler et al., 1975). The merged self-object which consists of a blended representation of self and mother ultimately, under a favorable environment of libidinal gratification and sufficient frustration, allows the nascent self-representation to emerge as intact, separate, and vital. A lifelong inner sense of self that is capable of integrating and recording the person's ongoing experiences is the result of a continuous refusion and differentiation of self and object representations under the predominance, but not exclusive cathexis, of libido (see Kernberg, 1976). Both the inner sense of self and the inner sense of the other are ultimately capable of ambivalence, that is, of an integration of both libidinal and aggressive cathexis. Both self and other are experienced with nuance and with "mixed" feeling.

The adopted person's importunate question, "Who am I?" is a reference to one half of the self/object dyad. "Who is my mother?" is a reference to the other half of the dyad, which is expressed through myriad variety from a tacit dismissal to clamoring obsession. For non-adopted individuals, differentiation and separation of self from mother often lags behind mature separation and fortification of the self-concept. People in psychotherapy or in daily life often report that a visit to their parents' home for the weekend reawakens a feeling of being a child and, with it, a reactivation of childhood behaviors long renounced or modified in the context of other adult relationships. It is easy to "slip" back into this experience and related behaviors because the self originally fused with the mother only very gradually and, under favorable conditions, differentiates from the primary object (Jacobson, 1954, 1964). These favorable conditions include a series of phase-appropriate, tolerable frustrations within the overall context of a positive, loving, libido-gratifying relationship. External experience with the mother is therefore a critical ingredient in this process. The loving mother, imbued with an adequate sense of empathy with the child's developmental needs, gratifies certain desires and frustrates others. The challenge to the adopted person's identity is obvious. Without real external contact with the birth mother, the object relation of adopted self to birth parent in all its varieties bypasses the normal process of cathexis-decathexis, fusion-separation-refusion of good and bad aspects of self and other that occurs as an individual synthesizes a sense of who they are. In other words, ongoing external contact with another person allows the representation of that person and the self in contact with that person to mature and become more integrated and capable of bearing mixed feelings. If the object representation of the birth parent has become centrally involved in the defensive network of the individual, the likelihood that the representation has been able to keep in step with the progression and development of other object and self-representations is reduced. Thus, clinicians frequently encounter the adopted patient, who appears to be productive and able to love and work, who nevertheless complains about a sense of not knowing who they are. The adopted individual is usually consciously aware only of a feeling of yearning. This yearning is the residue of the need to interact with the representation of the birth parent, who inhabits the internal world offering the adopted person no opportunity to gradually combine all-bad and all-good representations into whole objects capable of being loved and hated, that is, capable of being ambivalently cathected (Deeg, 1991). As I will discuss in a separate chapter, this process can be resurrected in treatment.

The adopted person often reveals and examines a desire to find and reunite with the birth parent. To a large extent, this can be understood as a derivative or manifestation of the adaptive drive toward identity consolidation (Deeg, 1991). If reunion occurs while the adopted person is in treatment, the experience can jolt the blocked sector of identity forward. Psychotherapeutic progress in this area can occur, however, in cases where reunion has not been possible or where reunion has been unfavorable. As I will discuss in a separate chapter, specific techniques and a specific emphasis in therapy can be helpful.

Perhaps most basically, the adopted person often feels a strong sense of hesitancy regarding the exploration and "making conscious" of their struggle with identity. The discomfort and pain of uncovering identity issues are not avoidable. When the seal of identity is cracked open, the adopted individual is led back to the primal object relation with the birth parent. Inevitably, and even in cases where there is a factual knowledge that the birth mother's actions were driven by love and concern, the adopted individual must allow access to their conscious awareness, the disavowed feelings of abandonment, sadness, or rage at being part of an original relationship which was, in most cases, permanently ruptured, and as once being part of an original unity which was cleaved.

Endnotes

Barnes, M.J. (1953). The working through process in dealing with anxiety around adoption. *American Journal of Orthopsychiatry*, 23, 605–621.

Barroso, R., & Barbosa-Ducharne, M. (2019). Adoption-related feelings, loss, and curiosity about origins in adopted adolescents. *Clinical Child Psychology and Psychiatry*, 24 (4), 876–891.

Bartram, P. (2003). Some oedipal problems in work with adopted children and their parents. *Journal of Child Psychotherapy*, 29, 21–36.

Berman, L.C., & Bufferd, R.K. (1986). Family treatment to address loss in adoptive families. *Social Casework*, 103, 3–11.

Blum, H.P. (1969). A psychoanalytic view of "who's afraid of Virginia Woolf?" *Journal of the American Psychoanalytic Association*, 17, 888–903.

DeCasper, A.J., & Fifer, W.P. (1980). Of human bonding: Newborns prefer their mother's voices. *Science*, 208, 1174–1176.

Deeg, C.F. (1989). On the adoptee's cathexis of the lost object. *Psychoanalysis and Psychotherapy*, 7, 152–161.

Deeg, C.F. (1990). Defensive functions of the adoptee's cathexis of the lost object. *Psychoanalysis and Psychotherapy*, 8, 35–46.

Deeg, C.F. (1991). On the adoptee's search for identity. *Psychoanalysis and Psychotherapy*, 9, 128–133.
Deeg, C.F. (2002). Issues of psychoanalytic technique with adoptees. *Journal of Social Distress and the Homeless*, 11, 193–205.
Derdeyn, A., & Graves, C. (1998). Clinical vicissitudes of adoption. *Child Adolescent Psychiatry*, 7, 373–388.
Eiduson, B.T., & Livermore, J.B. (1952). Complications in therapy with adopted children. *American Journal of Orthopsychiatry*, 23, 795–802.
Fenichel, O. (1945). *The Psychoanalytic Theory of Neurosis*. New York: Norton.
Freud, S. (1909). Family romances. *Standard Edition*, 9, 235–241.
Freud, S. (1933). Revision of dream-theory. *Standard Edition*, 22, 17.
Friegelman. W., & Silverman, A.R. (1986). Adoptive parents, adoptees, and the sealed record controversy. *Social Casework*, 106, 219–226.
Glenn, J. (1974). The adoption theme in Edward Albee's "Tiny Alice" and "The American Dream." *Psychoanalytic Study of the Child*, 29, 413–429.
Goodacre, I. (1966). *Adoption Policy and Practice*. London: George Allen & Unwin.
Grotevant, H.D., & Korff, L.V. (2011). Adoptive identity. In S.J. Schwartz, K. Luyckx, & V.S. Vigoles (Eds.), *Handbook of Identity Theory and Research* (pp. 585–601). New York: Springer Science + Business Media.
Hodges, J. (1984). Two crucial questions: Adopted children in psychoanalytic treatment. *Journal of Child Psychotherapy*, 10, 47–56.
Jacobson, E. (1964). *The Self and the Object World*. New York: International Universities Press.
Kernberg, O. (1976). *Object Relations Theory and Clinical Psychoanalysis*. New York: Jason Aronson.
Kisilevsky, B., Hains, S., Lee, H., Xie, X., Huang, H., Ye, H., & Wang, Z. (2003). Effects of experience on fetal voice recognition. *Psychological Science*, 14, 220–224.
Kohut, H. (1966). Forms and transformations of narcissism. *Journal of the American Psychoanalytic Association*, 14, 243–272.
Kohut, H. (1971). *The Analysis of the Self*. New York: International Universities Press.
Lifton, B.J. (2010). Ghosts in the adopted family. *Psychoanalytic Inquiry*, 30, 71–79.
Mahler, M.S. (1965). On the significance of the normal separation-individuation phase: With reference to research in symbiotic child psychosis. In M. Schur (Ed.), *Drives, Affects, Behavior* (pp. 161–169). New York: International Universities Press.
Mahler, M.S. (1968). *On Human Symbiosis and the Vicissitudes of Individuation*. New York: International Universities Press.
Mahler, M.S. (1975). *The Psychological Birth of the Human Infant*. New York: Basic Books.
Moon, C., & William, P. (2000). Evidence of transnatal auditory learning. *Journal of Perinatology*, 20, 537–544.
Moon, C., Lagercrantx, H., & Kuhl, P. (2013). Language experienced in utero affects vowel perception after birth: A two country study. *Acta Paediatrica*, 10, 156–160.
Neil, E. (2012). Making sense of adoption: Integration and differentiation from the perspective of adopted Children in middle childhood. *Children and Youth Services Review*, 34, 409–416.
Schechter, M.D. (1960) Observations on adopted children. *Archives of General Psychiatry*, 3, 21–32.
Stern, D.N. (1985). *The Interpersonal World of the Infant*. New York: Basic Books.
Tizard, B. (1977). *Adoption-A Second Chance*. London: Open Books.

7

BIRTH FATHERS IN ADOPTION

Into the Light

Gary Clapton, PhD

The Invisible Parent

Birth fathers have been called "phantom fathers," the "invisible parent," "shadowy figures," "an illusory entity," neglected from configurations of adoption as a triangle that features the child, the adoptive parents, and the birth mother. So much on the margins for many years that the prevailing notions of adoption convey that the child had only one biological parent (Salvo Agoglia & Herrera, 2021).

Before we discuss what we know of birth fathers and the implications for professionals, it is worth noting that fathers in general have traditionally had a marginal presence in the, for want of a better phrase, "psy-services": the traditional mental health fields of psychology and psychiatry and clinical social work, but also within the more general therapy, counselling, and social work services.

Fathers: The Forgotten Parents of Psychoanalytic Thought

For decades, leading lights in these professions have overconcentrated on and essentialized mothers, while marginalized fathers were cast out as irrelevant. We need look no further than Jung's (in)famous remark: 'one knows what comes out of the mother, but what is the use of the father?' (1954, p. 25). However, let's look a little further. Fink observes:

> If we hypothesize an initial child-mother unity (as a logical, i.e., structural, moment, if not a temporal one), the father, in a Western nuclear family, typically acts in such a way as to disrupt that unity, intervening therein as a third term – often perceived as foreign and even undesirable.
>
> (1995, p. 55)

The essentialization of mothers went hand in hand with such thinking. For instance, child psychiatrist Bruno Bettelheim remarked that "we must start with the realisation that, as much as women want to be good scientists or engineers, they want first and foremost to be womanly companions of men and to be mothers" (1965, in Siann, 1994, p. 81). John Bowlby's work on attachment and loss underpins a great deal of practice with children and their families, yet for him:

> In the young child's eyes, father plays second fiddle and his value increases only as the child becomes more able to stand alone. Nevertheless, fathers have their uses even in infancy . . . as the economic and social support of the mother.
> (1951, p. 16)

Another major figure in child and family psychiatry, Donald Winnicott, first coined the phrase "good-enough mothering" and was of the belief that the father's job was to support the mother, whose job, in turn, was to do the parenting. In *Home Is Where We Start From*, Winnicott asks that "fathers must allow me to use the term 'maternal' to describe the total attitude to babies and their care. The term 'paternal' must necessarily come a little later than 'maternal'" (1990, p. 154). Finally, *The Needs of Children* was written by influential child psychologist Mia Kellmer Pringle, and in it she writes that:

> Fathers cannot so readily serve as models for their sons; not only do most of them spend the major part of the child's waking life away from home, but also they do work which their sons can neither observe nor clearly comprehend.
> (1973, p. 26)

Notwithstanding that the remarks cited previously are specific to era and culture (i.e., fathers as the sole breadwinner in the relatively affluent Western societies of the 1950s and 1960s), they were then revised: Bowlby adjusted his views to incorporate the notion of the non-maternal primary caregiver. Overall, fathers have come later to the table than mothers in the attention paid by psychologists (O'Brien, 2005, p. 11). This has been noted intermittently throughout the twentieth century. See, for example, Nash's 1965 paper ("The father in contemporary culture and current psychological literature") and that of McCant's titled "The Cultural Contradiction of Fathers as Nonparent," in which he quotes a professor of psychology: "We didn't just forget fathers by accident; we ignored them on purpose because of our assumption that they were less important than mothers" (1987, p. 128). Then, calling attention to the persistence of father-related myopia, 40 years after Nash and 20 years after McCant, Freeman refers to the fathers as the "forgotten parent" of psychoanalytic thought (2008, p. 116).

A similar process of the historical neglect of fathers, fathering, and fatherhood has been traced elsewhere in human and social services, for instance, in maternity services (Goldman & Burgess, 2018), in parenting interventions (Panter-Brick et al., 2014), in child and family welfare and social services (Clapton, 2009), in psychotherapy (Barrows, 1999). Across these disciplines and professions, in the words of Zanoni et al. (2013), fathers have not been seen as "core business." When we concentrate our focus on adoption, we will see the same where the subject of fathers has been slow to attract interest. The neglect of adoptive fathers must await another discussion, because for now, attention is turned to what we know about birth fathers in adoption. Why? In short, there has been systemic exclusion of fathers from the processes leading up to and relinquishment of a child for adoption; therefore, there can be little in the record of his presence, his views, and his experiences (Neil et al., 2013). This makes for a mystery. And in adoption, there is a propensity for mysteries (and myths) to abound – unhelpfully. Adopted people regularly refer to their life as a jigsaw, with the missing pieces being that of their birth parents and family of origin. Shedding light on the birth father goes a long way to helping complete that jigsaw (although for adoptees who are no longer children, because of the many systemic problems over the decades, for example, access to records (Chapter 10), this may not be possible).

Birth Fathers' Experiences of Adoption

Past practices either ignored birth fathers or dissuaded them from participation in adoption (Sachdev, 1991; Trinder et al., 2004). Social workers and adoption professionals rarely inquired about the father, fathers' names were not recorded on the birth certificates, rarely were there efforts to inform them of their paternity or involve them in plans (one justification being that a father's involvement might delay the inexorable plans for adoption), along with pervasive stereotypical views of birth fathers being older and sexually exploitative. This made for, at best, a climate of disinterest in him or, worse, hostility (Passmore & Coles, 2009). More recently, much has been done in Australia to reach out to birth fathers in adoption, and the existence of birth fathers' pain and sense of loss has been acknowledged in a federal and state government process of developing apologies for past adoption practices. The report by the Parliament of New South Wales *Releasing the Past: Adoption Practices 1950–1998: Final Report* (Parliament of New South Wales Legislative Council Standing Committee on Social Issues, 2001) contains ample evidence of services' disempowerment of birth fathers. About the recording of the father's name on the birth certificate and other records, the report notes: "The treatment of those fathers who took an interest (in the adoption) was often poor and as most practitioners have acknowledged, very little consideration was given to their needs. Very little was done for fathers and they were rarely consulted" (Parliament of New South Wales Legislative Council Standing Committee on Social Issues, 2001, p. 114). The report goes on to conclude that:

> Fathers were disregarded and very little was done to consult or involve them during the birth and the postnatal period. . . . This failure to acknowledge

fathers was wrong and caused long-term harm to those involved. The failure to record the birth father's name . . . has also caused pain and suffering to them and to other people, including adoptees.

(ibid. p. 119)

Across the anglophone world, the same practices have been true (Baumann, 1999; Clapton, 2003; Kenny et al., 2012).

On the back of a rise in birth mothers speaking out about their adoption experiences throughout the 1970s, interest in birth fathers began to quicken in the late 1980s and 1990s (Clapton, 2019). As a result, we have an emerging picture of birth fathers that challenges the stereotypes of a vacuum where a person ought to be, of the absent and careless abandoner or sexually predatory older cad who gets a girl in trouble. Or all three.

Who Are These Men?

Most of the birth fathers were in their late teens or early 20s at the time of adoption (Triseliotis et al., 2005; Witney, 2004; Clapton, 2003; Cicchini, 1993; Deykin et al., 1988). Researchers have also found that instead of the popular notion of pregnancy following a one-night stand, the majority of these birth fathers were going steady with the birth mother. Witney (2004) found evidence of long-term relationships. In a US study, 83% of the fathers were "romantically involved," with just over half living together (Smith, 2007). Whitesel's secondary data analysis ($n = 149$) portrayed the typical birth father as a 25-year-old White man with slightly more than a college education who was earning a low income. Her findings also revealed that 84% of birth fathers reported knowing the birth mother "very well," and 72% had known the birth mother more than three years (2008).

What Were Their Attitudes toward the Adoption of Their Children?

When "invited in" and permitted to be involved with the plans, though most agreed with the decision to adopt, they continued to want to be involved, and some were present during the birth, though others were actively excluded (Witney, 2004; Triseliotis et al., 2005) or even physically ejected from the hospital (Clapton, 2003). Some struggled to see their child and were able to hold the baby. Others met the stereotype by not wanting to be involved with the pregnancy; these men are not a minority (Hughes & Logan, 1993), but neither are abandoning men a majority in the most significant birth fathers' studies to date (Deykin et al., 1988, Cicchini, 1993, Clapton, 2003, Witney, 2004, Cornefert, 2021). After the adoption, commonalities were found with the birth mother's experiences regarding grief reactions related to the relinquishment and bereavement (Clapton, 2003).

The Child in Their Lives: Out of Sight, Out of Mind?

The five most significant birth father studies point to the impact of the adoption experience in their lives and the presence of an enduring sense of connectedness to the child (Deykin et al., 1988; Cicchini, 1993; Clapton, 2003; Witney, 2004, Cornefert, 2021). In one of the studies (Cicchini, 1993), 13% said that this sense of a connectedness was constant. In the words of one man in Clapton's study: "The adoption rubbed me out legally but not emotionally" (2003, p. 122). Other studies have found enduring thoughts of their child and a deep sense of loss. In later life, many birth fathers, when asked the usual question of parents about the number of their children, were conflicted:

> What sort of person gives away a baby? Their own baby? Every time you meet someone and the conversation turned to "have you any children?" and "how many?", I would feel uneasy and ashamed.
> (Passmore & Coles, 2009, p. 8)

Or in the words of one man in Clapton (2003), "One is missing."

Most of the fathers in Cicchini (1993) reported that their own well-being was detrimentally affected. A minority of these fathers experienced continuing feelings of guilt and shame. Many of Witney's fathers indicated lasting damage to their self-esteem. Clapton reported that almost 50% of the participants in his study reported feelings of loss, anger, and powerlessness in the early weeks and months after the adoption, which eventually subsided (2003). Many felt unable to tell people outside the immediate family the story of their loss (Cicchini, 1993). Clapton also found that even those who had shared their story in outline had suppressed its full significance. This concealing of their experiences meant that their grief was disenfranchised (Witney, 2004). Many birth fathers experienced a profound sense of loss regarding their child's adoption and compared it to bereavement when someone dies. Some fathers spoke of a sense of persisting guilt and loss (Triseliotis et al., 2005). It was deemed as an ambiguous loss because the child, whilst lost to them, was living on elsewhere (Witney, 2004; Clapton, 2003). The absence of any accepted ceremony in which to contain and express grief made the experience more painful (Clapton, 2003). One participant in Clapton's study stated that he had been struck by feelings that something untoward had happened to his child and that he "had to let him go and pretend he was dead" (2003, p. 52). This device was necessary because to all intents and purposes his child's welfare was beyond his control. Many birth fathers felt a continuing sense of connection to the child. The adoption left uncompleted business, expunging the physical presence of the child but not the child's emotional presence in the birth father's mind (Clapton, 2003, p. 150). Most fathers thought about their child frequently or constantly (Cicchini, 1993; Witney, 2004). When the child came to mind, there was a continued feeling of fatherhood (Clapton, 2003).

Ultimately, the adoption issue remained "conflict ridden" for most of the fathers in the study by Deykin et al. (1988, p. 247) and cast a lifelong shadow. This contradicts the stereotype of birth fathers being "ghosts" or uninvolved. The powerful conclusion drawn in all the studies suggests that the relinquishment experience does not end at the time of adoption but has enduring effects throughout life. These effects emerge most clearly decades later in a desire to seek assurance that the child has thrived (Cicchini, 1993), and for some fathers, a wish to meet (Deykin et al., 1988).

In Sight and in Mind: Contact and Relationships between Birth Fathers and Adult Children

Based on a small sample of birth fathers, Passmore and Coles (2009) identified a range of contexts and characteristics of more- and less-satisfying meetings and subsequent relationships between birth fathers and their adult children. Lower satisfaction was associated with a mismatch between the needs of birth fathers and the needs of their sons or daughters, or if they reported having difficulty developing a relationship, such as when there were differing offers of degree of intimacy. In the study by Triseliotis et al. (2005) in which the sample is biased because it only includes birth fathers that were sought by their adopted children, 14 out of 15 fathers had met their children. Where a meeting had taken place, most fathers had found it life-enhancing and also helpful in enabling fathers to share their account of why the adoption had been decided upon. It seems, from the little we know from these few studies, that the relationships that result from later-life meetings of adopted adults and their birth fathers are more like friendships than father–child relationships (Cicchini, 1993; Triseliotis et al., 2005). One man's description in Clapton's work might sum this up when he drew a distinction between "being a father, but not a dad" (Clapton, 2003, p. 66). Notwithstanding this acknowledgment of the two realities of biology and social, the most recent study of birth fathers' experiences picks up on a suggestion in Clapton (2003) concerning the existence and persistence of feelings of attachment toward the child, regardless of never having parented the child (Cornefert, 2021). Whilst the majority of birth fathers in Cornefert's study had never seen the child they helped to conceive, he writes that:

> They appeared to experience a bond, frequently thinking about the child. There was evidence in the narratives of an ongoing connectedness to the child who had been adopted. For most birth fathers, this feeling of closeness never left them. There was always concern as to where the child had been placed, and whether they were happy and healthy.
>
> (ibid., p. 248–249)

He goes on to suggest that whilst there was no opportunity for the traditional development of attachment via hands-on care, nevertheless the men in his study experienced and maintained emotional ties. Clapton found that such maintenance of ties and feelings of a bond – in the absence of the child – was expressed through rituals, ceremonies, and acknowledgements on occasions, such as birthdays, Father's Days, and Christmases (2003).

Clapton's later work argues that enduring thoughts manifested in these such practices provide evidence for a birth fatherhood that holds in mind a "lost" child and disrupts narratives of fathering that regard fathering as "doing" and notions that once out of sight, a child is out of mind for a father. It is suggested that for birth fathers, "a diversity of feelings, but also behaviours, point to a form of continuing, lived fathering" (Clapton, 2019, p. 1). Ainsworth makes a difference between relationship bonds, which are dyadic, and affectional bonds, which can be experienced by the individual in absentia of the other (1991, p. 37), and this seems to be the best description of what these men feel. Later in life and in circumstances where meetings had taken place and a relationship formed, Cornefert reports that these bonds were developed between some birth fathers and their adopted child (2021).

Aside from blogposts and the like, a small handful of birth fathers have published accounts of their personal experiences. Ward adds a deeply personal but telling note to the experiences outlined earlier:

> Every year a period of subtle heaviness would arrive for a few days before his birthday and it would be harder to get out of bed in the morning. Then I would remember that the despondency had a cause. It was the impact of a birthday that was missing several people, without birthday cards and minus birthday presents. I was burdened by grief as I subconsciously counted the number of candles on an imaginary cake. The depression lifted when his birthday passed.
>
> (Ward, 2012, p. 32)

Likewise, but on a more upbeat note, Clapton writes:

> I might not have been her dad during all those years but being her father is so much part of my identity now that I no longer hesitate when asked how many kids I have: I proudly say that I have two boys and a girl.
>
> (in Clapton & Ward, 2013, p. 22)

In 2004, the Australian Gary Coles published *Ever After: Fathers and the Impact of Adoption*, which was the very first book of birth fathers' personal experiences. It features a painful autobiographical account of his continued attempts to meet with a son who was unwilling to meet him. The legacy of adoption is a "permanent scar" for him (2004, p. 96).

Clapton (2000) studied the experiences of 30 UK birth fathers, and among its appendices, it includes these two glimpses into the lives of the men he interviewed:

James

James was 20 at the time (1965) his girlfriend became pregnant. They had a steady relationship. The pregnancy was announced to friends and "claimed" by him. Then the pregnancy was denied by his girlfriend. Shortly afterward, they split up. He met his wife-to-be almost immediately after the breakup of this relationship. In his neighborhood, hints and rumors continued regarding a possible child. Two years later, he married, and within months, he reported that he was in a "part-time" relationship with his wife, who stayed with her parents every weekend (he was working nights during this period). This arrangement continued after a daughter was born four years after their marriage. Seventeen years after they married, they split up. Awareness of his wife's infidelity came out some years after the divorce. At the time of the divorce, he told his daughter that she might have a "half sister." About 7 years ago, 24 years after the pregnancy and birth of his first child, he had it confirmed by a local acquaintance that there had been a child, who was subsequently adopted. He has always lived in the same working-class neighborhood. It has strong community ties. About two years prior to the interview, he heard that this daughter was trying to get in touch with her birth mother but could not find out enough so as to meet her. He decided to initiate contact. A year after contact with the Social Work Department, he and his birth/adopted daughter finally met. This was six months before the research interview. He reports two significant moments. Firstly, seeing his name down as the father on official records in an early meeting in the Social Work Department and, secondly, meeting his birth daughter for the first time. She was accompanied by her partner. The social worker remained present throughout – to his dissatisfaction. He was over the moon. Since then, they have met once more, and there have been weekly phone calls and, until very recently, in relation to the interview. His birth daughter is pregnant with her second child. At the time of the interview, there had been no contact for three weeks. During the interview, James wondered whether his birth daughter and his daughter from marriage had spoken with each other (and that this had somehow prejudiced the birth daughter against him). His daughter from marriage appears to show little interest in his birth daughter. A particularly moving moment for him seems to have been when his birth daughter unexpectedly visited during a recent hospitalization. She introduced herself as his daughter, brought her husband and their son – his first grandchild.

Robert

He was a teenager and in a steady relationship with the birth mother. When she became pregnant, their greatest worry was telling their parents. Her mother was opposed to the baby and decided that the child would be adopted. The birth mother was placed in a mother-and-baby home. He visited regularly and was in the building when the baby was born. He remembers holding her and recalls that she was quite pretty. He and the birth mother split up shortly after. He feels that his daughter was stolen from him at that time. He feels that he had no options and was angry about the adoption. Within about three years, feelings about his daughter "began to grate." After that, his feelings remained intense. She was "just there on [his] brain." He proceeded to have three long-term relationships, all involving children, either his or young stepchildren. His wife (the first of these three long-term partners) and he had no children; however, he described a traumatic, full-term stillbirth. This event and its effect on his wife led to the breaking up of their marriage. His next partner was the mother of his first and only son. This partner had been in the same mother-and-baby home as the birth mother – and she, too, had given up a baby for adoption. Therefore, his son had two sisters he did not know about. At the time of the interview, his 15-year relationship with a third partner had come to an end. He had two other daughters from this relationship. He reports that he is very close and committed to all his children, including three stepchildren. Eight years ago, his feelings for his adopted birth daughter became so strong he reported that he had to do something about it. After some effort, he managed to have his name placed on file so that should she come looking, she would find him. She came looking six months before the interview. He received a letter from a post-adoption agency. He was so pleased he nearly fell off his seat! Their first telephone call lasted two and a half hours. They met two to three weeks after. He brought his adult son. She brought her daughter – his granddaughter – and her husband. In respect to his daughter, he reports that he has always taken her as "[his] daughter." He is very pleased that she refers to him as her daughter's granddad. Robert regularly referred to his daughter as having been stolen. She had "loomed large" all through his life. After the interview, he proudly showed photographs of his birth daughter and one of their first (adult) cuddles.

The preceding anecdote is a broad overview of what we know about birth fathers and their experiences. We know even less about how other adults in adoption perceive them, but for the purposes of this paper, the next section focuses solely upon what we know about how adopted people think of their birth fathers and their encounters with each other.

Adopted People's Encounters with, and Perceptions of, Their Birth Fathers

Sachdev (1991) reports on how birth fathers are perceived by other parties in the adoption process. The attitudes of birth mothers varied from grudging acceptance – in the best interests of the adopted child – of the importance of information about the birth father to hostility. The same study found that hostility toward the birth father was greater in adoptive parents. Of all three parties – adopted children, birth mothers, and adoptive parents – the adopted children were the most positive in their regard for information-sharing with their birth fathers, while adoptive parents were the most negative in their attitudes toward birth fathers.

It seems, from adopted people's accounts of searching and contact, that many adopted people have an interest in the birth father but that this, more often than not, follows contact with their birth mother. In the writings that deal with search activities of adopted people, there is a common theme of completing the jigsaw (usually once the birth mother has been contacted). *Preparing for Reunion Feast* records the thoughts of one woman which describe a major motivation for adoptees tracing both birth parents:

> I watched a programme on adoption, one of the adopted children who had found her birth mother said that now she felt a complete person – before she had found her mother, a part of her had been missing – but how can she feel whole until she has found her father?
>
> (1994, pp. 137–138)

In her study of adopted people's relationships with their birth mothers, March notes that adopted people appear to express "little interest in the birth father when they begin to search" (1995, p. 110), but that this lack of interest is replaced with a desire for contact with him during the search-and-contact process involving the birth mother (ibid.) Twenty-two respondents in March's study ($n = 60$) had met with their birth father. Types of contact were described as ranging from two who had felt rejected by their birth father to two who classified their relationship as "father–child." A majority of seven considered the contact to be "between friends." March also found that the adoptees' descriptions of adoptee–birth father interaction and outcome of contact resembled the accounts given for contact with the birth mother, that is, for both categories of birth parent (birth mother and birth father), there was a span of similar experiences reported by her adult adoptees (1995, p. 120).

Subsequent work involving March found that adopted women characterized unwed birth fathers who choose adoption as irresponsible and uncaring, while adopted men characterized birth fathers as either immature or not financially capable of fulfilling paternal responsibility. These perceptions exist despite the fact that respondents to a wider survey ($n = 706$) characterized men who make adoption plans as responsible, caring, and unselfish (Miall & March, 2003).

The adoption reunion literature certainly shows a spectrum of views following later-life contact. For adopted people, one woman declares: "You can't be my father, you are my biological father and there's no getting away from that, but you are not emotionally my father and you didn't bring me up" (Trinder et al., 2004, p. 66). Another (about her birth father): "[]}ven though someone conceived me and gave birth to me, those people can never be a parent and I've told them that. They can't be a parent because there's no history there" (Passmore & Chipuer, 2009, p. 98). The seven adopted people in the latter study were clear that their relationships with their birth fathers ranged from no relationship to distant relative to close friendship. After a reservation about the small sample size, Passmore and Chipuer go on to note that 'it is interesting that none of the adoptees regarded it as a father–daughter relationship" (ibid., p. 100). At the other end of the spectrum, there are instances of a conferring of both the title of dad and role by the adopted person: "me dad," as one person says in *Adoption Reunion Handbook* (Trinder et al., 2004, p. 62). An adopted male refers to his birth father as "my old man" (Clapton, 2003, p. 172). When first meeting her father in the Hughes study (2015, p. 163), the adopted woman thinks, "Well he can't be dad, so what do I call him?" (ibid., p. 158), but goes on to feel "easier" with him than with her biological mother and later still is "happy to call him 'dad' and herself 'his girl.'" Hughes counsels against any fixed conclusion to be drawn from this, preferring "precariousness" as a description of her adopted respondent's "new" relationships with her birth parents.

Whilst it is difficult to estimate prevalence, it is clear that "father" far outweighs "dad" in the language of adopted people – for example, in the study by Browning and Duncan (2005) of meetings and subsequent relationships between adopted adults and their birth parents, only 1 of the 20 adopted people uses the term *dad* to describe her birth father.

There is very little research available on sex-based differences in adopted people's assessment of their relationships with birth parents. One survey found that satisfaction with birth mothers and birth fathers was rated as between "somewhat dissatisfied and neutral." When responses were disaggregated, the assessment of the relationship with the birth mother was one of "very dissatisfied," and "neutral" regarding birth fathers (Baden et al., 2017, p. 212, emphasis in original). The authors do not speculate as to the difference; however, it may be that this is to do with the generally less-emotional freight that is devoted to fathers than mothers (Andrews et al., 2004).

It must be acknowledged that the little we know about birth fathers relates to the era of "closed" adoptions in which babies and infants were adopted with little effort to obtain information about birth fathers. Even less is known about how birth fathers negotiate current forms of adoption, such as open adoption (Ge et al., 2008; Clutter, 2020) or adoptions from state care, some of which will have been opposed by the birth father (Clifton, 2012). Furthermore, so far we have been discussing adults (birth fathers and adopted adults). What of the birth father–adopted adolescent dynamic?

The Birth Father in the Eyes and Mind of the Adopted Adolescent

Adolescence is a time and process during which young people explore their goals, values, and beliefs in order to develop a coherent sense of identity (Erikson, 1968). The adopted adolescent faces the extra task of finding answers to questions such as, "Who am I as an adopted person?" (Hoopes, 1990) and "What does being adopted mean to me, and how does this fit into my understanding of myself, relationships, family, and culture?" (Von Korff & Grotevant, 2011, p. 393). Freud's concept of the family romance fantasy as part of normal development for all children needs to be re-thought in the case of adopted children. In non-adoptive families, that in the "family romance" the child imagines and fantasizes about another set of "better" parents that have been replaced by her or his – flawed – real ones is a regular feature of growing up, how much more psychological work is required from adopted children who really do have another mother and father (Glassman, 2013)? For the purposes of this paper, how is it experienced by adolescents?

It seems that adolescence can be a period when an adolescent's adoptive status becomes more of a preoccupation than before. Over 80% ($n = 135$) of Kohler et al. (2002) reported thinking about their adoption at least once a month, with 27% reporting weekly frequency. They found that girls were more preoccupied with their adoptions than boys, regardless of how much contact they may have had with birth family members. The study by Wrobel and Dillon (2009) reported that 74% of the adolescents were "curious" about their birth fathers.

Pivnick suggests that "the central dilemma for the adopted child can be construed as the construction of a coherent, multi-stranded individual and family narrative, replete with twists and gaps in time" (2009, p. 5). Scholars have called for adoptive families to avoid concealment and to practice "adoption-related communication" (Wrobel et al., 2004), "adoption talk" (Jones & Hackett, 2007), and "communicative openness" (Von Korff & Grotevant, 2011; Santona et al., 2022). This is all very well, but what about the "adoption information gap?" (Wrobel & Grotevant, 2019, p. 29). That is, how is this possible when there is a difference, sometimes very large, between what an adopted person knows and what he or she desires to know regarding his or her adoption and the birth parents?

The Information Problem

The majority of adoptions today increasingly take two forms, with the "secret" (closed) adoptions of the twentieth century in decline (Siegel & Smith, 2012), although there are variations in law from country to country. The second is open adoption, in which birth parents and adoptive parents and the adopted child have ongoing contact either directly or indirectly with each other after the adoption. Yet despite the decades-long rise in the practice of open adoption, the consequent relationship that might develop between the adopted adolescent and her or his birth father has been examined in only two papers (Clutter, 2020; Ge et al., 2008). A third category of adoption relates to children collected from an invariably poorer country and taken to more advantaged countries in the Western world (United Nations, 2009). Here the adopted adolescent has little information about both their birth parents, and it is more than likely that whatever exists will relate to only the birth mother (Manley, 2006). So with regard to the lack of information about birth fathers, firstly, adoptees from the era of closed adoptions (which type of adoption continues in many states of the USA and elsewhere) will not have access to much information about the birth father; secondly, we know very little about the birth fathers' experiences within the open adoptions of today, especially with regard to their relationships with their adolescent children, and thirdly, we generally lack even the basics about the birth fathers of internationally adopted children. If adoption is a "fiction-generating machine" (Homans, 2006, p. 5), then for the adopted adolescent concerning their birth father, the conditions are ripe for speculation and fantasy but also for revilement and disapproval. None of this is helped by scanty records, partisan anecdotes, and shoulder-shrugging. This is an example of woefully inadequate training and skills of those handling adoptions, and also of the need for far higher and more consistent standards in the adoption field globally.

White (2013) cites Zoppi (2010), an American psychologist, who points out that most adoption stories do not include information about birth fathers. Zoppi argues that in the absence of information about the birth father, adoptive parents and therapists can assist adoptees in addressing the vacuum labelled "birth father" by encouraging the child to integrate his or her own fantasies about the birth father. She proposes that parents suggest "imagining what the birth father might be like as a father and as a man and integrating images of the birth father with images of other men." Doing this, she argues, will help the child develop more secure attachment and identity, develop stronger attachments to adoptive parents, maintain better connections to the past, and construct a more coherent life narrative

Elsewhere, Wrobel and Dillon argue that understanding and responding to "three phases of curiosity" are essential in navigating the rapids of growing up adopted. These phases, they claim, are the telling of the story to the adopted child, and then responding to their questioning, and then, in adolescence, they may be able to satisfy their curiosity by means of independent information-gathering (2009, p. 224). But in Chapter 10, Bertocci argues that for the adopted person, the term "curiosity" entirely misrepresents the actual internal experience and the meanings of it over time. For her or him, the alleged "three phases of curiosity" refer to the different occasions that the adoptee asks for information and, hopefully, receives authentic answers, if they are even available. These times of interest in having more information will depend largely on the circumstances in their lives at the time the need arises – more likely, in many cases, efforts to activate the search for information will come, if they do at all, later in young adulthood or even beyond. However, given the likelihood that it will continue that little or no information about birth fathers will be made available, unless adoption standards globally are significantly improved, any constructive approaches relating to the adolescents and their birth fathers must necessarily build in an assumption that loss will figure prominently (Brodzinsky, 2011; Barroso & Barbosa-Ducharne 2019).

Conclusion

This chapter began by referring to birth fathers in adoption as shadowy figures and ghosts. In *Ghostly Matters: Haunting and the Sociological Imagination*, Avery Gordon writes that while ghosts usually represent a traumatic loss, they also can simultaneously represent future possibilities and hope (2008). In the absence of, or presence of skewed, information about birth fathers, where can the possibilities for better practice begin? At home. We need to re-examine our reasons for dismissing the importance of the birth father and for not taking responsibility for learning what he means to the adopted child in adolescence and young adulthood. This will require a general shift in attitudes in the human services, but especially a major shift in adoption policies and practices globally. After all, why should mothers always bear all the responsibilities and emotional labor in adoption?

Endnotes

Ainsworth, M.D.S. (1991). Attachment and other affectional bonds across the life cycle. In C.M. Parkes, J. Stevenson-Hinde, & P. Marris (Eds.), *Attachment across the Life Cycle* (pp. 33–51). New York: Routledge.

Andrews, A.B., Luckey, I., Bolden, E., Whiting-Fickling, J., & Lind, K.A. (2004). Public perceptions about father involvement: Results of a statewide household survey. *Journal of Family Issues*, 25 (5), 603–633.

Baden, A.L., Kitchen, A., Mazza, J.R., Harrington, E.S., & White, E.E. (2017). Addressing adoption in counseling: A study of adult adoptees' counseling satisfaction. *Families in Society*, 98, 206–219.

Barroso, R., & Barbosa-Ducharne, M. (2019). Adoption-related feelings, loss, and curiosity about origins in adopted adolescents. *Clinical Child Psychology and Psychiatry*, 24 (4), 876–891.

Barrows P. (1999). The importance of fathers in parent-infant psychotherapy. *Infant Observation*, 3 (1), 74–88.

Baumann, C. (1999). Adoptive fathers and birthfathers: A study of attitudes. *Child & Adolescent Social Work Journal*, 16 (5), 373–391.

Bowlby J. (1951). *Child Care and the Growth of Love*. Geneva: World Health Organisation.

Brodzinsky, D. (2011). Children's understanding of adoption: Developmental and clinical implications. *Professional Psychology: Research and Practice*, 42 (2), 200–207.

Browning J., & Duncan G. (2005). Family membership in post-reunion adoption narratives. *Social Policy Journal of New Zealand*, 26, 151–172.

Cicchini, M. (1993). *Development of Responsibility: The Experience of Birth Fathers in Adoption*. Perth, Western Australia: Adoption Research and Counselling Service Inc.

Clapton, G. (2000). *Perceptions of Fatherhood: Birth Fathers and Their Adoption Experiences*. Unpublished PhD, University of Edinburgh, Edinburgh. https://era.ed.ac.uk/bitstream/handle/1842/7175/488475.pdf;jsessionid=4B6F9BA86B7BC038B4D2636CC1646DFD?sequence=1 Accessed 23 September 2022.

Clapton, G. (2003). *Birth Fathers and Their Adoption Experiences*. London: JKP.

Clapton, G. (2009). How and why social work fails fathers: Redressing an imbalance, social work's role and responsibility. *Practice: Social Work in Action*, 21 (1), 17–34.

Clapton, G. (2019). Against all odds? Birth fathers and enduring thoughts of the child lost to adoption. *Genealogy*, 3 (2). www.mdpi.com/2313-5778/3/2/13 Accessed 11 September 2022.

Clapton, G., & Ward, A. (2013). Adoption and birth fathers. *Therapy Today*, 20–25.

Clifton, J. (2012). Birth fathers and their adopted children: Fighting, withdrawing, and connecting. *Adoption & Fostering*, 36 (2), 43–56.

Clutter, L.B. (2020). Perceptions of birth fathers about their open adoption. *American Journal of Maternal/Child Nursing*, 45 (1), 26–32.

Coles, G. (2004). *Ever after: Fathers and the Impact of Adoption*. Melbourne, Australia: Clova Publications.

Cornefert, P-A. (2021). *Australian Birth Fathers of Adopted Children: Their Perspectives, Feelings, and Experiences about the Adoption of Their Child*. Doctoral thesis, University of New South Wales, Australia.

Deykin, E., Patti, P., & Ryan, J. (1988). Fathers of adopted children: a study of the impact of child surrender on birth fathers. *American Journal of Orthopsychiatry*, 58, 240–248.

Erikson, E.H. (1968). *Identity, Youth, and Crisis*. New York: Norton.

Feast, J. (1994). *Preparing for Reunion*. London: Children's Society.

Fink, B. (1995). *The Lacanian Subject: Between Language and Jouissance*. Princeton: Princeton University Press.

Freeman, T. (2008). Psychoanalytic concepts of fatherhood: Patriarchal paradoxes and the presence of an absent authority. *Studies in Gender and Sexuality*, 9 (2), 113–139.

Ge, X., Natsuaki, M.N., Martin, D.M., Leve, L.D., Neiderhiser, J.M., Shaw, D.S., Villareal, G., Scaramella, L., Reid, J.B., & Reiss, D. (2008). Bridging the divide: Openness in adoption and postadoption psychosocial adjustment among birth and adoptive parents. *Journal of Family Psychology*, 22 (3), 529–540.

Glassman N. (2013). Narrative, family romance fantasy, and the adoption triad. *Psychoanalytic Perspectives*, 10 (1), 116–119.

Goldman, R., & Burgess, A. (2018). *Where's the Daddy? Fathers and Father Figures in UK Datasets*. London: Fatherhood Institute.

Gordon, A. (2008). *Ghostly Matters: Haunting and the Sociological Imagination*. Minneapolis: University of Minnesota Press.

Homans, M. (2006). Adoption narratives, trauma, and origins. *Narrative*, 14 (1), 4–26.

Hoopes, J.L. (1990). Chapter 8: Adoption and identity formation. In D.M. Brodzinsky, & M.D. Schechter (Eds.), *The Psychology of Adoption*. New York: Oxford University Press, pp. 144–166.

Hughes, B., & Logan, J. (1993). *Birth Parents: The Hidden Dimension*. Manchester: University of Manchester.

Hughes E. (2015). "There's no such thing as a whole story": The Psychosocial implications of adopted women's experiences of finding their biological fathers in adulthood. *Studies in Gender and Sexuality*, 16 (3), 151–169.

Jones, C., & Hackett, S. (2007). Communicative openness within adoptive families: Adoptive parents' narrative accounts of the challenges of adoption talk and the approaches used to manage these challenges. *Adoption Quarterly*, 10 (3–4), 157–178.

Jung, C.G. (1954). *The Practice of Psychotherapy: Essays on the Psychology of the Transference and Other Subjects*. New York: Pantheon Books.

Kellmer Pringle, M. (1973). *The Needs of Children*. London: Hutchinson & Co. Ltd.

Kenny, P., Higgins, D., Soloff, C., & Sweid, R. (2012). *Past Adoption Experiences: National Research Study on the Service Response to Past Adoption Practices*. Canberra: Australian Institute of Family Studies/Australian Government.

Kohler, J.K., Grotevant, H.D., & McRoy, R.G. (2002). Adopted adolescents' preoccupation with adoption: The impact on adoptive family relationships. *Journal of Marriage and Family*, 64 (1), 93–104.

Manley, K.L. (2006). Birth parents: The forgotten members of the international adoption triad. *Capital University Law Review*, 35 (2), 627–664.

March, K. (1995). *The Stranger Who Bore Me: Adoptee-Birth Mother Relationships*. Toronto: University of Toronto Press.

McCant, J. (1987). The cultural contradiction of fathers as nonparents. *Family Law Quarterly*, 21 (1), 127–143.

Miall, C., & March, K. (2003). A comparison of biological and adoptive mothers and fathers: The relevance of biological kinship and gendered constructs of parenthood. *Adoption Quarterly*, 6 (4), 7–39.

Nash, J. (1965). The father in contemporary culture and current psychological literature. *Child Development*, 36 (1), 261–297.

Neil E, Beek, M., & Ward. E. (2013). *Contact after Adoption: A Follow up in Late Adolescence*. Norwich: University of East Anglia.

O'Brien, M. (2005). *Shared Caring: Bringing Fathers into the Frame* (Working Paper No. 18). London: Equal Opportunities Commission.

Panter-Brick, C., Burgess, A., Eggerman, M., McAllister, F., Pruett, K., & Leckman, J.F. (2014). Practitioner review: Engaging fathers – recommendations for a game change in parenting interventions based on a systematic review of the global evidence. *Journal of Child Psychology and Psychiatry*, 55 (11), 1187–1212.

Parliament of New South Wales Legislative Council Standing Committee on Social Issues. (2001). *Government Response to Releasing the Past: Adoption Practices 1950–1998*. www.parliament.nsw.gov.au/lcdocs/inquiries/2026/Report.PDF Accessed 23 September 2022.

Passmore, N., & Chipuer, H. (2009). Female adoptees' perceptions of contact with their birth fathers: Satisfactions and dissatisfactions with the process. *American Journal of Orthopsychiatry*, 79 (1), 93–102.

Passmore, N., & Coles, G. (2009). Birth fathers' perspectives on reunions with their relinquished children. In *Proceedings of 9th Annual Conference of the Australian Psychological Society's Psychology of Relationships Interest Group: Connecting Research and Practice in Relationships* (pp. 35–41), 7–8 November, Brisbane, Australia. Melbourne: Australian Psychological Society.

Pivnick, B.A. (2009). Left without a word: Learning rhythms, rhymes, and reasons in adoption. *Psychoanalytic Inquiry*, 30 (1), 3–24.

Sachdev, P. (1991). The birth father. A neglected element in the adoption equation. *Families in Society*, 72, 131–138.

Salvo Agoglia, I., & Herrera, F. (2021). 'I assumed he didn't exist': The birth father as the invisible member of the adoption kinship network. *Journal of Family Issues*, 42, 9841–1006.

Santona, A., Tognasso, G., Miscioscia, CL., Russo, D., & Gorla, L. (2022). Talking about the birth family since the beginning: The communicative openness in the new adoptive family. *International Journal of Environmental Research and Public Health*, 19 (3), 1203. https://pubmed.ncbi.nlm.nih.gov/35162222/ Accessed 21 September 2022.

Siann, G. (1994). *Gender, Sex, and Sexuality: Contemporary Psychological Perspectives*. Abingdon: Taylor & Francis.

Siegel, D., & Smith, S. (2012). *Openness in Adoption: From Secrecy and Stigma to Knowledge and Connections*. New York: Evan B. Donaldson Institute.

Smith, S. (2007). *Safeguarding the Rights and Well-Being of Birthparents in the Adoption Process*. New York: Evan B. Donaldson Institute.

Trinder, E., Feast, J., & Howe, D. (2004). *The Adoption Reunion Handbook*. London: BAAF.

Triseliotis, J., Feast J., & Kyle F. (2005). *The Adoption Triangle Revisited*. London: BAAF

United Nations. (2009). *Child Adoption: Trends and Policies*. New York: The Department of Economic and Social Affairs, United Nations.

Von Korff, L., & Grotevant, H.D. (2011). Contact in adoption and adoptive identity formation: the mediating role of family conversation. *Journal of Family Psychology*, 25 (3), 393–401.

Ward, A. (2012). *The Birth Father's Tale*. London: British Association for Adoption and Fostering.

White, J. (2013). Chapter 9: Adoptive parenting of teenagers and young adults. In V. Brabender, &V.A. Fallon (Eds.), *Working with Adoptive Parents: Research, Theory, and Therapeutic Interventions*. Hoboken: John Wiley & Sons, Incorporated, pp. 169–180.

Whitesel, A. (2008). *Post Adoption Adjustment of Birth Fathers: The Effects of Relationships with Birth Mothers and Family*. Unpublished PhD, Howard University, Washington, DC. www.proquest.com/openview/ce96dfac8384f396b360dff7510b8b77/1?pq-origsite=gscholar&cbl=18750&diss=y

Winnicott, D. (1990). *Home Is Where We Start from*. London: Penguin.

Witney, C. (2004). Original fathers: An exploration into the experiences of birth fathers involved in adoption in the mid-20th century. *Adoption and Fostering*, 28 (3), 52–61.

Wrobel, G., & Dillon, K. (2009). Chapter 10: Adopted adolescents: Who and what are they curious about? In G. Wrobel, & E. Neil (Eds.), *International Advances in Adoption Research for Practice*. New Jersey: John Wiley & Sons Ltd., pp. 217–244.

Wrobel, G., & Grotevant, H. (2019). Minding the (information) gap: What do emerging adult adoptees want to know about their birth parents? *Adoption Quarterly*, 22 (1), 29–52.

Wrobel, G., Grotevant, H.D., & McRoy, R.G. (2004). Adolescent search for birthparents: Who moves forward? *Journal of Adolescent Research*, 19 (1), 132–151.

Zanoni, L., Warburton, W., Bussey, K., & McMaugh, A. (2013). Fathers as 'core business' in child welfare practice and research: An interdisciplinary review. *Children and Youth Services Review*, 35 (7), 1055–1070.

Zoppi, J. (2010). Creating space for birth fathers in adoption stories: The significance of the fantasized birth father on attachment and identity development of adoptees. In V. Brabender, & A. Fallon (Eds.), *Working with Adoptive Parents: Research, Theory, and Therapeutic Interventions*. Hoboken, NJ: John Wiley & Sons.

8
GROWING UP ADOPTED IN INDIA – MENTAL HEALTH AND WELL-BEING

Implications for Therapeutic and Clinical Practice

Meera Oke, PhD; Sahana Mitra, PhD; and Valerie O'Brien, PhD

Introduction

India is a pluralistic, heterogeneous, democratic society with a rapidly growing economy in Southeast Asia. It has one-fifth of the world's population, with multiple subcultures, languages, and castes (Sanyal, 2015; Saraswathi & Dutta, 2010). Adoption is an age-old practice within India, surrounded by various preconceptions, practices, and norms coming from different cultures, subcultures, and communities (Makhnach, 2016). In this chapter, literature on Indian adoptees is examined with regard to kinship/non-kinship placements and the intersections of familial, social, cultural, and historical influences on adoptee mental health and well-being. The bio-ecological approach (Bronfenbrenner & Morris, 2006) to adoptees' mental health/well-being is utilized. We define *well-being* as "a state of complete physical, mental, and social well-being and not merely the absence of disease or infirmity" (WHO, 1946, p. 2). Through a "salutogenic" or holistic approach (Antonovsky, 1979; Simons & Baldwin, 2021), we see mental health as being more than the absence of pathology. Instead, we adapt a framework whereby adopted people's mental health is influenced by the interplay of four elements – the birth family, the adoptive family, the agency/institution, and adoptees' own personal and socio-emotional and psychological development. This is presented conceptually in Figure 8.1.

Furthermore, particular distal and proximal factors are discussed as part of sociocultural beliefs and changing socio-legal practices, which include the nature

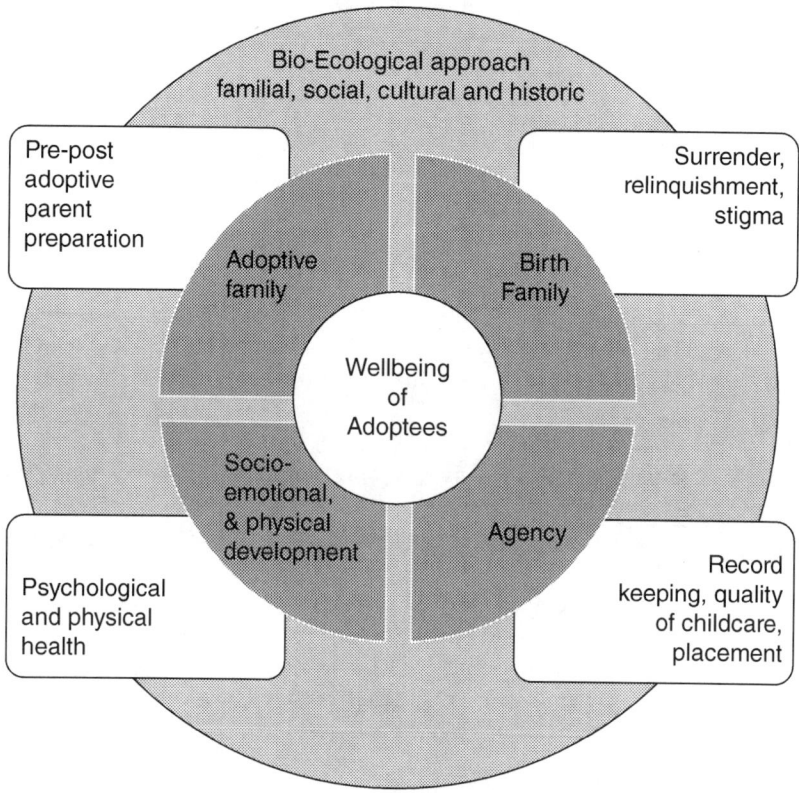

Figure 8.1 Conceptual framework – adoptees well-being in the Indian context.

of record-keeping, availability of birth-related information, and the quality of the childcare placement prior to adoption. This is achieved through accessing available Indian literature whilst drawing also on Irish adoption research and practice as one of the examples of Western adoption discourse. We also include information we have learned from adopted people themselves and agency workers. In conclusion, the implications are discussed for all involved in adoption as it relates to therapeutic and clinical services and practitioners.

Background of Adoption in India

The practice of placing children in extended kin and non-kinship adoptive families has a long history within the Hindu traditions (80% of the Indian population is Hindu – Census of India, 2011), as evidenced in myths and oral stories (Bajpai,

2021). We begin by outlining the historical lineage of community beliefs and practices around adoption and then discuss the socio-legal scenario that has shaped service availability.

Tracing Historical Underlying Sociocultural Beliefs and Practice of Indian Adoption

Historically, prior to the 1990s, there were two dominant sociocultural beliefs and norms that governed formal and informal "relinquishment" of children and the adoption process. There were cultural values that related to who is adoptable. *First*, the preference of a male child. In India, "the male enjoys culturally and scripturally sanctioned privileges" (Menon, 2017, p. 195). A belief in the "Hindu" tradition holds that only a male heir can carry the family name and perform the last rites for parents in order to achieve "moksha" (Appendix 1). Culturally, this sanctioned the preference of a male child for adoption. Moreover, the bloodline mattered, and due to the strong influence of a divisive caste system, most adoption arrangements were made between family members and relatives to keep the bloodline known and respected, while considering the process of giving away a child as a charitable act (Bhattacharya, 1990; Lilani, 1995).

The *second* belief centered on the importance of women's chastity and non-sexual relationships prior to marriage. While the cultural norm emphasizes fertility, the birth of a child was valued and sanctioned only after marriage (Bharadwaj, 2003), and society maintained highly conservative attitudes toward "unwed" mothers. Shame and stigma were very much attached to the conception of a child outside marriage. This often led to illegal abortions and the abandonment of babies. Although the Medical Termination of Pregnancy Act has been in place since 1971 in India, services and awareness for access to safe abortions were limited. Since the 1990s, with growing awareness of abortion and the availability of adoption services, there has been a reduction in the abandonment of children. In India, babies were in the main surrendered/relinquished in secrecy at the time of birth. In India, mothers returned to their community soon after making arrangements for their baby, so as to avoid shame and censure from society. For birth mothers, and sometimes for the children they surrendered, this remains a lifelong source of anguish. While some level of attitudinal change toward birth outside marriage has occurred, shame and stigma still remain.

In many ways, this social context is not unique to India. When we look at the history of adoption in Ireland, we find similar social pressures. Although differing in their faiths (India being predominantly Hindu and Ireland mostly Catholic Christian), both have similar sociopolitical backgrounds. In Ireland, both prior to and after the legalization of adoption in 1952, mothers and their children endured isolation, and "erring" women were consigned, along with their children, to mother-and-baby homes (Kelly, 2005; Sixsmith, 2009; O'Higgins, Sixsmith & Nic Gabhainn, 2010). While the situation began to change for unmarried mothers from the early 1970s, shame-based practices and the use of mother-and-baby homes continued up to the early 1990s (Government of Ireland, 2021). Change in Ireland was attributed to three major factors – the introduction of the unmarried mother's social protection payment in 1973; Ireland's membership of the EU in 1972, which propelled changing social attitudes; and women having greater control over their bodies through access to contraception and abortion (O'Brien & Mitra, 2018).

In both countries, greater emphasis was placed on the needs of the adoptive parents, with lesser importance being given to improving the quality of life of an "illegitimate" child or the mother giving birth outside marriage (Apparao, 1997; Government of Ireland, 2021). It is also a reminder of how disturbing the reality was for both unwed mothers and their children (O'Brien, 2016; O'Brien & Mitra, 2015). In terms of individual adopted persons, this historical piece is undoubtedly relevant for adoptees in their adolescence and emerging adulthood, as they comprehend how the circumstances and decision-making at the time of their adoption continue to influence their own and family identity across the life course.

Changing Socio-Legal Scenario as It Impacts Services for Adopted People

With a colonial history in India, much of the legislation around childcare and protection was regulated by policies and laws that favored denominational, biological, and religious connections over quality care and protection of all children. For example, the *Guardians and Wards Act (GAMA) of 1890* ensured guardianship rights to Muslim, Christian, Parsi, and Jewish communities. For Hindu, Buddhist, and Jain religious denominations/communities, the adoptive parent rights were provided for under the *Hindu Adoption and Maintenance Act (HAMA) of 1956* (Bhargava, 2005).

A similar kind of religious influence over adoption can also be traced in Irish adoptions. Section 12(2) of the *1952 Adoption Act* stated that no adoption order could be made unless the applicant(s) were of the same religion as the child and his or her biological parents(s) or the religion of mother, if the child was illegitimate (The Adoption Board, 1954). This was overruled by the subsequent 1974 Adoption Act that introduced a provision for adoption where adoptive parents and birth family could be of different religions, provided that the person consenting to the order was aware of this before giving consent (O'Brien & Mitra, 2019). Hence, the orthodoxy of religious morality in both countries significantly influenced nonfamily domestic adoptions (Appendix 2). These adoptions are also called "stranger" adoption or "non-relative" adoption (Mohanty et al., 2017; Sengupta, 2011).

Around the 1980s, India gained popularity as a "sending" country for intercountry adoption. In the process it witnessed a commodification of adoption, wherein there is evidence that a large number of international adoptions were illegal (Apparao, 1997). As a result, the Indian Supreme Court intervened in 1984 with a judgment which gave priority to domestic adoption by Indian adoptive parents (Indian Ministry of Women & Child Development, 2012). Advocacy groups built campaigns in India to increase awareness of "stranger" adoption as a win-win situation, where an orphan finds a home and prospective adopters – mostly infertile couples – have an option to build and complete a family. These factors led to an increase in the number of domestic adoptions. Placement agencies reported growing waiting lists of prospective domestic adoptive parents (Apparao, 1997). As the number of domestic adoptions rose, there was a corresponding strengthening of intercountry adoption procedures and safeguards. In 2003, India became a signatory to the 1993 Hague Convention, which helped reduce international child commodification. As a result, in the period 2010 to 2014 in India, there were ten domestic adoptions recorded for everyone intercountry adoption (Selman, 2020).

However, changes in domestic adoption also exerted pressure on the earlier open informal domestic adoptions, which were mostly kinship-based arrangements and which occurred largely outside the legal system. As part of the change, a "clean break" adoption system was perpetuated, where links between the adoptive and the birth families were severed and no identifying information was shared (Mitra et al., 2018; Momin, 2008). Interestingly, in India, this closed-system adoption was welcomed by non-kin domestic adoptive parents and birth families, as it incorporated "beliefs of secrecy over unwed motherhood and stigma related to adoption and the adopted child, into one model" (Mitra et al., 2019, p. 360; Wanglar, 2022). In other words, it meant no contact could be made with the birth family pre- or post-adoption (Gangopadhyay & Mathur, 2021).

The regime of closed adoption is found in the history of many Western countries (Neil & Howe, 2004), including Ireland. There is evidence that Irish practice has now transitioned to greater openness at a communication level, though it has not yet been underpinned in the legal code. In one study, McCaughren (2010) found that, while Irish adoptive parents tended to follow traditional closed models of adoption practice, they increasingly used discretion with regard to how and with whom they shared adoption stories. This shows that while "adoption is clearly being reformulated by those directly affected by it, these paradigm shifts are not always understood or reflected within wider society" (McCaughren & Lovett, 2014, p. 244). These similar shifts are evident among Indian adoptive families, where there is greater openness to talk about adoption. However, to a certain level, there is a reluctance to continue referring to the adoption story with the child and others. The decision to share the adoption story, and with whom to share, depends on the importance of the situation and the significance of the person in adopted families/adopted people's life (Mitra et al., 2019). There is a level of evidence that the educated urban family who occupies a position in a higher socioeconomic class may not be willing to disclose the adoptive status to the child (Mitra, 2017). Members of Child Welfare Committees dealing with adoption cases in North India shared that, even though many adopted people are happy and satisfied within their families, many have questions, and there is a limited opportunity to discuss these questions within the family.

In this cultural context, mental health professionals have limited training to deal with the feeling of adoptee loss, search, and root questions. Hence, the placement agencies have a significant role to play in providing counselling and information services to the adopted person and their families. They can provide a safe channel of communication and facilitate awareness and confidence to attend the post-adoption workshops and meetings and discuss the pertinent issues of sharing, bringing up, and management of adoption stories. However, there is no obligation for adoptive families to stay in touch with their placement agencies other than to send annual follow-up development reports of the child for five years; for some families, this route may not work.

This points to the need for better-informed mental health practitioners who may intersect with adopted young people and their families who attend for services. In these situations, adoption-related issues may be to the fore, but in other situations, the adoption may be more submerged and the reason for individual and family challenges may be constructed in a different way.

Distal and Proximal Aspects Influencing Well-Being of Adoptees in Their Adolescence and Emerging Adulthood

Utilizing a bio-ecological approach, the well-being of Indian adoptees is determined by several aspects. Key *proximal* aspects include description of circumstances that affect adoptees' immediate environment, such as parenting styles, levels of sensitivity, and awareness of adoptee concerns about their adoption in their immediate and extended families, neighborhood, and school surroundings. Predominantly, well-being is related to the openness in overall communication and talking about their adoption and feelings associated with the process. Key *distal* factors include the cultural beliefs about human rights, rights of adopted people, and beliefs related to contact with birth parent/family and record-keeping at placement agencies. The point to be noted here is that these distal and proximal factors influence the well-being of domestic and international adoptees differently. As part of the exploration, we show that, in an Indian context, children's pathways through care to adoption, parenting practices in general, and how these practices may relate to adoption can have a particular relevance.

Circumstances at the Time of Birth – Embedded Adversities

When children are born into traditionally wedded Indian families, they are welcomed with anticipation and great joy. However, children regularly enter the care system when traditional norms are not followed. The care pathways for children in India are varied: it can be through a referral from concerned individuals, such as the birth mother's extended family, local medical and social work practitioners, or from other institutions, such as the state homes for women (usually for destitute and abandoned women) or abandonment of the child (with no availability of birth information). About 3,500 children in childcare institutions (orphanages) (Appendix 3) are adopted legally each year domestically (Appendix 4). Recently, in a first of its kind, a retrospective study of birth family child intake records collected over four decades ($n = 3,709$) was conducted in association with BSSK, an Indian adoption agency established in 1979 (Oke & Lambert, 2021). The study included only those who legally surrendered their babies for care and adoption. The predominant reason for surrender was unwed pregnancy. The babies were/are taken into care soon after birth, with a two-month period for birth families to reconsider with counsel their decision to surrender. Babies are surrendered legally for care and protection only in circumstances where birth mothers are unable to rear their babies, and formal arrangements are made for permanent care through adoption.

The procedure for found/abandoned children who come into care in India includes advertising the particulars of the child (with photograph) in state-level newspapers within 72 hours of the time of receiving the child. Within 24 hours, the child must be produced before the Child Welfare Committee; a child below 2 years of age will be declared "legally free" for adoption within two months if the child's parent/s is/are not found. The birth-related information that is available when the child comes into care depends on if the child was surrendered by an unwed mother/family or if the mother was a minor, and also the circumstances under which the child was found (e.g., abandoned in a hospital, train, orphanage, etc.). Birth circumstances, and the kind of record-keeping conducted by agencies, have implications for the type of professional support available to adoptees if they initiate a search in their adolescence and early adulthood.

Experiences of Loss and Root Search – Thoughts and Emotions about Birth Parents

There has been limited empirical research into adoptees' experience of actual search and connection with birth families. As recently as 2017, within the framework of UN International Human/Children's Rights ratified by India in 1992, there are provisions in law (e.g., Sections 29(1) and (44) of Adoption Regulations India 2017) for "root search" (Ministry of Women & Child Development, 2022). This process can be initiated by persons over 18 years of age, but it does not amount to a legal right to original birth registration information. A new birth certificate is made for the child, based on the adoption order. In cases where the original birth certificate is available and parents have consented for it to be released to the child upon reaching adulthood, this information may be shared where the adoptee initiates a search. However, there is no legal provision to hold all this data centrally, and the proportion of birth mothers who permit contact is not known. Currently, only the placement agencies record the birth registration and parental consent, together with more detailed documentation related to genealogy and medical history.

It is also worth noting that, internationally, "root search" predominantly focusses on birth mothers, at least initially, while birth fathers have been, to a great extent, "least talked about figures" (Clapton, 2007; Mason, 1995). Evidence of the absence of birth fathers' information was noted in a recent Indian birth mothers study (Oke & Lambert, 2021), which highlighted that birth family data kept in placement agencies mainly included birth mother's age, health, marital status, nature of relationship with birth father, and occupation, whereas birth father biographical information was minimal.

In Western literature, major importance is attributed to search as a critical feature of identity development and the relief for adoptees knowing about their original birth families and reasons for being placed for adoption (Schechter & Bertocci, 1990; Brodzinsky et al., 1992; Kohler et al., 2002). In the Indian context, there is gap at both the research and practice level in terms of its importance for adoptees. Moreover, the root search–related questions and perceptions differ across domestic and international adoptees. Based on the limited domestic Indian data, Kalyanvala (2022) describes how many of the Indian domestic adoptees report satisfaction with their visits to the placement agency from where they were adopted. During the visit, they enjoyed spending time with the children, meeting staff, observing the agency activities, as well as seeing their adoption file. However, adoptees are often disappointed by how little information was left for them at the time of the placement. On the contrary, children adopted internationally are aware of their adoptive status much earlier as they are reared in families where adoption communication is more open and are more willing to search for their birth families by travelling to India (Damadoran & Mehta, 2000; Groza et al., 2014). This differentiation in openness and proximity to the place of their adoption may influence the adoptees psychologically. For adoptees, search can provide them with greater knowledge of physical health and inherited diseases, and also connections with birth family in terms of appearance, talents, and interests (Schechter & Bertocci, 1990). This is an areas that needs greater research, taking into account the particularities of the Indian context while providing greater training for mental health practitioners. Training needs to attune mental health practitioners to adoption-related issues for adoptees and their families and requires practitioners to expand their skill range while obtaining general and more Indian-specific adoption knowledge, in terms of sociocultural circumstances around adoptee birth and surrender, the nature of information available in the records, and what can be shared within the legal frameworks when the adoptee comes for search. This would be a necessary first step to provide more effective psychosocial support to adoptees at different stages of root search. Alongside this development of training, there is need to examine past and current record-keeping processes and practices.

Changes in Record-Keeping Practices

In India, there is a variation in the amount and quality of adoption record-keeping, with some agencies keeping detailed records of birth circumstances and the birth family, while others are restricted to birth mothers data only. It is important to note that, at the time of many children's admission to the agencies in the early 1980s, restrictive practices were in place related to information-gathering. Given the sociocultural context at that time, secrecy was critical for birth families. At that time, consent for surrender was frequently only verbal; having just given birth to a newborn in difficult circumstances, birth mothers were rarely in a frame of mind to discuss matters related to later-stage contact; in many cases, they were eager to have the process done with at the earliest. It is to be noted that agency practitioners did what many saw as in the best interest of birth families and children at the time of admission and worked on an individual basis to revisit the consent process.

It was convenient for some in the "stranger" adoption parent cohort not to know anything about the child's history, fearing that the birth mother might come back to claim her child or the child might make attempts to trace their birth mother. The difference in quality of information kept by adoption agencies at the time of child placement, combined with adoptive families' openness to adoption information, is a major determinant of subsequent outcomes. One must note that, because of poor recording practices in the past, for some individual adoptees now in their adolescence and adulthood, knowledge and contact with their birth family remain obtrusive.

Fortunately, over the years, record-keeping has evolved in India. These changes were influenced by agency workers' growing recognition of the need to collect data for future purposes. A new system of digitizing adoption information in India, enforced through Juvenile Justice (Care and Protection for Children) Act 2015, called "CARINGS," has created new opportunities to enhance future search. It is possible to upload through the new platform all relevant documents for an adoption, including prospective adoptive parents' home study report, photo, and medical/personal details of the child, matched with the family and details of the professionals involved (social workers, psychologists, agency workers, doctors, and district magistrate). CARINGS process provides greater transparency and enhances record-keeping. It is possible to keep track centrally on the number of children available for adoption and the parents on the waiting list (Mitra & Bhaskar, forthcoming). Though the record-keeping is now digitized, adoptee birth information may remain closed to the adoptee. This may continue to have a psychological impact for adoptees in their adolescent and young adulthood years. While domestic adoptees have greater access to the agencies and their records, the adult adoptees do not come forward to access biographical details of their individual records due to lack of openness or reluctance of the adoptive parents to talk about adoption on a regular basis (Sardesai, 2020). Instead, they use the knowledge of their placement agency, which is shared more openly by adoptive parents, to meet the adoption social workers and to undertake charity or volunteer work in the agency from where they were adopted. This helps them connect to their past without knowing who their birth parents were. This is psychologically gratifying for some domestic adoptees.

On the other hand, Indian adoptees adopted internationally have more immediate access to their birth records (non-identifying information) and agency institution from where they were adopted. As a result, placement agencies report that inquiries for "root search" come more frequently from international adoptees (S. Pawar (Social Worker) in discussion with the author October, 26th 2022).

Although differing in their needs, adoptees reared in a more closed system of adoption require more systematic psychological intervention programs. This can include emotion-focused coping, grief loss therapy, cognitive and family therapy, which takes account of the culturally diverse and a layered caste system within which the adoption occurs (Mitra, 2017). Currently, with a dearth of mental health professionals trained in the field of closed adoption (Corder, 2012) and a lack of more in-depth training for adoption agency workers, individualized counselling plans depend on what is available in the birth and adoptive records and workers' willingness to learn and use what is known about growing up in Indian adoptive families.

Features of Growing Up in Indian Adoptive Families

Traditionally, Indians follow a patriarchal pattern with multiple generations living in the same household and with close connections to an extended family network. With rapid economic development in India, there have been some shifts in family habitation patterns and parenting styles (Chaudhary & Shukla, 2020). Although multiple generations may not physically live in the same house, parents and children remain closely connected for all critical life events and practical life decisions. Indians place a high value on respect for parents, ancestors, and elders and academic success. In the context of adoption, this means adoptee loyalty and respect to adoptive parents are central. This may result in the adoptee not voicing their own emotional needs or asking questions they may have about their birth circumstances or their birth mothers, particularly during adolescence and emerging adulthood (Oke et al., 2015). It is not uncommon for parents to emphasize the importance of focusing on academic success above personal matters, particularly during adolescence. In the family, this is seen as a key life stage for the acquisition of skills and knowledge to enable performance of duties required for the next stage of householder life (Saraswathi & Oke, 2013). This priority impacts on the degree of openness available in the family for sharing and unravelling the adoption story and likely also impacts the adoptees voice and concerns.

Degree of Openness in Adoption Communication

Communicating about adoption with children is shrouded with complexity in the Indian context. Most adoptive parents choose either not to disclose the adoption story to their adopted child or share only when the child confronts them or are in their adolescence. Children are often aware of their adoptee status but do not have an environment that facilitates openness in communication. This results in a situation whereby many adoptees grow up not knowing, or knowing very little, about their adoption. Others, whilst knowing, may live in situations of heightened emotions about the reality of their adoption. Mohanty et al. (2017) studied 86 Indian adoptive parents, with the children in the median age of 5 years at the time of study. The findings indicated that few (12.8%) had disclosed the adoptee status to their children, while a little more than half (54.7%) declined to disclose the adoption status, and the remainder planned to tell the child (p 19). Furthermore, some of the parents considered that communication about the adoption was more a "one-time" event as opposed to a gradual process of sharing with the child (Mohanty, 2015). Another phenomenological study conducted with Indian adoptive parents found they encountered three kinds of dilemmas in relation to communication about adoption: first, a child-centered dilemma, which focused on parents not hurting the adoptee, with the knowledge that they were adopted and therefore born unwanted; the second centered on themselves as parents, experiencing a fear that their adoptive child will abandon them when they know about their adoptive status (these fears are in line with a cultural expectation that adult children are supposed to take care of their aging parents); and the third dilemma is that parents are overwhelmed and admit that they feel ill-equipped and lack the emotional strength to disclose the adoptive status to their child, as they feel they will be judged by society with regards to parenting behaviors and their decision to adopt, often in instances of infertility (Mitra et al., 2019). The process of disclosure is closely associated "with cultural parenting beliefs and practices" (Mohanty, 2015, p. 74).

These studies show that the cultural system in India promotes withholding and sharing of the adoption story till the child is older, usually during pre-adolescent and adolescent years. In this context, there is a belief that older children will cope better with loss and stigma associated with the adoption, within a more established and emotionally close and connected adoptive parent–child relationship. This is in contrast to Western literature, which emphasize the importance of open communication by adoptive parents right from the start. As domestic adoptees and family members negotiate the adoption and the complex issues related to it, many adoptees find it challenging to communicate with their adoptive parents. In a recent study, Kalyanvala (2022) interviewed 22 adult adoptees and their adoptive parents about growing up in adoption. She found that some adoptees who were told about their adoptive status in their early childhood felt that their adoption served as a barrier in developing a healthy relationship with their adoptive parents, whereas others felt that knowledge about their adoptive status did not influence their relationship. On other hand, international adoptees may be better supported by their adoptive parents, as the visible physical differences between the adopted child and adoptive parents generally propel greater levels of openness.

The important thing to note is that stability in adoptive family parent–child connectedness and circumstances determines how adult adoptees feel about their adoptive status, a topic which is revisited later in this chapter. Adoptees with emotionally close relationships and stable homes did not report issues and concerns about their adoptive status; in fact, they reported a sense of gratitude for their life trajectory (Kalyanvala, 2022).

Age of Adoption

Adoption literature indicates that another aspect influencing adoptee outcomes is the age at adoption. Western studies indicate that the younger the child is when adopted and the less time spent in institutional care, the fewer are emotional and social difficulties (Merz et al., 2013; Mitra, 2017). Bilson and Munro (2019) contend that the age of 5 years appears to be a significant cutoff point in mitigating long-term emotional and social consequences of early negative experiences. In India, a 2003 study by Groza and the BSSK team indicated the average age range of placement varies for domestic and international placements. Placements for children in domestic adoption is at a younger age (averaging in a range from 4 months to under 2 years), whereas those placed internationally are older (6.6 years).

Perhaps, critical to this discussion is the quality of experiences of adoptees prior to their adoption. Those adopted at older ages may experience greater difficulties and, as a result, require different kinds of therapeutic and clinical intervention. Hence, the age of adoption has implications for adoptees, adoptive families, as well as for the adoption agency social workers, who have an increased responsibility in preparing older children placed in adoptive families. In the main, clinicians have to work more intuitively with the children, as they may have little information about a child's origins and may also have limited information about the prospective adopters. There is usually very little, if any, preparation or inclusion by Indian agencies of international families adopting from Indian agencies, although a level of preparation may be undertaken by agencies in the adopters' own country.

These points highlight the need for a greater integrated support service to deal with the medical and mental health issues, and this is now generally recognized by those working in the adoption field. These developments must also be aligned with the provision of service for domestic adoptive parents – even if the children adopted are younger.

School and Peer Influences

Academic success, as indicated earlier, is highly valued in Indian families and society. If the child has low academic performance, this is usually attributed to the child's adoptive status in the adoptive family, whereas in education, adoptees tend to be perceived generally by teachers to be scholastically underachievers. In school settings, this can become a self-fulfilling prophecy. With misconceptions and prejudice about the adoptees (Best et al., 2021) regarding their background and behavioral concerns, schoolteachers often align with societal beliefs and expectations of poorer academic achievement from lower-class and lower-caste children. Teachers are not adequately trained to deal with or understand adoption in the classroom, as is perhaps the situation in many education systems. In the context of prevailing beliefs, Indian parents may be further propelled not to reveal the adoptive status of the child to the school. The findings from Mitra's 2017 study of Indian adoptive families reveal that adoptive parents did not generally share information at school.

However, as is indicated through many studies in Western contexts, in India adopted children may be anxious about disclosing their adoptive status to others. In Western countries, the reluctance is generally connected with their sense of difference (King, 2009), hesitation that teachers/others will be understanding of their needs, and fear of being bullied and experiencing other microaggressions associated with their adoption (Baden, 2016). Stress experienced by adoptees associated with a need to keep their adoption status secret may lead to the development of certain problematic behaviors. In an Indian study conducted by Dhavale et al. (2005), with 30 adopted and 30 non-adopted children aged 5 to 10 years, various behavioral outcome measures were assessed. Adopted children indicated more behavioral and school difficulties compared to the non-adopted children. Caution is required in interpreting these findings, given the small-scale nature of available studies and participation rates associated with the secrecy of many Indian adoptions.

Other studies carried out with Indian children adopted internationally have shown greater variation in results. For example, in a study with 192 children, 65% girls and 31% boys placed from Indian orphanages aged between 2 and 3 years and placed with 142 Norwegian families reported improvement in the language development and social skills of the child, but somatic complaints and anxiety also increased over time (Riley-Behringer et al., 2014). Barroso et al. (2017), through a systematic review of 258 studies carried out between January 2004 and June 2006, examined psychological adjustment in intercountry and domestic adopted adolescents. A key finding indicated that Indian children adopted internationally had a greater number of behavior and delinquency problems at schools compared to non-adopted children, indicating that adoptees experience more difficulties in schools. The authors concluded that difficulties faced by adoptees may be due to an intersection of the child's adoptive status and ethnicity, and this is an area that requires more detailed exploration (Reinoso et al., 2016).

In order to understand the needs of the adopted child more adequately, it is necessary to improve adoption awareness at the school level and change the prevailing simplistic belief that children will do well once they are adopted into a loving home (Adoption UK, 2014; Mitra, 2017). With not enough yet known about the educational experiences of adopted adolescents, it can mean that behaviors and symptoms stemming from their early experiences are overlooked (Golding, 2010) and that they remain "invisible" within the education system, especially when they internalize rather than externalize their feelings (Barratt, 2011, p. 141). School experiences of adoptees, no doubt, influence their well-being in the school environment. With the support of adoption-knowledgeable professionals, adoptees may cope better with the challenges they face across the contexts in which they live.

Adolescent and Adult Adoptee Voices

There are few studies which illustrate the voice of Indian adult adoptees. In fact, Stother et al. (2019) remark that the voice of adopted children are "strikingly absent" from Indian research (p. 437). Studying adoption outcomes, particularly in the area of emotional and mental well-being (Oke et al., 2015), has remained under researched. Insights and comparisons are drawn from the West to understand the developmental patterns in adopted adolescents and young adults associated with identity issues, feelings of loss and isolation, and relationships difficulties. In research, the nature and range of adoption outcomes are diverse (e.g., behavioral, emotional, academic, or social adjustment), and findings can vary based on many variables and factors, including research settings, samples used, and the timing of assessment (Holmgren & Elovainio, 2019). For example, adopted children may have issues with their identity in their emerging adulthood (Grotevant et al., 2017), but measuring identity concerns at some other point along the life course, such as during adolescence, might yield different results.

Earlier studies in the Indian context have indicated concerns and issues experienced by adult adoptees; for example, a study by Goodman and Kim (2000) indicated that adoptees reported medical difficulties (20%), social difficulties (11%), intellectual difficulties (9%), and emotional difficulties (5%), and these were significantly higher in female adoptees than male (83% versus 69%). In another study, Groza et al. (2012) studied 46 adult Indian adoptees in their adolescence who were aware of their adoptive status. Many had unanswered questions about their adoption, for example, why their birth parents left them, or their religious background. They wondered if they were not wanted because of gender, specifically in the case of girls. Almost 53% of the adoptees reported that they have thoughts about their birth families; they displayed a concern for the welfare of their birth mother but restrained themselves from talking about it so as to avoid emotionally hurting their adoptive parents and seeming disloyal to them.

Other, more recent Indian studies researching adoptee voices (Oke et al., 2015; Kalyanvala, 2022; Sardesai, 2020; Singh, 2021) have reported adoptees' deep curiosity or intense need to find more about their identity, a need to feel complete, to know about medical and genetic information, an urge to inform their birth family about their present life and express gratitude for making a good choice for them. Even though adoptees and their adoptive families see their adoption as generally positive both domestic (Groza et al., 2003) and International (Groza et al., 2005), they can still go through various stages of emotions, including grief, loss, anger, and acceptance, but may not share this with others. With their feelings of shame, guilt, anger, anxiety, conflict, fear, insecurity, and tension, regarding their birth and adoptive families, as well as prejudicial attitudes towards their skin color, they chose to remain silent. In both the scenarios, they look for mental health services from adoption professionals trained in the social, biological, political and economic, and psychological aspects of adoption (Kalyanvala, 2022).

Meera Oke, PhD; Sahana Mitra, PhD; and Valerie O'Brien, PhD

Appraisal of Existing Adoption-Related Services – Availability, Access, and Nature

Mental health services in India are provided by private and public health practitioners, by psychiatrists, psychiatric social workers, clinical psychologists, therapists, and counsellors. Public health services are provided by medical psychiatric services in state- and privately run hospitals, and the teams are generally multidisciplinary. Therapeutic and clinical support is provided mainly by private practitioners or by NGOs. In an environment where the general population is still hesitant to access mental health services openly and without stigma, providing specialist adoption-related support is complex. The complexity can be somewhat simplified if mental health professionals are trained in biological, sociocultural, psychological, and legal aspects of adoption practices. A well-coordinated system needs to be in place where medical and mental health professionals work with adoptees and adoptive and birth parents. We advocate the need for a more regulated system, specifying skill levels and credentials required for different settings and roles. This development requires to take into account the complexity of adoption.

In India, greater effort and resources are required to link the field of adoption with existing mental health professionals while also improving the training of those professionals currently working in adoption agencies. Furthermore, there is a need to ensure that professionals who intersect with adopted children and adults in their day-to-day work, that is, social workers, school counsellors, therapists, and clinical psychologists, develop and improve their adoption competence. Training needs to include the impact of cultural myths about adoption, stereotypical thinking and biases concerning infertility, childlessness, microaggressions experienced by adoptive people, and the meanings of blood ties. A particular emphasis should be centered on professionals' own attitudes and beliefs about adoption and how their views may be impacting in how people involved in adoption experience their services.

Implications for Future Support for Services for Adolescent and Emerging Adult Adoptees

Being adopted entails both gains and losses for adoptees, and coming to terms with these two antithetical features can be rather difficult (Reinoso et al., 2013). Socially prevailing cultural beliefs and stereotypes about the absence of relatedness and blood connection can negatively influence how adoption is experienced (Morgan & Langrehr, 2019). With changes in legal provisions and societal attitudes in India, there has been a greater openness to talk about adoption, with a result that adoptees and their families are looking for more support services.

We advocate the need for a strengths-based coherent approach to service provision, aimed at enhancing well-being right across the life span, for all parties involved in adoption. In Figure 8.2, we outline how a salutogenic (holistic) framework underpinned by an ecological approach and including supports and interventions could contribute to service development. The framework is inclusive of needs and

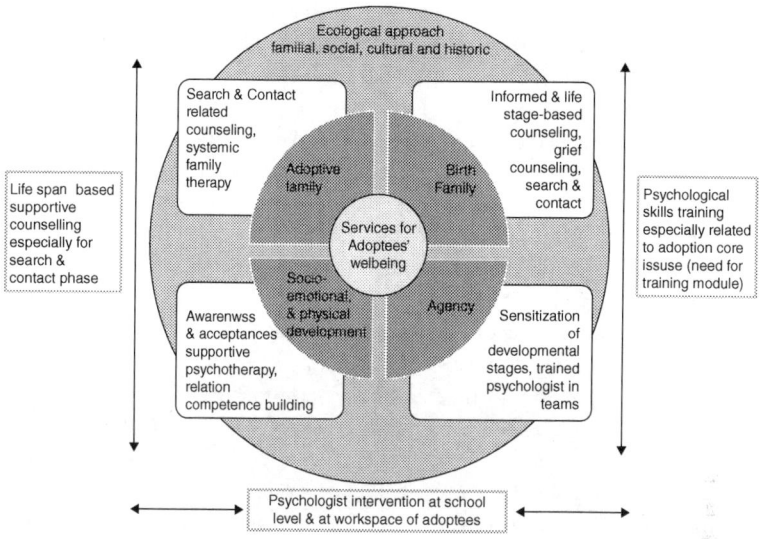

Figure 8.2 A salutogenic model to ecological, integrated, specialized adoption services.

services and is aimed at adoptees, adoptive and birth families, adoption professionals working in adoption agencies, and other professionals in the fields of mental and physical health, including school and higher education teachers. The type of knowledge and skills that may be required to effectively strengthen services is specified.

This framework is proposed to take account of gaps occurring in Indian society, including the limited articulation of adoption issues at a societal and media level. It also incorporates the universal finding that existing mental health professionals play a limited role in adoption-related issues in their clinical and research practice (Baden et al., 2013), and this is even more evident in India. In the main, developmental concerns experienced by adopted adolescents and adults are reduced to a problem that is largely managed by the parents within the family, or to a lesser extent by the adoption placement agency. It is generally seen as an individual issue, requiring individual attention.

Conclusion

As we research growing up in adoption, we learn how much a favorable environment can offset early difficulties and recognize a cultural strength of family and "parent–child connectedness" in India. With mental health professionals trained in the various dimensions of adoption, effective services can be provided to adoptees particularly in their adolescence and emerging adulthood as they negotiate their identity. While services are being developed for people currently involved in adoption, there is a need for a focus on the future needs of children currently on an adoption pathway. Social workers need to focus on creating and maintaining robust social and medical information that pertains to them and also their birth parents and family. These records will be vital for the adopted child and his/her family for their future use.

To conclude, the aim of the chapter has been to present how adoption is perceived and experienced by adopted adolescents and young adults in the Indian context. Most research has been carried out in Western countries, and Indian studies on the health and well-being of adoptees remain very limited. Through this chapter, it is clear that the limited knowledge and service provision mitigates against supporting the adoptee's adoptive and birth family unique developmental trajectory. At a more basic level, the evidence of continued parental reluctance to share the fact of adoption not only has implications for mental health interventions but also points to the need for change in adoption discourses at a wider sociopolitical and cultural level. In the meantime, there are sufficient people in need of service to point to the need to educate clinical practitioners toward greater adoption competence, including historical, cultural, bio-psychosocial aspects of Indian adoption. In this approach, lessons can be drawn from Western knowledge, but the particularities of the Indian and Asian contexts need to be held center stage.

Declaration of conflicting interests: The author(s) declare no potential conflicts of interest with respect to the research, authorship, and/or publication of this chapter. The author(s) received no financial support for the research, authorship, and/or publication of this chapter.

Endnotes

Adoption UK. (2014). *Adopted Children's Experiences of School.* www.adoptionuk.org/our-research

Antonovsky, A. (1979). *Health, Stress, And Coping.* San Francisco: Jossey-Bass.

Apparao, H. (1997). International adoption of children: The Indian scene. *International Journal of Behavioral Development, 20*(1), 3–16.

Baden, A.L. (2016). "Do you know your real parents?" and Other microaggressions. *Adoption Quarterly, 19*(1), 1–25.

Baden, A.L., Gibbons, J.L., Wilson, S.L., & McGinnis, H. (2013). International adoption: Counseling and the adoption triad. *Adoption Quarterly, 16*(3–4), 218–237.

Bajpai, L.M. (2021). *The Owl Delivered the Good News All Night Long: Folk Tales, Legends and Modern Lore of India.* New Delhi: Rupa Publications.

Barratt, S. (2011). Adopted children and education: The experiences of a specialist CAMHS team. *Clinical Child Psychology and Psychiatry, 17*(1), 141–150.

Barroso, R., Barbosa-Ducharne, M., Coelho, V., Costa, I., & Silva, A. (2017). Psychological adjustment in intercountry and domestic adopted adolescents: A systematic review. *Child and Adolescent Social Work Journal, 34,* 399–418.

Best, R., Cameron, C., & Hill, V. (2021). Exploring the educational experiences of children and young people adopted from care: Using the voices of children and parents to inform practice. *Adoption & Fostering, 45*(4), 359–381.

Bharadwaj, A. (2003). Why adoption is not an option in India: The visibility of infertility, the secrecy of donor insemination, and other cultural complexities. *Social Science & Medicine, 56*(9), 1867–1880.

Bhargava, V. (2005). *Adoption in India – Policies and Experiences.* New Delhi: Sage Publications India.

Bhattacharya, S. (1990). Motherhood in ancient India. *Review of Women Studies, Economic and Political Weekly*, 25(42–43), 50. www.epw.in/journal/1990/42-43/review-womens-studies-review-issues-specials/motherhood-ancient-india.html (last accessed on February 2022).

Bilson, A., & Munro, E.H. (2019). Adoption and child protection trends for children aged under five in England: Increasing investigations and hidden separation of children from their parents. *Children and Youth Services Review*, 96(C), 204–211.

Brodzinsky, D.M., Schechter, M.D., & Henig, R.M. (1992). *Being Adopted: The Lifelong Search for Self.* New York: Doubleday.

Bronfenbrenner, U., & Morris, P.A. (2006). The bioecological model of human development. In R.M. Lerner, & W. Damon (Eds.), *Handbook of Child Psychology: Theoretical Models of Human Development* (pp. 793–828). Hoboken: John Wiley & Sons Inc.

Clapton, G. (2007). The experiences and needs of birth fathers in adoption: What we know now and some practice implications. *Practice (Social Work in Action)*, 19(1), 61–71.

Census of India. (2011). *Census Tables*. https://censusindia.gov.in/census.website/data/census-tables (accessed on May 2022).

Chaudhary, N., & Shukla, S. (2019). Family, identity, and the individual in India. In G. Misra (Ed.), *Psychology: Volume 2: Individual and the Social: Processes and Issues* (pp. 143–189, Online ed). Oxford: Oxford Academic.

Corder, K. (2012). Counseling adult adoptees. *Family Journal: Counseling and Therapy for Couples and Families*, 20(4), 448–452.

Damadoran, A., & Mehta, N. (2000). Child adoption in India: An overview. In P. Selman (Ed.), *Intercountry Adoption; Development, Trends and Perspectives* (pp. 405–418). London: BAAF.

Dhavale, H., Bhagat, V., & Thakkar, P. (2005). A comparative study of behaviour problems between adopted and nonadopted children in India. *Journal of Child and Adolescent Mental Health*, 17(1), 27–30.

Gangopadhyay, J., & Mathur, K. (2021). Examining lived experiences of infertility and perceptions toward the adoption of children in Urban India. *Adoption Quarterly*, 24(3), 229–249.

Golding, K.S. (2010). Multi-agency and specialist working to meet the mental health needs of children in care and adopted. *Clinical Child Psychology and Psychiatry*, 15(4), 573–587. https://doi.org/10.1177/1359104510375933

Goodman, J.F., & Kim, S.S. (2000). "Outcomes" of adoptions of children from India: A subjective versus normative view of "success". *Adoption Quarterly*, 4(2), 3–27.

Government of Ireland. (2021). *Final Report of the Commission of Investigation into Mother and Baby Homes by Department of Children, Equality, Disability, Integration and Youth.* www.gov.ie/en/publication/d4b3d-final-report-of-the-commission-of-investigation-into-mother-and-baby-homes/ (last accessed on July 2022).

Grotevant, H.D., Lo, A.Y.H., Fiorenzo, L., & Dunbar, N.D. (2017). Adoptive identity and adjustment from adolescence to emerging adulthood: A person-centered approach. *Developmental Psychology*, 53(11), 2195–2204. https://doi.org/10.1037/dev0000352

Groza, V., Chenot, D., & Holtedahl, K. (2005). The adoption of indian children by norwegian parents. *International Journal of Child & Family Welfare*, 8(2–3), 98–113.

Groza, V., Kalyanvala, R., & BSSK Research Team. (2003). Indian families adopting Indian children. *Indian Journal of Social Work*, 64(1), 93–113. https://journals.tiss.edu/archive/index.php/ijswarchive/article/view/2821

Groza, V., Park, H., & Oke, M. (2012). *A Study of Adult Adoptees in India Placed Domestically in India through BSSK*, Pune. https://case.edu/socialwork/sites/case.edu.socialwork/files/201809/A_Study_of_Adopt_Adoptees_in_India_Final_Report.pdf

Groza, V., Park, H., Oke, M., Kalyanvala, R., & Shetty, M. (2014). Adoption and birth family issues: Adult adoptees in India placed through BSSK in Pune. *Indian Journal of Social Work, 75*(2), 285–300.

Holmgren, E., & Elovainio, M. (2019). Issues in interpreting the findings from adoption outcome studies: A checklist for practitioners. *Adoption & Fostering, 43*(2), 210–213.

Indian Ministry of Women & Child Development. (2012). *Annual Report 2012–2013.* http://wcd.nic.in/sites/default/files/AR2012-13.pdf (accessed on 20 August 2019).

Kalyanvala, R. (2022). *Growing up in Adoption: Stories from an Indian Perspective.* Tamil Nadu: Notion press.

Kelly, R.J. (2005). *Motherhood Silenced: The Experiences of Natural Mothers on Adoption Reunion.* Dublin: Liffey Press.

King, C.F. (2009). *Adopted Children and the Transition from Primary to Secondary School: An Examination of Pupil, Parent and Teacher Views.* Hampshire: Hampshire Educational Psychology Service.

Kohler, J.K., Grotevant, H.D., & McRoy, R.G. (2002). Adopted adolescents' preoccupation with adoption: The impact on adoptive family relationships. *Journal of Marriage and Family, 64*(1), 93–104.

Lilani, K. (1995). Adoption of children from India. In E.D. Jaffe (Ed.), *Intercountry Adoptions: Laws and Perspectives of Sending Countries* (pp. 23–37). Dordrecht: Martinus Nijhoff Publishers.

Makhnach, A.V. (2016). Medical and social models of orphanhood: Resilience of adopted children and adoptive families. In U. Kumar (Ed.), *The Routledge International Handbook of Psychosocial Resilience* (pp. 242–253). London: Routledge.

Mason, M. (1995). *Out of the Shadows: Birthfathers' Stories.* Edina, Minnesota: O.J. Howard Publishing.

McCaughren, S. (2010). *A Study of Open Adoption in Ireland through the Narratives of Adoptive Parents.* Unpublished PhD thesis, University College Cork, Ireland.

McCaughren, S., & Lovett, J. (2014). Domestic adoption in Ireland: A shifting paradigm? *Adoption & Fostering, 38*(3), 238–254.

Menon, S. (2017). The semiotics of parenthood in India: A lived experience. *Indian Journal of Gender Studies, 24*(2), 194–216.

Merz, E.C., McCall, R.B., & Groza, V. (2013). Parent-reported executive functioning in post institutionalized children: A follow-up study. *Journal of Clinical Child & Adolescent Psychology, 42*(5), 726–733.

Ministry of Women and Child Development. (2022, September 23). *Adoption Regulations 2022.* https://cara.nic.in/PDF/adoption%20regulations%202022%20english_27.pdf (accessed on April 2023) from https://cara.nic.in/

Mishra, R.C. (2013). Moksha and the Hindu worldview. *Psychology and Developing Societies, 25*(1), 21–42.

Mitra, S. (2017). *Parenthood through Adoption: An Indian Experience.* Unpublished PhD thesis, Tata Institute of Social Sciences, Mumbai.

Mitra, S., & Bhaskar, S. (forthcoming). Mapping the digitalization of child adoption in India: Challenges and future possibilities.

Mitra, S., Konantambigi, R., & Datta, V. (2018). A literature review of non-family domestic adoptions in India: Lessons from other countries. *Indian Journal of Social Work, 79*(4), 415–436.

Mitra, S., Konantambigi, R., & Datta, V. (2019). Adoption sharing in closed adoption system: Experiences of Indian adoptive parents. *Indian Journal of Social Work, 80*(3), 359–378.

Mohanty, J. (2015). Adoption disclosure and behavioral adjustment of domestic adoptees in India. *Family Science, 6*(1), 68–76.

Mohanty, J., Ahn, J., & Chokkanathan, S. (2017). Adoption disclosure: Experiences of Indian domestic adoptive parents. *Child & Family Social Work, 22,* 1–11.

Momin, E. (2008). *Sociology of Adoption.* Rawat Publications: Mumbai.

Morgan, S.K., & Langrehr, K.J. (2019). Transracially adoptive parents' colorblindness and discrimination recognition: Adoption stigma as moderator. *Cultural Diversity and Ethnic Minority Psychology, 25*(2), 242–252.

Neil, E., & Howe, D. Eds. (2004). *Contact in Adoption and Permanent Foster Care: Research, Theory and Practice.* London: BAAF.

O'Brien, V. (2016). Positioning and respectful professional interventions for working with the legacy of irish institutional care. In S. Barratt, & W. Lobatto (Eds.), *Surviving and Thriving in Care and Beyond. Personal and Professional Perspectives* (pp. 217–238). London: Karnac.

O'Brien, V., & Mitra, S. (2015). Search and reunion in adoption: The aftermath of the film 'Philomena' and an opportunity to shape change. *The Irish Social Worker,* 5–11.

O'Brien, V., & Mitra, S. (2019). *An Overview of Adoption Policy and Legislative Change in Ireland 1952–2017.* https://aai.gov.ie/images/Report_2_An_Overview_of_Policy_and_Legislative_Change_in_Ireland_1952_to_2017.pdf (last accessed on May 2022).

O'Brien, V., & Sahana, M. (2018, October). *Report 1 an audit of research on adoption in Ireland 1952 to 2017.* The Adoption Authority of Ireland. https://www.aai.gov.ie/images/Report_1_An_Audit_of_Research_on_Adoption_in_Ireland_1952_to_2017.pdf (last accessed on April 2023).

O'Higgins, S., Sixsmith, J., & Nic Gabhainn, S. (2010). Adolescents' perceptions of the words 'health' and 'happy'. *Health Education, 110*(5), 367–381.

Oke, M., Groza, V., Park, H., Kalyanvala, R., & Shetty, M. (2015). The perceptions of young adult adoptees in India on their emotional well-being. *Adoption & Fostering, 39*(4), 343–355.

Oke, M., & Lambert, J. (2021). What do we know about Birth Families: An exploration of birth parents records in relation to surrender of babies in the Indian and Irish context. *International Conference on Adoption Research,* 6–9 July, Milan, Italy.

Pawar, S. Personal communication with author, October 26th, 2022.

Reinoso, M., Juffer, F., & Tieman, W. (2013). Children's and parents' thoughts and feelings about adoption, birth culture identity and discrimination in families with internationally adopted children. *Child & Family Social Work, 18*(3), 264–274.

Reinoso, M., Pereda, N., Van den Dries, L., & Forero, C.G. (2016). Internationally adopted children's general and adoption-specific stressors, coping strategies and psychological adjustment. *Child & Family Social Work, 21,* 1–13.

Riley-Behringer, M., Groza, V., Tieman, W., & Juffer, F. (2014). Race and bicultural socialization in the Netherlands, Norway, and the United States of America in the adoptions of children from India. *Cultural Diversity and Ethnic Minority Psychology, 20*(2), 231–243.

Sanyal, S. (2015). *Incredible History of India's Geography.* London: Penguin Publishers.

Saraswathi, T.S., & Dutta, R. (2010). India. In M.H. Bornstein (Ed.), *Handbook of Cultural Developmental Science* (pp. 465–483). New York: Psychology Press.

Saraswathi, T.S., & Oke, M. (2013) Ecology of adolescence in India: Implications for policy and practice. *Psychological Studies, 58*(4), 353–364.

Sardesai, K. (2020). *Child Of My Heart: A Comprehensive Guide to Adoption in India.* India: Literature Publisher.

Schechter, M.D., & Bertocci, D. (1990). The meaning of the search. In D. M. Brodzinsky, & M. D. Schechter (Eds.), *The Psychology of Adoption* (pp. 62–90). New York: Oxford University Press.

Selman, P. (2020). International adoption from China and India 1992–2018. In G. Jianguo, B. Rajendra, G. Lakshmana, & C. Sheng-Li (Eds.), *Social Welfare in India and China* (pp. 393–415). London: Palgrave Macmillan.

Sengupta, N. (2011). *Babies from the Heart*. India: Random House Publishers.

Simons, G., & Baldwin, G.S. (2021). A critical review of the definition of 'wellbeing' for doctors and their patients in a post Covid 19 Era. *International Journal of Social Psychiatry*, 67(8), 984–991.

Singh, D.M. (2021). *Voices from the Heart: The Adoption Experience*. Mumbai: Twagaa International Publishers.

Sixsmith, M. (2009). *The Lost Child of Philomena Lee: A Mother, Her Son and a 50-Year Search*. Basingstoke: Macmillan.

Stother, A., Woods, K., & McIntosh, S. (2019). Evidence-based practice in relation to post-adoption support in educational settings. *Adoption & Fostering*, 43(4), 429–444.

The Adoption Board. (1954). *Adoption Board Annual Report*. Dublin: The Stationary Office.

Wanglar, E. (2022). Childcare institutions in India: Caregivers' solutions to challenges in childcare. *Child & Family Social Work*, 27(3), 381–391.

WHO [World Health Organization]. (1946). *Constitution of the World Health Organization*, New York, 22 July. https://treaties.un.org/doc/Treaties (last accessed on 01 July 2021).

APPENDIX

1. Mishra (2013) discusses "Moksha" as a moral and spiritual goal and reflects on the concept being related to everyday life rather than being an "otherworldly" reality – traditionally a concept that represents freedom from the "cycle of birth and death."
2. Those families who adopt a child who is not related to adoptive parents and "the adopted child becomes the lawful child of his/her adoptive parents with all the rights, privileges and responsibilities that are attached to a biological child" (Ministry of Women and Child Development, 2022).
3. Children in orphanages may not be orphans. They may be temporarily surrendered by poorer parents and, in this scenario, not available for adoption.
4. www.adoptionindia.nic.in.

PART III

Considerations in Medical Care

9
ADOPTION MEDICINE
Special Considerations in Pediatric and Adolescent Medicine and Young Adult Medical Care

Elaine E. Schulte, MD, MPH, and Laurie C. Miller, MD

Introduction

Adoptees have an increased risk of medical, developmental, and behavioral problems. Many of these problems relate to their complicated early lives, issues that can remain active during adolescence and early adulthood. This chapter focuses on the unique medical, developmental, and behavioral issues that physicians and other health-care providers need to consider when caring for adopted adolescents and young adults. The early life experiences contributing to these problems are also reviewed. Awareness of these issues is an important component of providing "adoption-friendly" health care to adoptees and their families during adolescence and early adulthood. Some of the issues are important across the life span.

What Is Adoption Medicine?

Adoption medicine is relatively new and was developed initially to address special medical issues in intercountry adoptions. The earliest adoption clinics were established over 35 years ago to address "exotic" infectious diseases in internationally adopted children (Johnson, 2005). As the number of newly arriving internationally adopted children increased in the early 2000s, adoption medicine physicians began to recognize that many of these children had additional medical problems beyond infectious diseases. The negative effects of prenatal and postnatal adversity (especially malnutrition and neglect) were increasingly recognized. Adoption medicine has expanded to include all adoptees, regardless of the type of placement (domestic infant, children in foster care who are adopted, intercountry adoptions). The impact of prior adversity, trauma, and the influence of "toxic stress" on physical and mental health was increasingly recognized (Gunnar, 2015), whether placed as newborns or from foster care.

Elaine E. Schulte, MD, MPH, and Laurie C. Miller, MD

As the number of adopted children increased, physicians began to recognize the need for specialized care for these children. A specific group of pediatricians, physician-members of the American Academy of Pediatrics (AAP), formed the "Section of Adoption Medicine" within the AAP in 2000, and the notion of "adoption medicine" as a medical specialty was established (now known as the Council on Foster Care, Adoption, and Kinship Care). Most physicians who practice "adoption medicine" are board-certified pediatricians who have a special interest in adopted children. Some are general pediatricians, while others are pediatric subspecialists (e.g., infectious disease or developmental-behavioral specialists). Some focus more on children who are internationally adopted, and others specialize in children adopted from (or living in) foster care. There are no certification requirements for a physician to practice adoption medicine. Adoption medicine physicians provide a range of services, including pre-adoption consultations, comprehensive post-adoption evaluations, and ongoing pediatric primary care or subspecialty pediatric care. Some provide all these services, while others provide select ones. Some provide pre-adoption consultation for free, or at nominal cost, while others charge a larger, onetime fee or use a "retainer" model (meaning, that parents can access them over a predetermined amount of time). For pre-adoption services, most adoption medicine physicians work with families remotely, although some meet families face-to-face when possible.

Once placed with their adoptive families, a best practice is for newly adopted children to undergo a comprehensive post-placement medical evaluation. This exam can be completed by an adoptive medicine physician in a specialized adoption clinic or by any pediatrician or family medicine provider (Long et al., 2018; Jones et al., 2019). Referrals to medical specialists and/or mental health providers may be necessary to manage specific problems identified in the evaluation.

Populations of Adopted Children

Approximately 2.4% of children in the United States are adopted, accounting for 2.1 million children (Jones et al., 2020). It is difficult to obtain exact numbers of annual adoptions, as data are compiled differently in each state and definitions of types of adoptions (public vs. private) vary. Overall, however, adoptions from foster care have remained relatively constant over the last ten years, while the number of children adopted internationally has decreased significantly. This decrease has been attributed to changing policies towards adoption and social change in several of the more frequent sending countries.

Children come into adoption through several pathways: domestically (as newborns or through the foster care system) or through intercountry adoption. The pre-adoption experience is quite different for each of these groups of adopted children. For example, foster care and international adoptees may spend time prior to placement with their birth families. For all children placed in adoptions, the birth parents and birth family are unable or unwilling to care for the child. Unfortunately,

Table 9.1 Possible Adverse Experiences Prior to Adoptive Placement

- Undernutrition
- Micronutrient deficiencies
- Emotional neglect
- Physical neglect
- Abuse (physical, sexual)
- Lack of medical care
- Exposure to infections

the early life histories of many adoptees are complicated by various prenatal and/or postnatal adversities (see Miller, 2005), which may have long-lasting effects. Table 9.1 presents the array of adverse experiences a child may experience prior to adoption.

The severity, duration, and timing of these adversities vary widely; likewise, the susceptibilities of individual children to these deprivations also vary.

There have been major changes in the women who place infants for adoption. It is not often an adolescent with an unplanned pregnancy, because most adolescents now decide to parent. Children adopted as domestic newborns are commonly born to women who live in high-stress situations, often with lack of social support, lack of access to medical care, and have frequent exposure to substances like tobacco, alcohol, marijuana, and opioids. Women who make an adoption plan are parenting other children but cannot parent another child.

Children adopted internationally typically have spent parts of their early life living in institutions, where they may have experienced malnutrition, exposure to infections, neglect, and/or physical, emotional, and sexual abuse. Frequent moves and orphanage policies may interfere with the development of healthy attachments and emotional bonds to caretakers. Experiences in institutions vary widely, depending on the overall size, the caregiver-to-child ratio, staff training and attitudes, material resources, the quality and quantity of nutrition, and access to medical care. A small number of internationally adopted children live in foster homes prior to placement; some of these children (notably in South Korea) benefit from consistent and attentive caregivers and regular, appropriate medical care. Over the last ten years, there has been an increase in the proportion of newly arriving internationally adopted children who have special medical needs. Common medical diagnoses include cleft lip, cleft palate, congenital heart disease, limb deformities, ear deformities, hemoglobinopathies, and gastrointestinal malformations. Some of these children have had surgical procedures prior to adoption. These medical special needs may pose additional challenges to the child and the adoptive family (Miller et al., 2021).

Children adopted from US foster care have usually been removed from parental care due to abuse or neglect. The average age of a foster child in the United States waiting to be adopted is 8.4 years. Children entering foster care wait an average of 32 months before adoption (US Department of Health and Human Services, 2020).

Many children in foster care suffer emotional neglect, rupture of attachments, and other negative experiences (Jones et al., 2020). Not surprisingly, children adopted from the US foster care system have a high prevalence of chronic medical, mental health, developmental, dental, and educational problems (Szilagyi et al., 2015).

Challenges Faced by Adoptees at Adolescence Related to Early Life Experiences

This section will review the issues faced by adoptees at adolescence related to their early life history and experiences. Infectious diseases, school issues, and behavior problems related to pre-adoption experiences may manifest for the first time in adolescence. The conditions may have been previously overlooked or come to medical attention after long latent periods or progression of symptoms. In other situations, problems emerge as the individual faces increasing challenges, such as at school or in social situations. It is difficult to know the true impact of early life experiences for adopted adolescents and young adults. There are many research gaps in identifying long-term outcomes of early medical and psychosocial conditions.

Infectious Diseases

Unrecognized infectious diseases are a concern for many intercountry adoptees; this is less common for domestically adopted newborns. Little is known about unrecognized infectious diseases in children adopted from foster care. Most international adoptees arrive before the age of 4 years. As described previously, the initial medical examination is designed to identify important infectious diseases at the time of entry into the United States (Long et al., 2018); if properly done, this screening greatly reduces the risk of an unrecognized infectious disease. However, occasionally, parts of the screening examination are not completed. As a consequence, the child may present in late childhood or adolescence with a previously unrecognized infectious disease. Some of these conditions have consequences not only for the individual but also for the child's family and for public health in general.

Tuberculosis (TB)

Roughly 23% of the world's population is infected with TB (Centers for Disease Control & Prevention, 2020b). Many of the sending countries for international adoption have endemic/widespread TB. Crowded orphanage conditions, combined with the lack of screening of orphanage staff, increase the likelihood of TB infection in international adoptees.

TB screening is mandated for all new arrivals, with the tuberculin skin test or with the newer IGRA (interferon-release assay) test (Long et al., 2018). Unfortunately, this screening may be overlooked; it may not be read or read correctly. TB screening should be repeated six or more months after the child's arrival to identify children who had "false negative" results at arrival. False negatives can be due to malnutrition, concurrent viral infection, or very recent exposure to TB. A study by Trehan et al. (2008), which has not been updated, found positive tuberculin skin tests in 20% of 191 intercountry adoptees who had had a negative skin test three months previously. When TB infection is missed, it usually remains in a latent state. However, the infection may become active. There is a lack of understanding and tools to predict who will and who will not progress from latent to active TB (Blumberg et al., 2016); it is known that the risk of TB activation increases if the infected person becomes immunocompromised. Once activated, the infection most commonly manifests in the lungs. Coughing can readily spread these pathogenic microbes, creating a public health hazard. Adolescents are considered to be more contagious than younger children, probably because of a more forceful cough and the higher sputum mycobacterial load (Piccini et al., 2017)). In a Swiss study of adolescent immigrants from TB-endemic regions who were not properly screened at arrival, latent TB infection was found in almost half of the individuals (Steppacher et al., 2014).

Chronic Viral Infections

Adoptees should be screened for hepatitis B, hepatitis C, and HIV at arrival (Long et al., 2018). As with TB, a best practice is for the tests for these three viral infections be done at arrival and repeated six months later, to account for the possibility of initial testing during "the seronegative window period" (a brief period after infection when diagnostic tests for these viruses may be negative). If this protocol is not followed, a chronic viral infection may go unrecognized and untreated. Untreated, long-term infection with any of these three viruses has serious consequences. Chronic infection with either hepatitis B or hepatitis C may result in progressive liver damage, cirrhosis, liver failure, or liver cancer. HIV infection leads to progressive immunodeficiency and is usually fatal without treatment.

Each of these three viruses is spread by body fluids (hepatitis B is by far the most contagious); the child may be the unwitting source of infection for others. This is especially important during adolescence, when many teens begin sexual activities. For children with a known chronic viral infection which has not responded to treatment, the pediatrician plays an important role in helping the infected teen understand how to navigate potentially difficult conversations with prospective sex partners.

Parasites

Intestinal parasites are the most common infection identified in newly arrived international adoptees. Most, but not all, of these parasites cause obvious symptoms, such as diarrhea, abdominal pain, flatulence, and poor appetite. With proper treatment and appropriate follow-up testing, most intestinal parasites can be readily eradicated.

However, parasites occasionally may evade detection. Overlooked parasite infection should be considered as a cause of persistent gastrointestinal symptoms in internationally adopted adolescents, regardless of earlier testing results.

Non-intestinal parasites may also be of concern. Neurocysticercosis results from infection with the pork tapeworm *Taenia solium* that is found in undercooked pork (Silver et al., 1996; Zammarchi et al., 2016). The tapeworm cysts settle in the brain. While this infection may lay dormant for decades, the cysts can cause seizures that can be misdiagnosed as idiopathic epilepsy if appropriate imaging studies are not done.

Chagas disease, or American trypanosomiasis, is a blood-borne (not primarily intestinal) infection which may not become symptomatic until many years after infection (Basile et al., 2011). Over time, up to 30% of chronically infected people develop cardiac alterations and up to 10% develop digestive, neurological, or mixed symptoms that may require specific treatment. Infected women may transmit the parasite to their unborn children. In later years, the infection can lead to sudden death due to cardiac arrhythmias or progressive heart failure caused by the destruction of the heart muscle and its nervous system. The disease is most often found in countries of Central and South America. Thus, this diagnosis should be considered in adolescent adoptees and young adults from these regions who develop unexplained neurologic, cardiac, gastrointestinal, or other unexplained symptoms.

School Issues

Most children adopted from foster care or internationally have some type of developmental delay upon arrival into their adopted families (Schulte, 2021). Although many of these children make developmental gains after adoption, it is impossible to predict which children will catch up quickly and which will have ongoing learning needs and attentional and other psychological challenges. Pre-adoption and post-adoption factors both contribute to a child's developmental trajectory (Szilagyi et al., 2015; Jones et al., 2020). Compounding past maltreatment, disrupted home, and educational experiences, children adopted from foster care have a greater prevalence of prenatal alcohol and substance exposure. These cause neurodevelopmental disabilities which increase the risk for learning and behavioral challenges (Jones et al., 2019) (discussed in detail next).

Learning Disorders (LD)

The American Academy of Pediatrics describes a *learning disorder* (LD) as a range of learning problems (Silver et al., 2010) related to the way the brain receives, uses, stores, and transmits information. Children with LDs may have trouble with one or more of the following skills: reading, writing, listening, speaking, reasoning, abstract and critical thinking, and math. As many as 15% of children in the general population have an LD. An LD can appear at any point in time, not just when a child starts school. Many children find ways to work around their academic challenges, until, at some point, the schoolwork just becomes too hard. For some children, an LD is first diagnosed during adolescence.

Children adopted internationally often arrive with language delays in their birth language, usually because there were limited interactions with adults. A child adopted from foster care may have delays caused by inconsistent care or education. Early language delays can place an adopted child at risk for language-based learning difficulties.

Attention-Deficit/Hyperactivity Disorder (ADHD)

Depending on the source, estimates indicate that somewhere between 6% and 15% of school-aged children have some sort of attention challenge (Centers for Disease Control & Prevention, 2020a). The proportion of adopted children diagnosed with ADHD is not known with certainty, but research suggests that it is more common in this population compared to non-adopted children (Abrines, 2012). This biologically based developmental disorder affects a child's behavior, attention, and ability to learn.

Recognizing ADHD in the adopted child is important. Making the diagnosis is relatively straightforward, using standardized instruments such as the Connors Comprehensive Rating Scales or NICHQ Vanderbilt Assessment Scales. The causes of ADHD are unknown; risk factors for ADHD include genetics (Thapar et al., 2013), prematurity (Franz et al., 2018), and prenatal exposure to alcohol (Infante et al., 2015). In adoptees, understanding the cause(s) is complicated due to limited or lack of birth history or family medical history.

ADHD is not a learning disorder, yet it can make it hard for a child to do well in school. ADHD can coexist with learning disabilities as well as mental health challenges, such as anxiety and depression. Oppositional defiant disorder or conduct disorder occur in up to 27% of children with ADHD (Infante et al., 2015). This type of coexisting condition is more common among children with the primarily hyperactive and impulsive and combination types of ADHD.

Additionally, there are a number of conditions that may mimic symptoms of ADHD. A child with a learning disability may have difficulties attending to and mastering specific skills, such as reading and math. A pragmatic language disorder may not show up with standard tests of language and look like a problem with attention. Sensory processing disorder can also mimic ADHD. Children with depression or anxiety may first present with inability to attend and be misdiagnosed. The adopted teen may have a history of posttraumatic stress disorder that can also mimic or overlap symptoms of ADHD. Trauma can affect a child's working memory, inhibitory control, and cognitive flexibility (Spann et al., 2012).

Stimulant medications are most commonly prescribed, along with age-appropriate therapy. Parents may also want to consider parenting courses to help understand their child's ADHD and help with coping strategies. Many helpful resources are available online (https://chadd.org/for-parents/overview/ or https://wwwhealthy-children.org/English/health-issues/conditions/adhd/Pages/default.aspx).

Late Manifestations of Early Exposure to Lead

Lead is a hazardous neurotoxin; children may be exposed both pre- and postnatally to lead. Elevated lead levels have been associated with attention deficits, increased impulsivity, reduced school performance, aggression, and delinquent behavior. Targeted lead screening is recommended between 12 and 24 months of age in all children, and for children adopted from foster care, and in all newly placed international adoptees. Even if elevated lead levels are identified and treated appropriately, an increased risk of neurodevelopmental and behavioral problems in adolescence and adulthood has been reported in several studies (Sampson et al., 2018; Desrochers-Couture et al., 2019; Shadbegian et al., 2019). Furthermore, fetal exposure to maternal cumulative lead burden may influence long-term epigenetic programming and disease susceptibility in the child throughout the life course (Pilsner et al., 2009).

Prenatal Exposures

Understanding the precise etiology of the school and behavior problems experienced by adoptees is incomplete. However, adverse prenatal exposures have been linked to several of these outcomes. Some evidence suggests that adoptees are at increased risk of adverse prenatal exposures to substances, including alcohol and illicit drugs. In addition, it is likely that many birth mothers of children placed in adoptions experience elevated levels of depression and stress during the pregnancy. These adverse prenatal exposures increase the risk of complicated neurobehavioral outcomes in childhood and adolescence and, accordingly, may affect the adaptation and function of adoptees as teens and young adults. Additionally, adoptive parents often wish to know if prenatal exposure to substance abuse increases the risk that the child will also abuse the substance.

Prenatal Exposure to Alcohol (PEA)

Alcohol use during pregnancy occurs worldwide, despite its recognition as an important fetal teratogen. The most severe form is fetal alcohol syndrome (FAS): this is characterized by obvious facial dysmorphology, growth delays, especially microcephaly, and many psycho-behavioral problems. When physical signs are absent but behavioral and/or cognitive effects and a history of PEA are present, the diagnosis alcohol-related neurodevelopmental disorder (ARND) is applied (Coles et al., 2020). Maternal history of alcohol intake during pregnancy is usually not available. In a recent study from an Israeli adoption clinic, 72% of 89 foster care children being placed in adoptions had signs of PEA, but only 18 of the children had histories confirming maternal alcohol use during pregnancy (Tenenbaum et al., 2020).

Numerous cognitive and behavioral problems have been identified in association with PEA. Issues related to global intelligence, language, academic achievement, executive function, arousal (irritability), coordination, state and sensory regulation have been recognized in young children with prenatal alcohol exposure (Rodriguez et al., 2009, Doyle et al., 2019, Lees et al., 2020, Mitchell et al., 2020, Nissinen et al., 2021). Many of these problems persist into adolescence and adulthood. Some researchers have stated that as many as 90% of individuals with PEA have mental health problems (Streissguth et al., 1994); these include internalizing and externalizing behaviors, conduct disorders, psychosis, suicidality, and substance abuse. During adolescence and young adulthood, these problems may become more challenging (Easey et al., 2019, Easey et al., 2020, Flannigan et al., 2020). Major cognitive impairments may worsen: in one study, a median IQ of 86 in childhood declined significantly to 71 by adulthood (Landgren et al., 2019). Serious suicide attempts in males with PEA are >19 times the US national norms (O'Connor et al., 2019). Mental health problems create many difficulties in the individual's ability to function: in a recent report from Australia, the prevalence of PEA was 10–40 times higher among specialized populations (correctional facilities, residential care, etc.) than in the general population (Popova et al., 2019).

Family context is an important factor in the neurobehavioral outcomes of individuals with PEA. Some research suggests an increased risk of substance abuse by adolescents with PEA (Pfinder et al., 2013). For example, in a Swedish registry study, including >18,000 adoptees. Alcohol use disorders in the adoptees were significantly predicted by alcohol use disorders in the biological parents (OR 1.46; 95% CI, 1.29–1.66) and siblings (OR 1.94; 95% CI, 1.55–2.44), but also the adoptive parents (OR 1.40; 95% CI, 1.09–1.80) (Kendler et al., 2015). Prior studies have shown that children with PEA who lived with their biological parents had worse behavior problems and worse developmental delays than children with PEA who were adopted at birth (Koponen et al., 2009, 2013). In a recent adoption study of individuals with PEA, rates of difficulty with the law were lower among those living with adoptive or other family members compared with those living in child welfare care. However, the rate of mood disorders was higher among those living with adoptive/other family members compared with child welfare care (Burns et al., 2021). The authors speculate that mental health problems may be more closely monitored and treated in the child welfare setting. As an alternative hypothesis, adoptive/other family members may have been more vigilant in identifying problems and seeking diagnoses and treatments for their children. Regardless, individuals with suspected PEA deserve careful pediatric follow-up and prospective family guidance.

Prenatal Drug Exposure (PDE)

Overall, PDE increases the likelihood that offspring will exhibit symptoms of ADHD, externalizing behaviors (Sagiv et al., 2013), and learning disabilities (Leppert et al., 2019). Notably, in a study of 233 children evaluated ~8 years after domestic adoption (Barth et al., 2000), those with PDE (n = 121, various combinations of cocaine, heroin, marijuana, PCP, as well as alcohol [85%] and tobacco [90%]) were twice as likely to be enrolled in classes for the learning-disabled, compared to those without PDE. However, their adoptive parents reported similar closeness, quality of family relations, and satisfaction with the adoption as the parents of non-drug-exposed children.

The risk of illicit drug use in adoptees with PDE seems to be low and more closely related to issues in the adoptive family (divorce, psychiatric disturbances) and older age at placement (>5 months, in this study) than the prenatal exposure (Cadoret et al., 1995). Drug abuse was highly correlated with an antisocial personality, which was predicted by an antisocial birth parent (information retrieved from adoption agency records) (Cadoret et al., 1995). Clearly, behavior, cognitive, and emotional disturbances in some individuals with PDE could predispose to substance abuse, as confirmed in a recent Norwegian survey of 45 international adoptees. Depression and ADHD were particular risk factors for substance abuse by PDE adolescents (Askeland et al., 2018).

Prenatal Exposure to Stress

Prenatal exposure to stress is another important driver of long-term outcomes. Pregnant women may experience many forms of stress, including emotional and physical. Birth mothers in difficult situations which result in the adoptive placement of their children are especially likely to experience excess stress during pregnancy. The fetus is particularly vulnerable to the mother's stress. Even prenatal exposure to an isolated adverse weather event (e.g., Quebec ice storm, hurricanes, volcano eruptions) has been linked to adverse and long-term mental health outcomes, including increased risks of autism, depression, and schizophrenia (Watson et al., 1999, Kinney et al., 2008, King et al., 2012).

Individuals exposed to prenatal stress have persistent alterations in their hormonal regulation of stress (hypothalamic-pituitary-adrenal [HPA] axis function). Children placed in adoptions after early institutionalization have aberrant regulation of cortisol responses (Fries et al., 2008, Kroupina et al., 2012, Hostinar et al., 2015, Shirtcliff et al., 2021). Results from the Bucharest Early Intervention Project support both the persistence of these findings and the relationship to institutionalization: 12-year-olds assigned to "Care as Usual" (e.g., who remained institutionalized) had blunted stress responses measured both by autonomic and HPA axis reactivity, while children randomized to a foster care intervention had more normative responses (and those randomized to foster care before 24 months of age did not differ from age-matched community controls) (Cameron et al., 2017).

In other studies, a history of institutional rearing has been associated with broad changes in cortical volume even after controlling for variability in head size. The prefrontal cortex is especially susceptible to early adversity, with significant reductions in volume (driven primarily by differences in surface area rather than cortical thickness) in post-institutionalized youth. Hippocampal volumes are associated with duration of institutional care: later-adopted children have the smallest volumes relative to non-adopted controls. Altered amygdala volumes have been found in some but not all post-institutionalized children (Tottenham et al., 2010, Hodel et al., 2015). Also to be considered would be the birth mother's stress, while pregnant, regarding the anticipated separation from her unborn child.

Prenatal maternal stress is sometimes accompanied by maternal undernutrition. Multiple studies of humanitarian disasters, such as the Dutch Hunger Winter, Chinese Great Leap Forward Famine, Leningrad Siege, Biafran Famine, and World War II–related food deprivation in France (reviewed in (Mink et al., 2020), have highlighted the links between prenatal exposure to maternal undernutrition and later development in the offspring of non-communicable diseases (e.g., insulin resistance, dyslipidemia, type 2 diabetes, obesity, metabolic syndrome, and schizophrenia). More severe outcomes are associated with adverse exposures early in gestation. A similar cardiometabolic risk profile (e.g., higher systolic blood pressure, total cholesterol, low-density lipoprotein cholesterol, triglycerides, and insulin levels) has been documented in post-institutionalized children (Reid et al., 2018). Although specific screening for these conditions is not currently recommended for adolescents with suspected prenatal exposure to stress or other adversities, the risk of these non-communicable diseases should be kept in mind by the caring physician.

Physician's Approach to Adolescent and Young Adult Adoptees

Most health-care providers know that conversations with teenagers can be challenging, regardless of adoption status. Providers must first establish trust with the teen, and eventually, the adolescent will develop a sense of comfort with the provider. When approaching an adopted adolescent patient for the first time, it is important that providers speak from a sense of curiosity and support, rather than a position of authority. Asking open-ended questions about birth history, family of origin medical history, and any past medical history will help build trust.

Occasionally, a health-care provider may encounter a teen who knows very little about their adoption history. In these instances, using neutral language is the best approach (e.g., "Tell me what you know about your family of origin," "What do you know about your adoption?" or "What questions do you have about your family of origin or your adoption?"). For example, adopted teens may not know anything about their birth family's medical histories. They may have questions about their own medical (e.g., asthma) or mental health issues (e.g., depression) and whether these conditions were inherited, and what the likelihood might be that such conditions would be passed on to their own children. It can be uncomfortable and awkward when the adolescent doesn't know or have the complete story about her past. This presents an opportunity for the provider to share statements of empathy (e.g., "It must be hard not knowing information about your birth families' health. What do you wish you understood?")

Other topics that may come up in conversation during a medical visit might include a discussion about the teen's adoptive parent(s) or sibling(s). If an adoptive family member is confronted with a medical issue, the teen may be terrified about losing this member of their family. Even if the medical issue is not serious, the degree of concern may seem excessive. Concern about an ill parent or grandparent may trigger behavioral outbursts. Reactions to the death of grandparents or relatives may be extreme. These anxieties relate to the teen's early (likely pre-verbal) experience of separation and loss.

Some adoptees may be particularly anxious about their own medical conditions. The rash that won't go away may be perceived as "deadly." Or the chronic headaches may be interpreted as "I must have a brain tumor." When family medical issues arise, the adopted adolescent may wonder how the illness or condition might affect her. For example, if her adoptive father has a heart attack, she may wonder about her own risk factors for heart disease. The provider can use these situations as opportunities to provide medical education and anticipatory guidance, in a very straightforward and objective manner, while being very sensitive to the fact that the adolescent may have enhanced underlying worries about her own mortality as well as that of members of her birth family, along with underlying anxiety.

Adolescent Adjustment

Adolescence is a challenging period for all young people; adoption renders these challenges even more complicated. While age at adoption and pre-adoption experiences vary widely, all adoptees share the loss of their birth families. This loss may be felt differently at various stages of life. Adoptees may experience periods of loss and grief for their family of origin and self-questioning as they traverse certain challenges in adolescence and young adulthood. They may wonder not only about birth parents but also of birth siblings and other biologically related relatives. Such periods of questioning have been called "normative crises" of adoption (Pavao, 2005). These episodes require emotional support and should not be evaluated as pathological; they are a typical part of adoptee developmental adjustment.

However, there are concerns that may not have been recognized when an adopted person is young that become prominent during adolescence and young adulthood. These are new or worsening behavior problems.

Several reviews and meta-analyses have highlighted an increase in both internalizing and externalizing behavior problems among adoptees (e.g., Juffer et al., 2005; Dekker et al., 2017; Melero et al., 2017). Early institutional rearing has been associated with long-lasting brain structural abnormalities, particularly in areas associated with emotional regulation (prefrontal cortex, hippocampus, amygdala) (Tottenham et al., 2010, Sheridan et al., 2012, Hodel et al., 2015, VanTieghem et al., 2021). Several registry studies have highlighted the increased prevalence of behavior problems in adoptees but have also emphasized that most adoptees do well (Hjern et al., 2002, Melero et al., 2017, van Ginkel et al., 2018, Strand et al., 2020). Some studies suggest that behavior problems persist; others find that behavior problems decrease over time (Gunnar et al., 2007, Melero et al., 2017, Hjern et al., 2020). These differences likely can be explained by the different populations observed. Further details about behavior problems and adjustment in adopted adolescents are found in other chapters.

Health-Care Management

The AAP provides standard recommendations for initial medical screenings of children who are adopted or in foster care (Long et al., 2018). These screenings include tests for medical conditions, as well as developmental screening. Newly adopted children are also assessed for immunization status. It is important to know that most newly adopted children will have at least one undiagnosed medical condition at the time of adoption (Jones et al., 2019). Between 60 and 80% of children adopted from foster care will have at least one medical condition at the time of adoption (Szilagyi et al., 2015).

Regardless of when the adoption occurred, the medical provider must be aware of specific medical issues, in addition to routine health-care maintenance, as adopted children become adolescents. Providers must be cognizant of the possibility of diseases of long latency, missed diagnoses, or progression of symptoms. For example, anemia or lead poisoning at arrival could contribute to school problems, while pre-adoption sexual abuse may manifest as behavioral disorders in adolescence.

An additional medical consideration that may occur as internationally adopted children grow and develop is early entry into puberty (medically described as "precocious puberty"). Some (Teilmann et al., 2006, Soriano-Guillén et al., 2010) but not all reports (Hayes, 2013) suggest that this condition is more common among adoptees. A study in Spain suggested that adoptees had ~28-fold higher relative risk of precocious puberty than either non-adoptees; for immigrants, the risk was 1.55-fold higher than non-adoptees (Soriano-Guillén et al., 2010). The condition is more common in females than in males, and it is more common among females who were adopted at a later age. There are multiple factors that influence the onset of puberty, including the shift from a low-protein diet to a balanced diet, exposure to toxins, psychologic factors, and rapid weight-for-height recovery (Miller, 2005). Children who are adopted are frequently much smaller than their aged-matched peers on arrival; the typical rapid catch-up growth seen in most children may be a trigger for early onset of puberty and its associated early menarche and premature cessation of bone growth (Mason, 2014).

Puberty can be medically delayed, which will help the child continue to grow, maximizing the final adult height. Treatment should be left up to the primary care provider with the guidance of pediatric endocrinologists. Occasionally, the question of age assignment may arise, and this further complicates the management.

In addition to medical specialists, mental health providers may also be needed to provide support to both the child and the parents.

Based on the increased likelihood of adopted children having medical and emotional challenges, it is important that families work with a health-care provider who can provide a "medical home" for the child. A medical home offers comprehensive medical care, with care coordination to medical subspecialists and mental health professionals as needed. After the adoptive placement, the primary care provider will schedule regular visits to ensure that growth and development are progressing in an age-appropriate manner, to monitor for any issues, and to be available for child and family support.

Health-care providers should be prepared to address additional, often challenging topics, during these conversations with adopted adolescents and their parents. Some adolescents struggle with gastrointestinal issues and disordered eating (Strand et al., 2020), weight management, sexual health, pregnancy prevention, intimacy and attachment issues, behavior problems, and gender identity (Shumer et al., 2017).

For the adopted teen, any type of transition (e.g., graduating from middle school and going onto high school, moving into a new home), while exciting, can trigger strong, unwanted feelings of change that may trigger old, subconscious feelings of separation and loss. While many adolescents wrestle with self-esteem issues as part of typical development (Mohanty, 2013), a meta-analysis showed that adopted teens do not lack self-esteem (Juffer et al., 2007). However, adopted teens are more likely to struggle with mental health challenges and high-risk behaviors.

The primary care provider may be one of the adults outside the family in whom the adopted teen can confide. Ideally, the patient, and their family, have developed an ongoing relationship with the provider over time. For this reason, the teen may be more likely to share intimate thoughts and feelings with their doctor. The doctor should be prepared for the adopted adolescent to raise questions about searching for members of their birth family. Adopted adolescents are typically reluctant to discuss search with their adoptive parents because they don't want to hurt their feelings. However, adopted teens often search on the internet for members of their families of origin, sometimes without the knowledge or support of their adoptive parents.

The physician should also be prepared to talk with the adopted adolescent about issues related to peer relationships, stigma, microaggressions, and discrimination (Sue et al., 2007, Baden, 2016, Miller et al., 2020, Miller et al., 2021). Many of these difficult situations play out in the school environment. Occasionally, lack of sensitivity of school personnel (teachers, administrators) may result in inappropriate comments or projects (e.g., "family tree"). Comments – intentional or not – from peers can result in the child feeling bullied. When aware, parents can be wonderful advocates for their child. If the teen discloses to the physician, the physician may want to refer to the "Observe/Why?/Think/Feel/Desire" (OWTFD) approach to help the teen handle inappropriate comments (Sotto-Santiago et al., 2020).

Conclusions

Adolescent adoptees, whether adopted domestically as newborns, from foster care, or internationally, are at high risk for consequences from early adversity. Long-term effects of emotional and physical deprivation, poor nutrition, and increased risk of infectious diseases may manifest in adolescence. Medical professionals, mental health providers, and educators must provide "adoption-friendly" and adoption-informed support to adopted adolescents and their families to ensure their adjustment and well-being.

Endnotes

Abrines, N. (2012). ADHD-like symptoms and attachment in internationally adopted children. Attachment & Human Development, 14(4): 405–423.

Askeland, K.G., B. Sivertsen, J.C. Skogen, A.M. La Greca, G.S. Tell, L.E. Aarø and M. Hysing. (2018). Alcohol and drug use among internationally adopted adolescents: Results from a Norwegian population-based study. American Journal of Orthopsychiatry, 88(2): 226–235.

Baden, A. (2016). "Do you know your real parents?" And other adoption microaggressions. Adoption Quarterly, 19(1): 1–25.

Barth, R.P. and D. Brooks. (2000). Outcomes for drug-exposed children eight years post-adoption. In R. P. Barth, M. Freundlich and D. Brodzinsky (Eds.), Adoption and Prenatal Alcohol and Drug Exposure. Washington, DC: Child Welfare League of America, pp. 23–58.

Basile, L., J. Jansa, Y., Carlier, D.D. Salamanca, A. Angheben, A. Bartoloni, J. Seixas, T. Van Gool, C. Cañavate and M. Flores-Chávez. (2011). Chagas disease in European countries: the challenge of a surveillance system. Eurosurveillance, 16(37): 19968.

Blumberg, H.M. and J.D. Ernst. (2016). The challenge of latent TB infection. Jama, 316(9): 931–933.

Burns, J., D.E. Badry, K.D. Harding, N. Roberts, K. Unsworth and J.L. Cook. (2021). Comparing outcomes of children and youth with fetal alcohol spectrum disorder (FASD) in the child welfare system to those in other living situations in Canada: Results from the Canadian national FASD database. Child: Care, Health and Development, 47(1): 77–84.

Cadoret, R.J., W.R. Yates, G. Woodworth and M.A. Stewart. (1995). Genetic-environmental interaction in the genesis of aggressivity and conduct disorders. Archives of General Psychiatry, 52(11): 916–924.

Cameron, J.L., K L. Eagleson, N.A. Fox, T.K. Hensch and P. Levitt (2017). Social Origins of Developmental Risk for Mental and Physical Illness. The Journal of Neuroscience, 37(45): 10783–10791.

Centers for Disease Control and Prevention. (2020a). ADHD. Retrieved November 16, 2020, from Error! Hyperlink reference not valid.

Centers for Disease Control and Prevention. (2020b). Tuberculosis. Retrieved April 17, 2021, from Error! Hyperlink reference not valid.

Coles, C.D., W. Kalberg, J.A. Kable, B. Tabachnick, P.A. May and C.D. Chambers. (2020). Characterizing alcohol-related neurodevelopmental disorder: Prenatal alcohol exposure and the spectrum of outcomes. Alcoholism: Clinical and Experimental Research, 44(6): 1245–1260.

Dekker, M.C., W. Tieman, A.G., Vinke, J. van der Ende, F.C. Verhulst and F. Juffer. (2017). Mental health problems of Dutch young adult domestic adoptees compared to non-adopted peers and international adoptees. International Social Work, 60(5): 1201–1217.

Desrochers-Couture, M.Y., Courtemanche, N. Forget-Dubois, R.E. Bélanger, O. Boucher, P. Ayotte, S. Cordier, J.L. Jacobson, S.W. Jacobson and G. Muckle. (2019). Association between early lead exposure and externalizing behaviors in adolescence: A developmental cascade. Environmental Research, 178: 108679.

Doyle, L.R., L. Glass, J.R.Wozniak, J.A. Kable, E.P. Riley, C.D. Coles, E.R. Sowell, K.L. Jones, S.N. Mattson and T. CIFASD. (2019). Relation between oppositional/conduct behaviors and executive function among youth with histories of heavy prenatal alcohol exposure. Alcoholism: Clinical and Experimental Research, 43(6): 1135–1144.

Easey, K.E., M.L. Dyer, N.J. Timpson and M.R. Munafò. (2019). Prenatal alcohol exposure and offspring mental health: A systematic review. Drug and Alcohol Dependence, 197: 344–353.

Easey, K.E., N.J. Timpson and M.R. Munafò. (2020). Association of prenatal alcohol exposure and offspring depression: A negative control analysis of maternal and partner consumption. Alcoholism: Clinical and Experimental Research, 44(5): 1132–1140.

Flannigan, K., K.D. Coons-Harding, T. Anderson, L. Wolfson, A. Campbell, M. Mela and J. Pei. (2020). A systematic review of interventions to improve mental health and substance use outcomes for individuals with prenatal alcohol exposure and fetal alcohol spectrum disorder. Alcoholism: Clinical and Experimental Research, 44(12): 2401–2430.

Franz, A.P., G.U. Bolat, H. Bolat, A. Matijasevich, I.S. Santos, R.C. Silveira, R.S. Procianoy, L. A. Rohde and C.R. Moreira-Maia. (2018). Attention-deficit/hyperactivity disorder and very preterm/very low birth weight: A meta-analysis. Pediatrics, 141(1).

Fries, A.B.W., E.A. Shirtcliff and S.D. Pollak. (2008). Neuroendocrine dysregulation following early social deprivation in children. Developmental Psychobiology, 50(6): 588–599.

Gunnar, M.R. (2015). The effects of early life stress on neurobehavioral development in children and adolescents: Mediation by the HPA axis. Psychoneuroendocrinology, 61: 3.

Gunnar, M.R. and M.H. Van Dulmen. (2007). Behavior problems in postinstitutionalized internationally adopted children. Development and Psychopathology, 19(1): 129–148.

Hayes, P. (2013). International adoption,"early" puberty, and underrecorded age. Pediatrics, 131(6): 1029–1031.

Hjern, A., F. Lindblad and B. Vinnerljung. (2002). Suicide, psychiatric illness, and social maladjustment in intercountry adoptees in Sweden: A cohort study. The Lancet, 360(9331): 443–448.

Hjern, A., J. Palacios, B. Vinnerljung, H. Manhica and F. Lindblad. (2020). Increased risk of suicidal behaviour in non-European international adoptees decreases with age – A Swedish national cohort study. EClinicalMedicine, 29–30: 100643.

Hodel, A.S., R.H. Hunt, R.A. Cowell, S.E. Van Den Heuvel, M.R. Gunnar and K.M. Thomas. (2015). Duration of early adversity and structural brain development in post-institutionalized adolescents. NeuroImage, 105: 112–119.

Hostinar, C.E., A.E. Johnson and M.R. Gunnar. (2015). Early social deprivation and the social buffering of cortisol stress responses in late childhood: An experimental study. Developmental Psychology, 51(11): 1597.

Infante, M.A., E.M. Moore, T.T. Nguyen, N. Fourligas, S.N. Mattson and E.P. Riley. (2015). Objective assessment of ADHD core symptoms in children with heavy prenatal alcohol exposure. Physiology & Behavior, 148: 45–50.

Johnson, D.E. (2005). International adoption: What is fact, what is fiction, and what is the future? Pediatric Clinics of North America, 52(5): 1221–1246, v.

Jones, V.F., E.E. Schulte, A. Council On Foster Care and C. Kinship. (2019). Comprehensive health evaluation of the newly adopted child. Pediatrics, 143(5).

Jones, V.F., E.E. Schulte, D. Waite, A. Council On Foster Care and C. Kinship. (2020). Pediatrician guidance in supporting families of children who are adopted, fostered, or in kinship care. Pediatrics, 146(6).

Juffer, F. and M.H. van IJzendoorn. (2005). Behavior problems and mental health referrals of international adoptees: A meta-analysis. JAMA, 293(20): 2501–2515.

Juffer, F. and M.H. Van IJzendoorn. (2007). Adoptees do not lack self-esteem: A meta-analysis of studies on self-esteem of transracial, international, and domestic adoptees. Psychological Bulletin, 133(6): 1067.

Kendler, K.S., J. Ji, A.C. Edwards, H. Ohlsson, J. Sundquist and K. Sundquist. (2015). An extended swedish national adoption study of alcohol use disorder. JAMA Psychiatry, 72(3): 211–218.

King, S., K. Dancause, A.M. Turcotte-Tremblay, F. Veru and D.P. Laplante. (2012). Using natural disasters to study the effects of prenatal maternal stress on child health and development. Birth Defects Research Part C: Embryo Today: Reviews, 96(4): 273–288.

Kinney, D.K., K.M. Munir, D.J. Crowley and A.M. Miller. (2008). Prenatal stress and risk for autism. Neuroscience & Biobehavioral Reviews, 32(8): 1519–1532.

Koponen, A.M., M. Kalland and I. Autti-Rämö. (2009). Caregiving environment and socioemotional development of foster-placed FASD-children. Children and Youth Services Review, 31(9): 1049–1056.

Koponen, A.M., M. Kalland, I. Autti-Rämö, R. Laamanen and S. Suominen. (2013). Socioemotional development of children with foetal alcohol spectrum disorders in long-term foster family care: A qualitative study. Nordic Social Work Research, 3(1): 38–58.

Kroupina, M.G., A.J. Fuglestad, S.L. Iverson, J.H. Himes, P.W. Mason, M.R. Gunnar, B.S. Miller, A. Petryk and D.E. Johnson. (2012). Adoption as an intervention for institutionally reared children: HPA functioning and developmental status. Infant Behavior and Development, 35(4): 829–837.

Landgren, V., L. Svensson, E. Gyllencreutz, E. Aring, M.A. Grönlund and M. Landgren. (2019). Fetal alcohol spectrum disorders from childhood to adulthood: A Swedish population-based naturalistic cohort study of adoptees from Eastern Europe. BMJ Open, 9(10): e032407.

Lees, B., L. Mewton, J. Jacobus, E.A. Valadez, L.A. Stapinski, M. Teesson, S.F. Tapert and L.M. Squeglia. (2020). Association of prenatal alcohol exposure with psychological, behavioral, and neurodevelopmental outcomes in children from the adolescent brain cognitive development study. American Journal of Psychiatry, 177(11): 1060–1072.

Leppert, B., A. Havdahl, L. Riglin, H.J. Jones, J. Zheng, G. Davey Smith, K. Tilling, A. Thapar, T. Reichborn-Kjennerud and E. Stergiakouli. (2019). Association of maternal neurodevelopmental risk alleles with early-life exposures. JAMA Psychiatry, 76(8): 834–842.

Long, S.S., Brady, M.T., Jackson, M.A., & Kimberlin, D.W. (2018). Red Book 2018: Report of the Committee on Infectious Diseases. DuPage County, Illinois: American Academy of Pediatrics.

Mason, P.W. (2014). Long-term growth and puberty concerns for adopted children. In P.W. Mason, D.E. Johnson and L.A. Prock (Eds.), Adoption Medicine: Caring for Children and Families. Itasca: American Academy of Pediatrics.

Melero, S. and Y. Sánchez-Sandoval. (2017). Mental health and psychological adjustment in adults who were adopted during their childhood: A systematic review. Children and Youth Services Review, 77: 188–196.

Miller, L.C. (2005). The Handbook of International Adoption Medicine: A Guide for Physicians, Parents, and Providers. New York: Oxford University Press.

Miller, L.C., E. Pinderhughes, M.O. P. de Montclos, J. Matthews, J. Chomilier, J. Peyre, J. Vaugelade, F. Sorge, J.V. de Monléon and A. de Truchis. (2021). Feelings and perceptions of French parents of internationally adopted children with special needs (SN): Navigating the triple stigma of foreignness, adoption, and disability. Children and Youth Services Review, 120: 105633.

Miller, L.C., M.O.P. de Montclos, J. Matthews, J. Peyre, J. Vaugelade, O. Baubin, J. Chomilier, J.V. de Monleon, A. de Truchis and F. Sorge. (2020). Microaggressions experienced by adoptive families and internationally adopted adolescents in France. Adoption Quarterly, 23(2): 135–161.

Mink, J., M.C. Boutron-Ruault, M.A. Charles, O. Allais and G. Fagherazzi. (2020). Associations between early-life food deprivation during World War II and risk of hypertension and type 2 diabetes at adulthood. Scientific Reports, 10(1): 5741.

Mitchell, J.M., F.J. Jeffri, G.M. Maher, A.S. Khashan and F.P. McCarthy. (2020). Prenatal alcohol exposure and risk of attention deficit hyperactivity disorder in offspring: A retrospective analysis of the millennium cohort study. Journal of Affective Disorders, 269: 94–100.

Mohanty, J. (2013). Ethnic and racial socialization and self-esteem of Asian adoptees: The mediating role of multiple identities. Journal of Adolescence, 36(1): 161–170.

Nissinen, N.M., M. Gissler, T. Sarkola, H. Kahila, I. Autti-Rämö and A.M. Koponen. (2021). Completed secondary education among youth with prenatal substance exposure: A longitudinal register-based matched cohort study. Journal of Adolescence, 86: 15–27.

O'Connor, M.J., L.C. Portnoff, M. Lebsack-Coleman and K.M. Dipple. (2019). Suicide risk in adolescents with fetal alcohol spectrum disorders. Birth Defects Research, 111(12): 822–828.

Pavao, J.M. (2005). The Family of Adoption. Boston: Beacon Press.

Pfinder, M., S. Liebig and R. Feldmann. (2013). Adolescents' use of alcohol, tobacco and illicit drugs in relation to prenatal alcohol exposure: Modifications by gender and ethnicity. Alcohol and Alcoholism, 49(2): 143–153.

Piccini, P., E. Venturini, L. Bianchi, S. Baretti, P. Filidei, L. Paliaga, F. Mazzoli, E. Chiappini, M. de Martino and L. Galli. (2017). The risk of Mycobacterium tuberculosis transmission from pediatric index cases to school pupils. The Pediatric Infectious Disease Journal, 36(5): 525–528.

Pilsner, J.R., H. Hu, A. Ettinger, N. Sánchez Brisa, O. Wright Robert, D. Cantonwine, A. Lazarus, H. Lamadrid-Figueroa, A. Mercado-García, M. Téllez-Rojo Martha and M. Hernández-Avila. (2009). Influence of prenatal lead exposure on genomic methylation of cord blood DNA. Environmental Health Perspectives, 117(9): 1466–1471.

Popova, S., S. Lange, K. Shield, L. Burd and J. Rehm. (2019). Prevalence of fetal alcohol spectrum disorder among special subpopulations: A systematic review and meta-analysis. Addiction, 114(7): 1150–1172.

Reid, B.M., M.M. Harbin, J.L. Arend, A.S. Kelly, D.R. Dengel and M.R. Gunnar. (2018). Early life adversity with height stunting is associated with cardiometabolic risk in adolescents independent of body mass index. The Journal of Pediatrics, 202: 143–149.

Rodriguez, A., J. Olsen, A.J. Kotimaa, M. Kaakinen, I. Moilanen, T.B. Henriksen, K.M. Linnet, J. Miettunen, C. Obel, A. Taanila, H. Ebeling and M.R. Järvelin. (2009). Is prenatal alcohol exposure related to inattention and hyperactivity symptoms in children? Disentangling the effects of social adversity. Journal of Child Psychology and Psychiatry, 50(9): 1073–1083.

Sagiv, S.K., J.N. Epstein, D.C. Bellinger and S.A. Korrick. (2013). Pre- and postnatal risk factors for ADHD in a nonclinical pediatric population. Journal of Attention Disorders, 17(1): 47–57.

Sampson, R.J. and A.S. Winter (2018). Poisoned development: Assessing childhood lead exposure as a cause of crime in a birth cohort followed through adolescence. Criminology, 56(2): 269–301.

Schulte, E.E. (2021). Adoption: An Overview. Waltham: UpToDate.

Shadbegian, R., D. Guignet, H. Klemick and L. Bui. (2019). Early childhood lead exposure and the persistence of educational consequences into adolescence. Environmental Research, 178: 108643.

Sheridan, M.A., N.A. Fox, C.H. Zeanah, K.A. McLaughlin and C.A. Nelson. (2012). Variation in neural development as a result of exposure to institutionalization early in childhood. Proceedings of the National Academy of Sciences, 109(32): 12927–12932.

Shirtcliff, E.A., J.L. Hanson, J.M. Phan, P.L. Ruttle and S.D. Pollak. (2021). Hyper-and hypo-cortisol functioning in post-institutionalized adolescents: The role of severity of neglect and context. Psychoneuroendocrinology, 124: 105067.

Shumer, D.E., A. Abrha, H.A. Feldman and J. Carswell. (2017). Overrepresentation of adopted adolescents at a hospital-based gender dysphoria clinic. Transgender Health, 2(1): 76–79.

Silver, L.B. and D.L. Silver. (2010). Guide to Learning Disabilities for Primary Care: How to Screen, Identify, Manage, and Advocate for Children with Learning Disabilities. Itasca: American Academy of Pediatrics.

Silver, S.A., Y.S. Erozan and R.H. Hruban (1996). Cerebral cysticercosis mimicking malignant glioma: a case report. Acta Cytologica, 40(2): 351–357.

Soriano-Guillén, L., R. Corripio, J.I. Labarta, R. Cañete, L. Castro-Feijóo, R. Espino and J. Argente. (2010). Central precocious puberty in children living in Spain: incidence, prevalence, and influence of adoption and immigration. The Journal of Clinical Endocrinology & Metabolism, 95(9): 4305–4313.

Sotto-Santiago, S., J. Mac, F. Duncan and J. Smith. (2020). "I didn't know what to say": Responding to racism, discrimination, and microaggressions with the OWTFD approach. MedEdPORTAL, 16: 10971.

Spann, M.N., L.C. Mayes, J.H. Kalmar, J. Guiney, F.Y. Womer, B. Pittman, C.M. Mazure, R. Sinha and H.P. Blumberg. (2012). Childhood abuse and neglect and cognitive flexibility in adolescents. Child Neuropsychology, 18(2): 182–189.

Steppacher, A., I. Scheer, C. Relly, B. Zacek, A. Turk, E. Altpeter, C. Berger and D. Nadal. (2014). Unrecognized pediatric adult-type tuberculosis puts school contacts at risk. The Pediatric Infectious Disease Journal, 33(3): 325–328.

Strand, M., R. Zhang, L.M. Thornton, A. Birgegård, B.M.D'Onofrio and C.M. Bulik. (2020). Risk of eating disorders in international adoptees: a cohort study using Swedish national population registers. Epidemiology and Psychiatric Sciences, 29: e131.

Streissguth, A.P., H.M. Barr, P.D. Sampson and F.L. Bookstein. (1994). Prenatal alcohol and offspring development: the first fourteen years. Drug & Alcohol Dependence, 36(2): 89–99.

Sue, D.W., C.M. Capodilupo, G.C. Torino, J.M. Bucceri, A.M.B. Holder, K.L. Nadal and M. Esquilin. (2007). Racial microaggressions in everyday life: Implications for clinical practice. American Psychologist, 62: 271–286.

Szilagyi, M.A., D.S. Rosen, D. Rubin and S. Zlotnik. (2015). Health care issues for children and adolescents in foster care and kinship care. Pediatrics, 136(4): e1142–e1166.

Teilmann, G., C.B. Pedersen, N.E. Skakkebaek and T.K. Jensen. (2006). Increased risk of precocious puberty in internationally adopted children in Denmark. Pediatrics, 118(2): e391–e399.

Tenenbaum, A., A. Mandel, T. Dor, A. Sapir, O. Sapir-Bodnaro, P. Hertz and I.D. Wexler. (2020). Fetal alcohol spectrum disorder among pre-adopted and foster children. BMC Pediatrics, 20(1): 275–275.

Thapar, A., M. Cooper, O. Eyre and K. Langley. (2013). Practitioner review: what have we learnt about the causes of ADHD? Journal of Child Psychology and Psychiatry, 54(1): 3–16.

Tottenham, N., T.A. Hare, B.T. Quinn, T.W. McCarry, M. Nurse, T. Gilhooly, A. Millner, A. Galvan, M.C. Davidson and I.M. Eigsti. (2010). Prolonged institutional rearing is associated with atypically large amygdala volume and difficulties in emotion regulation. Developmental Science, 13(1): 46–61.

Trehan, I., J.K. Meinzen-Derr, L. Jamison and M.A. Staat. (2008). Tuberculosis screening in internationally adopted children: The need for initial and repeat testing. Pediatrics, 122(1): e7–e14.

U.S. Department of Health and Human Services. (2020). Preliminary Estimates for FY2019 as of June 23. Washington, DC: Y. A. F. Administration on Children, Children's Bureau.

van Ginkel, J.R., F. Juffer, M.J. Bakermans-Kranenburg and M.H. van Ijzendoorn. (2018). Young offenders caught in the act: A population-based cohort study comparing internationally adopted and non-adopted adolescents. Children and Youth Services Review, 95: 32–41.

VanTieghem, M., M. Korom, J. Flannery, T. Choy, C. Caldera, K.L. Humphreys, L. Gabard-Durnam, B. Goff, D.G. Gee and E.H. Telzer. (2021). Longitudinal changes in amygdala, hippocampus and cortisol development following early caregiving adversity. Developmental Cognitive Neuroscience, 48: 100916.

Watson, J.B., S.A. Mednick, M. Huttunen and X. Wang. (1999). Prenatal teratogens and the development of adult mental illness. Development and Psychopathology, 11(3): 457–466.

Zammarchi, L., A. Angheben, F. Gobbi, G. Zavarise, A. Requena-Mendez, V. Marchese, C. Montagnani, L. Galli, Z. Bisoffi and A. Bartoloni. (2016). Profile of adult and pediatric neurocysticercosis cases observed in five Southern European centers. Neurological Sciences, 37(8): 1349–1355.

PART IV

The Spectrum of Search and Reunion

10
REVISITING THE MEANING OF THE SEARCH

Doris Bertocci, LCSW

Introduction

Mental health practitioners are increasingly seeing adopted clients, or adoptive parents regarding their children in high school or college, who reveal their thoughts of seeking information about their birth families or hoping to actually meet them. This may be either the presenting concern or a topic that comes up in the course of ongoing treatment. Since the latter third of the twentieth century, there has been a groundswell of advocacy, especially in the United Kingdom and the United States, for challenging the sealing of the adoption records that dates to the 1930s (USA). Although the internet has been helpful for many searchers (Whitesel & Howard, 2013; Shier, 2021), if those born in states (USA) with sealed records return to the source of their adoption, they are typically faced with a long wait for "non-identifying information," allegedly due to the large volume of requests from adopted adults. The long wait is in fact due to agencies' views that the adopted person's request for information is not sufficiently "legitimate" to warrant provision of adequate staff time for this purpose. Most notably, while the adopted person is at their most vulnerable, they are provided little or no service. Some American agencies offer a few in-person meetings, but otherwise, despite online services generally being available, the agencies handling these requests say they can only mail out brief summaries. Adopted people experience this as a baffling and profound betrayal, while the sources of adoption information, such as agency social workers, do not conceptualize the adopted person as being eligible for more than the most perfunctory effort. Reformers view this practice as unethical on humanitarian grounds but this has never been considered, much less actively addressed.

The sealing of the records, beginning with the original birth certificate, was intended to protect the privacy of the birth parents and the adoptive family; however, the adoption field took the liberty of defining "full confidentiality" to include the child, not only at the time of relinquishment, but also for the duration of the child's life. Although evidence demonstrates that this was never specified in the relinquishment papers (Samuels, 2001, 2013), adoption personnel have long treated their interpretation of "full confidentiality" as law and as pertaining to their own records as well. In short, the US adoption culture continues to hold adopted adults to its original naïve assumptions and errors since the early part of the twentieth century. As a related problem, many social workers also believe it is their role to mediate the adopted person's pursuit of information or reunion (Shier, 2021), even if the adopted person has acquired their own birth certificate. Missing altogether in their thinking, and in legal debates, is the concept of basic human rights of children, including adopted persons of any age, to information important for their personal identities and medical care. The non-adopted population takes both for granted, benefiting greatly from access to their own personal information, while for the adopted person, the adoption culture dismisses its significance altogether.

In recent decades, the sealing of the record has been consistently challenged by massive activism vis-à-vis state/provincial and national legislatures and other legal entities, with varying results and large numbers of reunions with birth relatives despite the prohibitions of law (Triseliotis, 1973, 2005; Evan B. Donaldson Adoption Institute, 2010). In the 1980s, the director of a prominent American adoption agency was heard by the author to refer to searching adoptees as "criminals." This captures the degree to which adoption personnel have long felt threatened, typically with an underlying anxiety and resentment toward adopted persons for disrupting the *status quo*. From the volume of anecdotal information about the experience adopted people have had with agencies and welfare departments, they say that adoption workers seem to be on the alert that the adopted person might disturb or even harm those they may find. In other words, workers' own anger is attributed to the adopted person, and they see their role as "damage control." For this reason, many agencies require the adopted adult to undergo preliminary coaching sessions "to be sure they have thought through the issues." This comes at a time that the adopted person is typically in an emotional crisis. In effect, the adopted person is left feeling abandoned (again), rejected (again), devalued (again), and patronized. A number of American agencies have shifted to acknowledging the need to provide services, typically under the label of "post-adoption services," even when it is long after the placement. Or the staff, even with various master's degrees, including those who are members of the triad themselves, often do not have, or attempt to acquire, advanced training for the level and specialty of treatment required. Beyond this, it is left to the adopted person and their families to seek ongoing help from the community where therapists are not likely to be adequately trained in this field. As a generalization to date, neither the adoption nor the social service/social work fields have yet come to terms with their biases, with their conflicts of interest, or with their concepts of professional standards.

Revisiting the Meaning of the Search

Background for Mental Health Professionals

Meeting the desires of infertile couples was not supposed to have resulted in so many profound complications. In the United States and Canada, and to some extent, Australia, in the 1930s, as settlement houses were struggling with massive immigrant populations, and while fledgling child welfare efforts were attending to young children who had lost their families due to illness, accident, poverty, and death, the law stepped in to try to regulate practices, with some input from the child welfare workers of the day called "social workers," who usually had little training at a professional level. In the United States, they imagined that shifting children without families from the immigrant ghettos into a country setting in the West, or away from urban life, could mean elimination of their grimy past and secret transition into a new family to which the child would automatically transfer all attachments, form a new identity with an altered name and birth certificate, and never look back.

The orphan trains of the earlier part of the twentieth century in the United States (Paton, 1968) had a twofold agenda that had similarities to some of the adoption field's values and assumptions in the decades that followed, that is, not only could the children potentially have a better quality of life, as many but not all did, but they could also earn their board by providing labor on the new frontier. Although the latter was eventually changed by child labor laws, adoption policy and practice came of an idea that was relatively simple, clean, well-meaning, and expedient. But in overall child welfare in the twentieth century, and still in many places in the twenty-first century, the problem with these good intentions is that they have not had an adequate foundation in human or child development, least of all in the early years. Further, child labor laws notwithstanding, the "best interests of the child" continues to have little meaning in American family law, for the "sealed adoption record" then and now, as in child custody litigation, is based on concepts of property law (Derdeyn, 1979) and on justifications for denying children their human rights in favor of adults' entitlement (Appendix 2), the overriding motive being economic (Hansen, 2020) rather than humanitarian.

To the adopted person, this is a form of discrimination and "second-class citizenship." It has been observed that the only other group in the United States to be denied birth certificates were the Black American slaves, who were also bound by property law, that is, commodities to be used by their owners. Added to this is the adoption culture's evident socio-legal indifference to their continuing burdens that so many adopted people say they experience socially, emotionally, and physically/medically. In addition to the United States, there were parallel attempts to change the sealed record laws in Canada (Strong-Boeg, 2006), Australia (Chapter 3), and New Zealand. Just as social science researchers' curiosity was leading them to ask questions about what subgroups of "adoptees" engaged in "search behavior," and about the outcomes for all members of the adoption triad, uncomfortable therapists were questioning their adopted clients considering a search whether they had considered the possible results, that is, the feelings and rights of others who might be affected. Such questions have a subtext that is not lost on their client. Especially if the adopted person is not living independently, this is an example of the therapist's countertransferential identification with the adoptive parents, which may be a risk if the therapist links the concern about the search with being paid by the parents.

Ironically, it was from the upper classes of the British realm, with its hallowed practices of separating children (boys) from their mothers by age 7 for the discipline of boarding school life, that John Bowlby began his observations on separation, loss, and attachment (1969, 1973, 1980), in concert with the many other pioneers in early childhood development who focused as well on the exquisite emotional sensitivity and vulnerability of babies and, for older children, on the powerful influence of the incipient unconscious (see Dedication). This is an example of strong cultural traditions, in this case British colonialism, that is, taking young boys from their mothers in order to prepare them for military service, with the goal of establishing British colonies around the world ("expanding the empire"), that served as a background for John Bowlby's thinking. Thus, in the late 1940s, it was the impact of war on children, especially *separation from their parents*, that over time culminated in his theories of loss and attachment. For the larger context, as this was being quietly developed through the decades that followed, at the "macro" level, it was also the span of time for reckoning with the impact of the atom bomb, and at the "micro" level, with the significance of the unconscious in human emotion and behavior. For entirely different reasons, Western society reacted to both with shock and disbelief, as with any discovery that profoundly threatens the social order.

Laws sealing adoption records occurred long before the full implications of the more recent psychological discoveries could be recognized. Along with so many notions, assumptions, and cultural norms imposed on those lacking the power to speak for themselves, laws do not usually change for many decades or even generations. And so it was, with the transition of ownership of the child (Derdeyn, 1979) from the birth mother/birth family to the people "wanting to build their families," records of the child's biological (human) connections and original identity were locked away in health departments in perpetuity, without their knowledge or consent. Quite literally, it was never anticipated that adopted children would grow up, with their own unique blend of identities and needs and their own perspectives on what had happened to them (Perry & Winfrey, 2021).

In the 1970s, the adoption records were being opened in the UK amidst much apprehension, loud debate, and dire warnings, but in the end, the opening of the records was virtually free of the imagined hazards and damage to family life that had been predicted and on which the "sealed record" had been based earlier in the twentieth century (Triseliotis, 1973; Triseliotis et al., 2005; Evan B. Donaldson Adoption Institute, 2010). In addition to the UK and some Canadian provinces, Australia and New Zealand followed in the next decade (Spark & Cuthbert, 2009). Ireland and India have had their own versions of loosening restrictions on access to information: India is "semi-open," that is, identifying information is still sealed (Chapter 8). In countries claiming to have "semi-open" adoption records, identifying information is still sealed, thus the material given is undoubtedly helpful but the adoption record is still closed. The United States, with its massive, rapid, and recent mix of national origins, ethnicities, races, and cultures, relative to Western/Eastern Europe and Asia, was only starting to take its turn with the mounting social and legal turmoil around adopted adults' demand for their own (original) birth certificates. This was parallel with rising protest from courageous birth mothers, upon whom alleged "confidentiality" from the child and community had been legally forced at the behest of adoption workers, at a time of their greatest confusion and vulnerability (Samuels, 2001, 2013; Madden et al., 2020). Meanwhile, in the United States, the field most involved with adoption practice, increasingly professionalized social work, remained for decades – through the latter part of the twentieth century – steadfastly threatened by the very children, albeit now grown up, that they imagined they had rescued. Since the 1970s, while social workers remained silent in the halls of the state legislatures with pending bills for opening the record, "adoptees" actually became persons who insisted on recognition of their full human and civil rights. With their being denied access to information needed to protect them in their health care and to consolidate their full identities, they proved not to be very grateful.

At the same time, the discipline of professional social work increased its breadth and, as an offshoot from the mainstream, also developed a significant clinical depth, benefitting from its strong alliance with psychiatry that, in the era of the 1960s to the 1990s, emphasized psychodynamic understandings of emotions and behavior. From the last quarter of the twentieth century, this perspective came to greatly benefit services within the private adoption agencies but has not been incorporated into the knowledge base of personnel representing the other "pathways to adoption." Clinical social workers, understanding much more about the internal complexities of life as an adopted person, joined psychiatrists and clinical psychologists in taking a growing interest in the *psychology* of adoption. They also advocated for social work to engage in some serious soul-searching about its outdated policies and practices (Sorosky et al., 1978). For the few who dared, unofficial apologies were made to birth mothers and adopted adults, while the adoption/social work culture was confronted for its naïve assumptions and practices without the support of any evidence. For example, the contention was that neither the birth mother nor the child should ever have any reason to think further about each other, and that the child's sense of personal identity was supposed to come entirely from the adoptive family. Unfortunately, the latter idea has pervaded the thinking in the traditional mental health field. In the current century, the shift to considering the internal, as well as external, complexities in the adopted person's development has been taken up in both the United States and the United Kingdom (Hindle & Shulman, 2008; Zilberstein, 2011; Festinger & Jaccard, 2012; Buckwalter et al., 2018).

However, in the domain of treatment, the structure and relative expedience of cognitive-behavioral and DBT formats, the limited focus of trainings in trauma and attachment, and the mental health field's apparent lack of interest in learning about the unique complexities in *being* adopted result in adopted persons being unable to find psychotherapists and advanced clinicians who are adequately trained to work with them. Especially in the areas of search and reunion, therapists may be more likely to continue with their clients without availing themselves of additional training or without considering referral to a specialist.

In the meantime, while the need of adopted persons to search has been explicitly questioned, or even implicitly condemned historically, in contrast for the non-adopted world, biological ties to past and current generations, nations, and cultures via DNA and genealogical searches continue to be celebrated and encouraged as adding potentially beneficial, even joyful, discoveries and experiences with their extended family. It is said that these come through forming "ties" with new relatives, with additional benefits for their personal health (family medical history), and a richer, fuller sense of personal and family identity (Bettinger, 2019). The latter author, an attorney and expert in genetic genealogy, speaks publicly about his own personal genealogical search and all that it meant to him when he discovered a close relative that he had never known about. There is something to be said for the secret indiscretions throughout human history that undoubtedly have resulted, sooner or later, in the existence of each of us.

What It All Means for Health and Mental Health

The effort here is to step back and attempt to understand the many layers of meaning in the adopted person's thoughts, fantasies, memories, fears, literally indescribable needs, and conscious-level intentions and hopes underlying the phenomenon known as the adopted person's search for the birth family. By definition, these *internal* dimensions, that is, the psychology of *being* adopted, are not addressed in quantitative research in fields that generally see the meanings of search in terms of specific demographic groups, cultural factors, and cognitive "reasons" or "motives," such as obtaining a medical history (May, 2018), along with concern about the impact of the adopted person's search on other people. Also, it has typically been assumed by social workers that the adopted searcher will (that is, *should*) have discussed their intentions with their adoptive parents, as though it is an obligation: it is part of the psychology of being adopted that, in the way they feel they have been treated, "the adoptee is always a child" whom the adoption culture believes it must oversee and intervene with even throughout their adulthood. But when the search is undertaken in adulthood it cannot be assumed what the circumstances may be for either the adopted person or the adoptive parents.

> *In the middle of my search, my mother needed a hysterectomy, and there was no way I would upset her by bringing up my hope to find my birth parents.*

But fundamentally, the odyssey of self-discovery and healthy self-determination, two of the original tenets of social work practice, belongs solely to the adopted person, and concerns about what the search may mean for the adoptive parents sometimes need to wait until the turmoil settles.

As most important from a *clinical/psychodynamic* perspective, the search does not begin with a phone call or conversation or with any other concrete action. It begins symbolically, subconsciously, and in fantasy over time, *once the adopted person is informed of the existence of birth parents and begins to try to conceptualize them*. It is important to note that some children have been told they are "adopted," but without reference to birth parents, who were conveniently left out of the adoption narrative in the 1940s and 1950s (Wasson, 1939). Likewise unmentioned in some cases were the complexities of pregnancy and birth that *may have* become included in the parents' story gradually over time. The problem came with the adoption culture's unwillingness to hire personnel trained in early childhood development, which accounts for their unstudied assumption that "early telling from the beginning" would be best for all children. But this involved information that could not be understood by a very young child without introducing additional *internal* confusion, potentially threatening the child's early development of self-esteem, security, and mutual attachment within the adoptive family (Wieder, 2001). In the development of any child, the timing is essential for presenting new and potentially unsettling information, that is, there is a certain risk what course the given narrative may take in a very young child's imagination. The parents may believe the impact on the child did not seem significant, but they cannot know the actual impact internally, which is entirely different and depends on multiple variables.

I came out of another lady's tummy, and then I was put on a plane, even though I didn't know how to fly yet, but anyway, that's how I ended up here.

Simple formulas for parents tend to endure, as do impulses to tell "too much too soon," especially when they relieve guilt and anxiety for them. However, very young children can only think and respond to adults' explanations from the limited perspective of their own very limited cognitive and emotional world. Since they do not have the maturity to comprehend complex information or to have developed reasoning capacities, there is no way of knowing if, or to what degree, any particular child may experience a narcissistic injury from learning that the parents to whom the child was born decided not to raise them – or, worse, "rejected" or "abandoned" them. In some cases, the latter is accepted at face value and then conveyed to the child. The point is to resist simple formulas because every family needs to consider its own circumstances and, hopefully, avail themselves of adoption knowledgeable professional assistance with the difficult questions, just as they might consult a physician or lawyer for medical or legal matters.

The existing literature relating to search and reunion tends to treat these topics as a series of behavioral steps without including the underlying foundation of multiple demographic data about the adopted person, as described in Chapter 4, but also without including the source of the adoption and details of the family narrative (Chapter 5), as well as the internal meanings to the adopted person. The search may remain at an unconscious level, as in career decisions and indecisions, or symbolically represented in dreams, reading preferences, experimentation with a new skill, or even behavioral oddities based on the enduring struggle with loss that they experience such as sleepwalking.

> *I often have dreams that I'm in a strange place like a hotel, rushing to pack to leave for the airport, but I can't figure out what city I'm in, and I can't remember how I even got there. I look frantically for my ticket and can't find it. I realize I had made the reservations months earlier, so I can't remember the name of the airline, but for this reason, I don't know where in the airport I should go. I'm very upset that I'm likely to miss my plane, but then I can't even remember where I'm flying to or why. Sometimes it's not a plane but a train that I watch leaving without me. Usually, I don't even recognize where I am, much less where I'm going. These dreams are very stressful, and I'm still having them — I suppose they may have something to do with my being adopted — but what I don't understand is that I completed my search a long time ago.*

Such a dream represents the feeling that the adopted person, in this case a young woman, is "missing something," that is, feels "lost" and always in a state of suspension, with no name, no sense of being permanently anywhere, and having no way of getting where she wanted to be, if she could figure it out, because she did not have a ticket (i.e., birth certificate). She had no way of knowing who or where she was, and she has an impaired sense of her future. We might wonder whether such a dream replayed a form of dissociative amnesia, that is, her earliest history, of frequent changes in caretaking, but also how the adoptive family narrative was handled. On the other hand, the adopted client's occasional sense of disorientation as the search proceeds, experiencing themselves to be straddling two worlds, needs to be distinguished from a form of clinical dissociation because there is no shift in consciousness.

> *How can I make any plans for the future if I can't even imagine having one?*

> *I sometimes feel "spaced out" [what some adopted writers have referred to as "the fog" (Merritt, 2022)] and suspended in time because I don't know anything about my past or where I came from.*

> *I go back and forth between thinking about my life as I've experienced it, while imagining what my life might have been like otherwise, and knowing that if I find my birth family, my life as I've know it will be forever changed.*

Such internal confusion may become organized around the conscious wishful fantasy, based on specific needs (instinctual), relating to the virtually universal "seeing someone who looks like me." A sense of frustration around missing information may be triggered by a look in the mirror at any age, by comments on the color of their skin or eyes, or by inquiries into their unclear plans for study, their choices of work and career, their interests in social and love relationships, or in whether they want to marry and have children themselves.

> *I feel like I can't figure out what I want to do with my life unless I can first know what my birth family did, or what they were interested in.*

They feel the need for a frame of reference in their biological relatives for a sense of comfort and security when up against the unknown. In other words, for the adopted person, especially in adolescence and young adulthood, life-defining decisions can be heavily "loaded" by unresolved areas of anxiety and internal confusion. But for this very reason, they can become the most powerful areas in which the therapist can help the adopted client develop the healthiest trajectory for their future life. It should be noted, however, that the aforementioned dream also reveals that completion of the search does not mean that the impact of early trauma can be assumed to be over.

When the complex psychological issues underlying the adopted person's search are better understood, it becomes clearer that it is inaccurate and misleading to say that search interests are based on "normal curiosity." First, there is nothing "normal" about the vacuum of information that infiltrates the adopted person's life or about the "adjustments" that adoptive status requires of them. Second, "curiosity" is a term from common speech that is used by researchers who do not work with the benefit of a clinical (psychodynamic) knowledge base (Simmonds, 2008; Wrobel & Dillon, 2009; Wrobel & Grotevant, 2012; Wrobel et al., 2013; Barroso & Barbosa-Ducharne, 2019). In the context of search and reunion, such a knowledge base provides a foundation in the great neuropsychological and instinctual complexity of how the search, conscious and unconscious, is experienced *internally* by adopted people. The sociological perspective refers to the "subjective experience" of research subjects and their "search behavior," which is sometimes misunderstood in simple lay terms, such as "filling holes" and "minding the gap" (Wrobel & Grotevant, 2019). However, in the effort to "normalize" the search, it borders on trivializing a very complex phenomenon that is rooted in the early part of life. Such terms do not contribute to a clinical understanding, but of course, this was not their intent. Yet lay references such as to "curiosity" are also used by adopted persons themselves because they are part of the same behaviorally oriented culture that is not trained to think with a deeper emotional and psychodynamic vocabulary for understanding the multiple meanings of search phenomena. This includes interconnections of thought patterns, fantasies, dreams, memories, associations, and complex feelings that they experience, even though many are hard to describe. This puts them at a disadvantage if the validity of the adopted person's need to search is being weighed or debated (Leighton, 2013).

It remains that there is little yet in the way of study of what the completed search appears to represent, resolve, complicate, confound, or liberate in the adopted person's internal experience and *alternate* development over time (Affleck & Steed, 2001). Because of the complexity and layers of processing and integration, it does not help for researchers to think in terms of "a primary motive" or "mechanism." This approach may derive from the protocols of medical/pediatric research, but also from the inclination to seek a "primary reason" in order to simplify an equally valenced multidetermined phenomenon. To complicate this, there are many reasons adopted people give, but some that they may not understand themselves. These vary a good deal because the detailed circumstances for adopted persons vary so greatly, *especially in combination*, they are always multi-layered psychologically, and the adopted population itself is so diverse. Social scientists are oriented toward observing, quantifying, and documenting the external contexts of "search behavior" and, not surprisingly, given the historical focus and anxiety within the adoption field, its impact on other members of the triad. However, clinicians in mental health begin by asking different and far more detailed questions, not only about specific facts of the person's adoption (Chapter 11, Appendix 3A and 3B), but also about their inner thoughts and feelings over time. In short, it is maintained that the therapist's evaluation and treatment are exponentially enriched by their investment in advanced psychodynamic training that helps inform not only with external, concrete data but also with what it may actually mean to the client emotionally. This, after all, is what the clinical level of psychotherapy is intended to do. It must carefully explore the different facets of the client's affective life and distinguish between the variations that are normative for adopted persons, and those that may meet full clinical criteria for an affective disorder or for confused or fragmented identity (Schore, 2003).

An allied field addresses the ethical issues in adoption, most recently in the context of alternate reproductive methods. It basically asks the questions, "How is access to information about the genetic parents to be valued?" and "How are the various claimed needs of the different parties to be measured and weighed?" (Leighton, 2013). This author (DB) asks the same questions but inserts the importance of understanding the psychology of *being* adopted, although it may carry as little weight in ethical discourse as in family law. Overall, this handbook is a call for greater collaboration between different systems of focus and inquiry, regardless of orientation or discipline. As one remarkable example, there has never been any research on adopted adolescents' and adults' earlier or recent medical histories or their sequelae (e.g., gastrointestinal, pulmonary, cardiac, psychosomatic, and neuropsychological), much less the details of their experiences with various counselors and mental health professionals.

In particular, the author refers to the neglect of the American CDC (Centers for Disease Control) and NIMH (National Institute of Mental Health), both of which appear to have absorbed the notion from the adoption culture that adoption is (only) about children. Thus, any disproportionately found medical or adjustment problems, including a few in child psychology case studies, are likely about asthma, food allergies, stomach aches, sleep disturbances, anxiety about school, ADHD and conduct disorders. The lack of funding for qualitative and quantitative studies is particularly troubling, given what we are learning about the connection between "early childhood adversity" (complex trauma) and vulnerability to serious health problems that can extend into adulthood (Lanius et al., 2010). We therefore have no information about the likely variations in prevalence and severity of specific health and mental health conditions, both singly and in combination, for adopted adolescents and young adults, depending on multiple variables, including the six demographic factors discussed in Chapter 4.

The American Experience with the Search, with Review of the Clinically Relevant Literature

For the Americans, it was as the Vietnam War was winding down that preoccupations could now turn to more immediate domestic matters, including the new "access to information" laws and the genetic discoveries of inheritable disease, that the earliest meetings were being organized in various cities across the country for adopted adults who were increasingly determined to confront the state laws sealing the adoption records (Fisher, 1973; Lifton, 1979, 1994, 2009). The publication of "The Meaning of the Search" (Schechter & Bertocci, 1990) was the first attempt to provide both psychosocial and clinical perspectives on the internal processes underlying the search that could be distilled from a large survey of adopted adults. In an effort to categorize the thought processes and related emotional needs (as compared to cognitive "motives") that were expressed by the subjects, the findings highlighted the specific themes of the adopted person's search for the birth parents as representing (1) an effort to repair their sense of loss, deficiency, or inadequacy in their life experience which came to be organized around adoption-related issues, that is, the search represents an effort to relieve their sense of disadvantage, that is, of envious resentment vis-à-vis people who are born rather than adopted, that is, as compared with themselves being left to wonder about their origins, that is, being deprived of their genetic inheritance (Sants, 1964), specifically, they refer to the primary narcissistic injury of being unable to experience physical similarities with their adoptive family; the theme in these reports is so common, intense, and determined that it seems akin to an inner unconscious, survival-based drive, that is, instinct); (2) an effort to consolidate the various fragments of their physical, social, racial, ethnic, and psychological identity involving two or more families, not one; (3) a determination to take charge of their lives in the form of actively pursuing answers to their questions rather than passively accepting their sense of disadvantage and injustice (Chapter 3); (4) particularly in the case of adopted females, a greater ability than reported for males (which may partly account for the majority of searchers in our study being young adult females) to identify with the birth mother's difficult physical and emotional experience throughout pregnancy, birth, and relinquishment, and a wish to resolve what is sensed to be their sorrow by undoing their mutual loss;

> *In a way, I was doing my search as much for my birth mother as for myself. And when I did finally find her, she told me that all these years she had been following me through my horoscope, even through dabbling in astrology, to be sure I was still all right.*

(5) reconciliation of the cognitive dissonance that the adopted person often experiences regarding contradictory information they are given, such as narratives about the birth mother "loving them so much" that she chose to "give them away"; (6) particularly for the older subjects, concern about having inherited a vulnerability to certain diseases, such as cancer or heart disease; (7) discarding their sense of being "unreal" or artificial in comparison with those who are born into their birth families, that is, restoring their sense of authenticity through feeling for the first time a sense of "wholeness" and "human connectedness" (to be distinguished from the seeking of object attachment) if they can encounter someone biologically related to them (Bertocci & Schechter, 1991).

An American literary scholar writes a cerebral but richly explored account, based on multiple sources, of the impact of narratives from the adoption field on many adopted persons' struggles with the concepts of what is "real" (biological) and what is "fictional" (related to adoption) but still questions some of their assumptions (illusions) about search and reunion (Homans, 2015).

Literature informing *clinical* practice around search and reunion is rare relative to the profusion of autobiographies and/or anthologies and journalistic accounts (Fisher, 1973; Lifton, 1979, 1994, 2009; Keum-Cox, 1999; Strickland, 2013; Eldridge, 2015;. Glaser, 2021). Some have been published or self-published by adopted authors (LaCure, 1992, 1995, 2018; Keum-Cox, 1999; Slaton, 2012; Strickland, 2013; Eldridge, 2015; O'Connor et al., 2016). Other venues address changes within the adoption field and in society (Pertman, 2011; Evan B. Donaldson Adoption Institute) and psychoeducational books written by knowledgeable adoptive parents or by adoptive family educators, often a combination of the two (Verrier, 2003; Riley, 2006; Schooler & Atwood, 2008). Most publications are intended primarily for a readership of adoptive parents, social service personnel, and generic professionals (Roszia & Maxon, 2019), but some are in the scholarly literature relating more generally to search and reunion (Sachdev, 1992; Trinder et al., 2004) and to specific subgroups of adopted people, such as those placed in transracial and/or international adoptions (Gordon et al., 2014; Walton, 2012). Researchers in social science have, to a limited degree, sampled adopted adolescents and young adults to learn about "information seeking" and "motives" for activating the search, and hopes and expectations for completing their search, that is, reunion (Affleck & Steed, 2001; Koskinen et al., 2019). However, there is little in the way of clinically focused publications (to be distinguished from sociology/social work, search autobiographies, and guidebooks) by mental health professionals on their experience treating adopted patients. This refers in particular to their observations on the multiple *internal meanings* for particular patients of search and reunion, its impact emotionally and developmentally both during the search process and subsequently over time, and any thoughts on handling the treatment *process* in this context.

Overall, from the latter part of the twentieth century into the twenty-first, the focus of international research has primarily been on the continuing problems of children in foster care ("in care") (Henry, 2012; Roszia & Maxon, 2019; Pinto, 2019), with particular recognition of those disadvantaged by poverty, race, and culture (Jackson & Samuels, 2019); on complexities and special considerations in international/transnational and transracial/interracial/cross-cultural adoptions (Fong & McRoy, 2016); and on the benefits and complexities of open adoption (Baran & Pannor, 1990; Grotevant et al., 2005; Von Korff et al., 2006; Grotevant et al., 2007; Ge et al., 2008; Wolfgram, 2008; Grotevant, 2020; Gordon et al. 2014, 2020). But all this has, in effect, eclipsed the plight of the current majority left behind, that is, those adopted people still struggling with the continuing fallout from closed adoption over the decades. For example, when there is reference to only 5% of adoptions in the United States being closed, this refers only to current placements of children (Evan B. Donaldson Adoption Institute, 2010). The recent changes in state laws allowing access only if the birth mother gave written permission at the time of relinquishment was not offered before the 1980s. Even then, she was not provided the information she needed in order to make an informed decision. This is complicated by the fact that at the time of relinquishment, most birth mothers have been too overwhelmed to process what was happening and therefore have been left vulnerable to the forces pressuring them to relinquish their children. Thus, for its part, adoption law continues to divide the adopted population between those with certain rights and those without, varying by locale.

There are also the numbers of adopted people placed internationally, now adolescents and young adults, whose adoptive parents were provided little information at the time of placement because the source, for a variety of reasons, did not or could not obtain the information that the child may later need; they were probably unaware of its importance. Further, there has been little in the way of continuing or substantive help for the adoptive family following placement (Welsh, 2007), with agencies offering at most brief follow-up consultations. In particular, studies are needed of international adoption programs' and agencies' "post-adoption" referral practices, and of outcomes, when adoptive families with different socioeconomic circumstances see further help.

Adoption reformers point out that when adopted adults seek information, the typical, limited response on the part of agencies, welfare departments, and international placement programs is a reflection of the broader societal perspective of children as commodities for the domestic and international market, without human rights of their own, including a full, consolidated personal identity. This explains the reason that adoption placement programs assisting potential adopters view their services as exclusively for both sets of parents rather than for the child her/himself. Hoksbergen (Chapter 2) explains that in the Netherlands, birth mothers have been given highly idealized rather than realistic information about what life for the adopted child would probably be like. This is part of the adoption culture's nearly exclusive investment, notwithstanding their occasional claims of primary concern for the child, in appealing to the desires of potential parents, that is, by typically not allowing anything to threaten the relinquishment. But to provide some ballast to this observation, there are also the far greater numbers of people we have all been acquainted with whose suffering from neglect and abuse throughout their youths was ignored by their communities. This has continued in large numbers to the present time partly because of the pervasive overemphasis on "parents' rights" that, in many cases, are actually at the greater expense of the human rights of their children, I.e., the children have been denied the chance to grow up with well-attuned adoptive parents, with whom many should have been placed, when a pattern of neglect or abuse became known in the school and community.

There are also important intergenerational considerations in the current century, that is, expressions of need for information from adopted adults' own children and grandchildren. Those adopted internationally, or from poor families with limited education, are particularly at a disadvantage since the success of DNA searches depends entirely on whether a birth relative has contributed to the database (Cashen et al., 2019). While we cannot know, or even estimate, the proportions of adopted adults who have used DNA technology or the internet (Howard, 2012; Shier, 2021) to find biological relatives, or who have succeeded, a study sponsored by the Evan B. Donaldson Adoption Institute in the United States (Appendix 3) found that, among the greatest challenges encountered by adopted adults using the internet to locate birth relatives was the combination of lacking their own original birth certificates and the lack of uniformity in state laws, that is, the problem that there are no nationally – or internationally – consistent terms, meanings, or standards (Whitesel & Howard, 2013).

The Common Themes for Psychotherapists, with Commentary

1. Questions about Who Searches and Why

There was a time, in the 1970s and 1980s, that uneasy social workers, and even a prominent American child psychiatrist affiliated with an adoption agency (Chapter 1), ventured the notion, as they chose to see it at that time, that adopted people who activated the search for birth relatives were only the relatively few who had "probably" had unsatisfactory experiences in their adoptive families. Even if this had been accurate, there was no expressed interest or concern about how or why this might have been their experience. Some social workers imagined adopted people to be angry about being relinquished, the search representing perhaps a wish to "confront the birth parent" – or a resentful wish to have been kept in the first place, or both, neither of which had any backing in evidence or even support at an anecdotal level. This is an example of anxious fantasies of adoption workers lacking sufficient and updated training that become assumptions and belief systems.

In the 1970s and 1980s, adopted people advocating for access to their birth certificates may have been the noisier ones, as occurs with all social movements, but we now know that the activated search is not only commonplace but even also viewed by some therapists as a rite of passage developmentally (Baden & Wiley, 2007) as adopted individuals seek to dismantle the power over them of secrets and unknowns, to rid themselves of what they experience as "holes" in their lives, that is, not only the lack of information, but also externally imposed deficiencies in their understanding of themselves and of the different components of their identities and health. Interviews with adopted people, or their publications and presentations at conferences, reveal that in most cases, their search becomes a great act of courage, a concept with limited currency in clinical formulations that insufficiently consider strengths. That is, rather than passively (masochistically) surrendering to external forces imposed only on adopted people in closed adoptions, they are both confronting their sense of helplessness and internalizing the locus of control (Seligman,

1978, 1992) in an active effort toward consolidating their sense of personal identity and "wholeness" (Lifton, 1994).

Especially in young adulthood, the adopted individual reflects back on how long they have felt stuck in the "forever kind of wondering" (Colaner & Kranstuber, 2010) and decides to try to put an end to it because it has become a chronic irritant that is experienced as "holding them back." This has been implied in a given formula of "stuck places" in the experience of adopted youth (Riley & Meeks, 2006), but the *internal* complexities discussed in this handbook warrant recognition that it is actually a more profound and emotionally consuming experience of being at an impasse in their life development: as they face their arrival into the adult world, they come to realize that their adoption-related preoccupations are interfering with their health, emotional, and social life, that is, with their ability to make sound decisions in education, work, and interpersonal relationships.

Especially in young adulthood, the adopted person decides, finally, to try to obtain the information that, they acknowledge, they still want and now feel entitled to know. The need they may have felt throughout their adolescence that they had intermittently been aware of, but could not articulate, has not gone away, and the system's control over them becomes, as they experience it, the dragon they still have to slay. The dragon is not to be misinterpreted as the birth mother, as the earlier social workers exposed to psychoanalysis might have ventured, but the gnawing ambiguity and unknowns about themselves. Many searchers may have also experienced microaggressions regarding their adoptive status (Garber, 2020), so that for them the search would likely represent an active attempt to confront and eliminate sources of low self-esteem. A small study from Finland found that the desire for parenthood played an important role in intensifying interest in searching, that those in reunion spoke of gaining an important sense of coherence and continuity, and that their ability to communicate with the adoptive parents on adoption-related issues played an important role also (Koskinen & Book, 2019).

Similar findings are reported in an American study of adopted young adults (Farr et al., 2014). At this juncture, as the meaning of the search is being contemplated, it is essential for the therapist to examine their own countertransference (Chapter 15) and to remain focused on their therapeutic role, but as suggested earlier, perhaps consider having a consultation with a specialist so that their work with such a client can be better informed and appropriate clinically. It is expected that this will increasingly become available through online resources. At the same time, it is anticipated that most therapists will resist doing this because of their belief that they can handle it themselves, preferring instead to "learn as I go." This choice, of course, is evidence of their resistance to taking the time to acquire the necessary knowledge base (to which the adopted patient is entitled from the beginning), which has serious ethical implications.

Throughout childhood and adolescence, the adopted individual typically experiences much in the way of feeling-laden fantasy and thought processes, sometimes inexplicable sensations deriving from anxiety (Hindle & Shulman, 2008) that are unknown to the vast majority of the population that is not adopted, and therefore unknown to the vast majority of psychotherapists. If clinical empathy, an internal sense of being genuinely moved emotionally, does not develop in the therapist, it is likely to jeopardize the patient's engagement in the treatment. Also, many of the adopted person's reactions are tied in with the body, that is, in somatically based "implicit memory," or in an adoption-specific "latent trauma" (Merritt, 2022), as well as the mind and a variety of emotions, for which the adopted person, particularly in closed adoption, has no point of reference, that is, no direct encounters with biological relatives, no way of anticipating their bodily changes over time, or of knowing their family medical histories, which become more important with age, as is evident every time they meet with their physicians. They experience the vacuum of information as forcing them to sail, sometimes through turbulent waters, without a rudder. On the other hand, the belief that information about the birth relatives is needed in order to figure out the decisions they must make for their future lives can also be pursued in treatment as a likely overdetermined illusion. There are notable luminaries throughout history whose earliest lives were disrupted by separation and loss of their birth parents and who went on to forge remarkable careers, for example, Alexander Hamilton, the American patriot; Steve Jobs, the co-founder of the multinational technology company Apple Inc.; and the actress Frances McDormand. Not in this rare group, however, are the far greater numbers who grew up with stepparents or within the extended family, their psychology and development being different from those in non-kinship families.

2. Conjectures about Early Development and the Role of Instinct

For survival, nature endowed all mammals with primary sensory capacities that were critical for new mothers and their young offspring in order to identify, recognize, and bond with each other, that is, *so that they could never be lost from each other*. From mammals through the other primates, that sensory capacity was primarily olfactory, auditory, and tactile. However, in the evolution of the human species, while those remained important, vision became critical: not only tactile sensations from touching and nuzzling but also seeing and touching the body of the other, beginning with the eyes and facial recognition. It should not be a long leap to understanding that one of the most frequently, if not universally, stated needs and enormous longings that adopted people – especially those separated from their birth mothers prior to memory, that is, within "the first thousand days" (Schore, 2001, 2002, 2013, 2015; Schore & Schore, 2008) – attempt to explain that babies generally experience "mirroring," or the exchange and reinforcement of recognition as part of the infant's bonding with the birth mother and, by extension within the first year, the father, whose role is to provide support and protection but also to begin a mutual attachment process within the first year (Chapter 7). It is this experience that adopted people, especially those placed in families of another race than their own (Gordon et al., 2014; Godon-Decoteau & Ramsey, 2020), express the great need for visually acquired information. This is because, without the mutual reinforcement of bonding through touch, smell, and vision, some have expressed a sense of being suspended in time and space and, beneath all the normal intrafamilial and interpersonal connections, still a stranger on the periphery in being barred from information, including visual, or "in a fog" (Merritt, 2022). It is as though searchers feel their maturation is being held up unless and until they can finally satisfy this craving and experience some inner safety – eliminate anxiety about themselves, about their "real" identity and place in the world – that they have a hard time explaining even to themselves, and that the law, being cerebral in its nature and limits, cannot understand. Nature compels it, regardless. The paradox is that, if they had any doubts about their human roots, they are demonstrating them in their need to search.

> *I'd give anything just to be able to see someone who looks like me – not someone who may vaguely resemble me, like my brother, although we aren't related, but someone who really is part of me, who has the same coloring, or hair, or eyes, maybe even the same talent, who is actually genetically connected to me, and I'm connected to them. I don't care whether they want a relationship with me – if they do, that would be a bonus – but I just want to be able to see what they look like, most of all their face, but also their body shape and skin, how they sound when they talk.*

> *It's hard to explain how often I automatically look for somebody who resembles me when I walk down the street. Sometimes I see some feature in them that I keep staring at, but then I get embarrassed and look away, then the excitement disappears when I have to remind myself – again – that there's no way (we're related). They're just another stranger.*

In short, it is proposed here that this sense of "connectedness" through *visual* recognition was mandatory for physical survival of the *human* species, and similarly, the critical importance of visual engagement between infant and mother is emphasized in neurobiological studies by the pioneers bridging the twentieth and twenty-first centuries (Schore, 1994, 2001, 2008, 2013, 2015). Taking this into account, consider the implications for the development of adopted people who were never able to experience this, that is, who were separated from their birth mothers in the early days, weeks, months, or years of life. Thus, there is a driving, internal sense of emotional starvation described by some adopted persons, particularly those who grew up in closed adoptions, which had become universal in the twentieth century until the advent of open adoption a generation ago. When adopted people attempt to explain these great longings and sensations to the non-adopted, they know they will not be understood. Thus, "being understood," which represents another form of connection, becomes a theme and another sense of great longing, and of "belonging," in their emotional and social development – and in their psychotherapy (Chapter 15).

Doris Bertocci, LCSW

3. The Importance of Distinctions and Timing

Extending this observation, there is a full spectrum of what the adopted person may, or may not, have experienced in the way of an empathic connection with one or both adoptive parents, which reflects a process of understanding and being understood, of being empathized with *emotionally* (affectively, not cognitively). This is one of the most essential areas for the psychotherapist to explore in detail, as with any clients. For example, it is observed more generally that, with current adoption placement practices, adoptive parents represent the same full spectrum of psychosocial health, disease, and character structures as the general population. Further, they bring with them the internalized communication patterns and parenting styles from their own original families (Alexander et al., 2004).

> *When I was a teenager, if I had any complaints, my mother would say, "Beggars can't be choosers." I remember thinking at that time that maybe in her day, that was just a common saying. But as I thought more about it, underneath I still felt hurt. I realized that since I came from nowhere, she thought of me as just a beggar – she was really saying that I should feel lucky for what I had, that I wasn't entitled to whatever it was that I wanted. But maybe what she said was not because I was adopted; maybe she would have said the same thing to any child. But I was never sure about this.*

To those accustomed to their adoptive parents' rational, concrete thinking and to life being limited to the most basic, practical requirements, typical of survivors of disadvantaged circumstances, an empathic connection may not be understood or expressed by a parent if they themselves had never previously experienced it. Thus, it is an important part of treatment of the adopted client, or any client, to explore whether and to what extent this may have been part of the adopted client's experience developmentally. Consider the following, typical accounts of a subgroup of adopted young adults:

> *My mother was from a poor family whose Sunday suppers, she would say, consisted of milk toast. Her parents had both died when she was in her early 20s, and I suspect the adoption workers felt sorry for her. She was a very practical and responsible person, but any expression of feelings at all seemed to threaten and embarrass her. Neither of my parents had really known what affection was in their own families, and I never saw any between them – or with me. Actually, throughout my growing up, this has made my life pretty painful. People would tell me I never expressed my feelings, that I seemed cold. But this is what I knew as normal. I feel guilty about seeming critical of my parents, but it was really the welfare workers who were clueless.*

> *All those years I assumed he was my father because he was married to my mother. I could never figure out why, so often, he couldn't even remember my name or why he didn't seem to do the kinds of things my friends' fathers did.*

My parents tried to do the basic things, but as I became an adult, it kept crossing my mind: "What were those welfare workers thinking?"

Thus, it is a basic mandate that the therapist take the time, and put in the work within themselves, to develop an empathic capacity that the adopted client can actually feel, which cannot be gauged well unless it is carefully inquired about. For this, the right words and timing need consideration, along with ways to "decode" hidden meanings if the adopted client makes cryptic or vague statements, as they have learned to do for self-protection. Again, the therapist might have a clinical consultation with a specialist, perhaps online, which could potentially be very helpful. At a suitable time, the therapist might say, "It's common for an adopted person sometimes to feel that, deep down, they aren't really being understood, or that they're not being 'heard.' I'm wondering how well you feel I really understand you, or if there is something I may have missed or not quite gotten right." Even if this is shrugged off (a defense) or if the client's affect is not actively engaged in the therapy, the therapist's sensitivity and concern may still have registered, and there may be another time when there can be more of an exchange, enabling more affect, about how the client is experiencing their (mutual) relationship.

Depending on what the client selects as possible goals for treatment, such as dysfunctional habits like procrastination, or strategies for containing anxiety, for which cognitive behavioral approaches may be sufficient at the time, the therapist needs to be aware of the larger context (clinically) of the specific presenting difficulty. If the client can be encouraged to think more broadly in order to understand and change long-standing, painful symptoms of anxiety or depression, which require careful differential diagnosis, or dysfunctional patterns in personality functioning (e.g., difficulty trusting, chronic low self-esteem, low-grade depression, a pattern of self-sabotage, repeated episodes of interpersonal conflict, or anger management problems), this warrants highly skilled treatment that has the option of extending into ongoing treatment. This is the reason for emphasizing the benefits of a psychodynamic approach which, unlike the more common cognitive-behavioral formats, requires of the therapist a good deal of self-knowledge at the emotional as well as intellectual level in order to work with the transference and countertransference as powerful vehicles of permanent change for the patient (Zuckerman & Buchsbaum, 2007; Chapter 15). But it is also the reason for emphasizing the important role of any psychotherapist to provide the necessary information for the adopted adolescent or young adult that will help them make an informed decision about the form of treatment that would be most suitable at a particular time, depending on various factors and circumstances in the client's life. This is an important aspect of timing, and ethically, every health practitioner needs to know whether and when to refer the patient to a colleague with different or advanced skills. For example, therapists in college counseling services may see an adopted college student from time to time (Appendix 4) and will need to discuss what is possible to accomplish within the briefer form of treatment on campus, but also what is possible in a later treatment with an adoption-knowledgeable therapist (i.e., one who is trained in the psychology of *being* adopted) after they graduate.

Regardless of the therapist's attempts to invite further discussion of the patient's personal experience with adoption, it may be responded to dismissively with "I haven't really thought about it that much." The therapist might handle this by commenting that sometimes "not knowing what to say" or "having no thoughts" can mean something is blocking their memory, or perhaps there is a lot more to say but "now" is not the time, that is, the therapist leaves the invitation open and then listens for subtle opportunities in future sessions. As an example, an adopted male graduate student in architecture specialized in the properties of antique wood and, as he referred to it, its "provenance," but he was too frightened to discuss with his therapist the possible meaning of his (dissociated) anger in not knowing anything about his own origins. The therapist needs great sensitivity and patience, recognizing that, because of early fears and anxiety that paralyze their memories or confuse their sense of chronology, some adopted patients take longer to fully engage in treatment than the therapist is accustomed to with their other patients.

4. The Need for the Development of "Best Practices"

Views of "best practices" in the treatment of adopted adolescents and young adults vary according to adoption specialists' training, experience, skill sets of their discipline, and setting in which they work. There is a significant difference between the work of social service and adoption professionals on the one hand and therapeutic work at the advanced clinical level that is based on psychological theories of personality development with the goals of deeper, more encompassing, and potentially more permanent change. Most importantly, this can still be done within a short time frame because the richness of the psychodynamic perspective helps therapists "listen faster" in more rapidly developing their understanding of the client and in providing well-focused treatment. Both approaches are of equal value, validity, and importance, depending on the nature of the setting, on the client's needs and also capacities for self-reflection, and on what they feel ready to undertake. However, the client needs enough explanation from the therapist so that they can make an informed decision about the approach that would be most useful for them.

Marriage and family therapists emphasize the interplay and communication patterns of family life between and among its members, but they are unlikely to have been trained in the psychology of being adopted or in understanding the relevance of the birth family in the internal lives of all family members. Counseling psychologists refer to the importance of validating strengths and using positive role models in order to demonstrate alternate or new ways for the adopted client to react to limitations in their life experience. This includes addressing "negative self-attributions" (habits in thought processes reflecting low self-esteem) and cognitive strategies for encouraging the client to become more flexible about trying new skills, such as in their social lives (Baden & Wiley, 2007). These are versions of the original roles that have been taught in professional social work dating to the 1950s, while "counseling" in general is a broader term with less-defined skill sets and parameters for practice. Clinical psychologists may have the possible advantage of training in psychological testing, although for many it is typically long forgotten, while some of the best of the protocols for testing personality and the underlying meanings of thought processes (e.g., projectives) are usually no longer taught in the United States because of insufficiently pursued questions about their validity, perhaps also because priority has been increasingly given to evaluating neuropsychological problems and cognitive testing for school achievement.

Regardless, all skilled therapists incorporate psychoeducation and support as part of their work. Psychodynamically trained therapists explore relevant underlying (subconscious or unconscious) material, helping the client learn what is "behind the curtain" in the way they interpret, or misinterpret, the underlying meanings of manifest material that the patient shares, such as sensitivity to rejection, difficulties with anger management, and confusion about the meanings and intents of others' behavior. Those observed by the author include the inadequate attention given to assessing clients' capacities for self-reflection (Sharp & Bevington, 2022), and the level of their desire to learn more about themselves and the "tunnel vision" within each subdiscipline of the mental health field (probably serving as self-justification). This typically results in insufficient training in distinguishing, working with, and benefiting from the skill sets of different disciplines and approaches, treatment goals, and referral practices.

5. Some Comments on "Genetic Sexual Attraction"

Psychotherapists are alerted that "genetic sexual attraction," originally discussed in a publication by two British psychiatrists (Greenberg & Littlewood, 1995), is a rarely reported phenomenon that, soon after an adopted adult was reunited with a biological relative, they experienced sexual arousal, or even felt a temptation to act on it; also rare are similar reports of arousal in birth relatives. It has been conjectured – but broadly misinterpreted in current trainings for the social service field – that there is a genetic component to the arousal response, as though the shared genes work magnetically by sparking sexual arousal when the search is completed. One proposed explanation refers simply to an attraction to encountering similar body features, "a recognition of oneself in the other" (ibid, p. 29). A pamphlet by the Cumbria County Council (UK), available online, repeats the basic warnings and includes another explanation as "missed bonding." Perhaps, but they did not account for the adopted person's age when separated from the birth mother: In the UK, where adoptive placements tend to be of children already "in care," the bonding process in infancy should have already occurred with the birth mother, unless she was minimally involved in the child's care and/or unless she herself had difficulties with attachment (Buckwalter et al., 2018). This, of course, has implications for the trauma of later being separated from her. But most relevant of all, there is no scientifically derived evidence of a genetic component that could account for the intensity of the reunion, particularly if it involves sexual arousal, for which reason the commonly referenced concept of "GSA" has no validity.

A more reasoned way to conceptualize it is to consider, and recognize, the high level of neuropsychological excitement experienced by the adopted person when finally, *in vivo*, encountering a biological relative for the first time, especially if it is a birth parent. An adopted young woman referred to her reunion with her birth mother as "an orgasm of the soul" because the experience was so powerful, although she never experienced sexual arousal and did not see any physical similarities until a later time, in old photographs. Clients may need to be prepared for the possibility that the physical similarities they yearn to see may not turn out to be evident at all. In any case, it is not so far-fetched to view any arousal as a powerful neuropsychological and neurophysiological response that becomes diverted or confused, for reasons presently unknown, and briefly experienced psychosexually. In the rare instances to date that the arousal may continue beyond the initial experience with reunion, the therapist may want to consider boundary problems in the client. Most important, it would be understandable if it is underreported and it is likely followed by re-emergence of shame and bewilderment that must be addressed in the therapy.

Overall, it should be understood as evidence of the complexity and power of unconscious and conscious "events" that converge at a critical time, and of the great intensity of the felt need to be rejoined (if separated very early, perhaps merged, as in early infancy) with the lost object, which is also experienced as the joyful retrieval of a missing part of the self. Siblings and other biological relatives may be responded to similarly as extensions in the birth family. But most importantly, it is neither "romance" nor "incest," as suggested in passing in some publications. The primary point here is that therapists should not underestimate the significance of the internal excitement to the adopted person, however it is experienced, even though therapists themselves will not be able to identify with it because it is so unique to this context.

Observations on Therapeutic Responses to Clients' Search

The adopted client's expressed interest in activating a search for birth relatives, or her/his request for the therapist's help with the emotional turbulence they are experiencing after it is underway, or at the critical time that a birth relative is found, constitutes a psychological crisis for the patient that the therapist needs to recognize immediately and respond to as such. But it is also a challenge for the therapist in carefully monitoring her/his countertransference. This, then, may involve the risk of the therapist's personal reactions (e.g., "fascination with an unusual case" or a certain level of their own excitement or narcissistic pleasure when the client finds a birth relative) is that therapists often recommend readings for a client, such as about "the search," without themselves being familiar with the materials they are recommending and, more troubling, without having obtained at least a foundation in the psychology of adoption before taking on an adopted patient to treat. This especially pertains at the critical time of the client finding a birth relative and typically being in crisis: The patient does not have time for the therapist to educate themselves at the last minute. Indeed, the therapist's lack of knowledge and understanding is a very common complaint of adopted clients more generally:

> *I could tell right off that each therapist I saw didn't really know much about what it's like to be adopted, and I got very tired of having to teach them.*

> *It's easy to pick up that the therapist doesn't really know much about adoption; they use the wrong terms, ask about the wrong things, and make automatic assumptions that are just plain wrong, basically revealing how little they actually know.*

> *Therapists have failed me my whole life. Either they never brought up my adoption or they swept it under the rug and wouldn't talk about it.*

As a further clarification, it is not the therapist's role in any way to encourage or recommend that the client search for the birth family. Rather, the therapist's role is to be a therapist: to listen and then to know the right questions to ask regarding the complex meanings of their thoughts, fantasies, memories, felt needs throughout their development. The therapist also needs a knowledge base to share with the client as may be appropriate to the context, including review of their possible future needs, regardless of what he/she decides about activating a search. For example, there are life decisions they will want to make for themselves that could be, for better or worse, influenced by adoption-related themes in their development, including choices in love relationships and potential complications in health if they lack a family medical history: what seems unimportant at one stage of life can become of great importance at a later time, and vice versa. In the context of this chapter, the therapist can reveal their awareness that some adopted people do search for birth relatives and that, from a large amount of anecdotal information along with limited research (Evan B. Donaldson Adoption Institute), they have reported primarily positive experiences with it despite any complications or disappointments (Koskinen & Book, 2019). In other words, the more the therapist has learned about *being* adopted, and the more they become interested, the easier it will be to know how to explore various areas of the client's experience, but the therapist must become authentically interested. That is, the therapist's revelation of what they are aware of from the literature and/or from any training can be used in therapy as a means of reassuring the client that the therapist is already knowledgeable; it is also a means of recognizing and opening topics for further discussion.

Psychotherapists who are themselves adopted have differing practices and views on the topic of the therapist's self-disclosure of being adopted and on the timing of revealing it to a client. From a clinical perspective, particularly one that is psychodynamically informed, any personal information is best shared, if at all, only after the therapist has enough clinical knowledge about the patient to be clear about the purpose and goal of any personal disclosures the therapist may consider making: Generally, the therapist needs to be aware that self-disclosure is risky and can sometimes have the opposite effect from the one intended. Psychotherapists who are adoptive parents will be particularly challenged on the issue of self-disclosure and certainly in the countertransference. Both topics would likely be useful areas for further study.

Depending on how the client responds to the initial discussion of search, he/she can be told that there is a wide range of search experiences, the only certainty being a good deal of anxiety if reunion is the goal, and there are many reasons for this. They include, typically, whether they will be "rejected again," even though the chances are, on the basis of massive anecdotal information from those who have counseled birth mothers, that the child was never "rejected" in the first place but, rather, the birth mother was forced by her circumstances at that time. Especially in international adoptions, the theme of the child being "abandoned" may be commonly mentioned, typically out of expedience, but it lacks information about the birth mother's actual internal experience. For the adopted person, there may also be concerns about finding that a birth parent has died, that is, they must come to terms with the possibility that they may have to face a permanent loss – again. Some adopted people approach their search in an intermittent way, taking various steps and then stopping for some amount of time, which gives them a greater sense of control over the process. Other searchers get underway and find it "taking over their lives" in a way that can be confusing or even somewhat disorienting, but this should not be confused with a dissociative process.

> *I started to feel great sadness and frustration as I tried to step back in time and imagine what it must have been like for her [birth mother] in those days. I wanted to go back to her at the time she was pregnant with me. I took an interest in seeing movies and photographs from that period, and I thought about how alone she must have felt. I tried so hard [the subconscious yearning to "return to the beginning"] that it was sometimes hard to get back to my daily life because my world was changing. I knew that if I found her, I would never be the same again.*

This is a common experience reflecting the sense that they are embarking, as some have expressed, on a form of "giving birth to themselves emotionally." They are starting over, but this time with real information, and this time they are the active agent. Regarding outcomes, occasionally the adopted person in reunion expresses disappointment with some of the results, or with not having fully realized the complexities involved in meeting birth relatives or in sharing information with their adoptive families, but it is also typical for both adopted people and birth mothers to express enormous relief, a sense of peace from "all the wondering" about the other, and even the idea that, regardless of any "unpleasant surprises" or "sad discoveries" from their experience, their lives are markedly changed for the better. But in essence, if activated search for birth relatives is on the client's mind, their decision should be an informed one, and unlike so many other life-impacting decisions that were made for them, it needs to be entirely theirs alone to make. Further, "search issues should be normalized as part of development yet not required" (Baden & Wiley, 2007, p. 894). Regardless of the decision, there is likely much to gain and lose either way that has profound significance. This encapsulates a good deal of the adopted young adult's inner experience prior to searching, a pattern of uncertainty, paralysis, perhaps problematic relationships, and anxiety about their own endurance, the search representing their need for relief by putting an end to years of frustration.

> By the time I found my birth mother, she was in her 70s and, except for her son, my brother, all her family had died. Throughout the time I was a teenager and in my 20s, I had several medical complications for which my doctors asked about my family history. Of course there was nothing I could tell them. But ironically, when I finally found my birth mother, I came away without much of a family medical history after all.

This chapter ends on one of the themes within the psychology of being adopted: ambiguity.

Summary

This chapter follows up the author's collaboration with a colleague in the late 1980s, then writing the first account of adopted adults' experience searching for birth relatives, not the "motives" that is the common focus of cognitively oriented researchers, but the *internal* emotional struggles that their searches attempted to resolve, and their expressions and the nuances of what search and reunion either meant to them or had accomplished for them. The findings, summarized here, were consistent with all themes reported in self-published accounts of adopted adults, only some of them mentioned in professional publications. To further our understanding, while there will continue to be many variations on these themes, much more is needed in the way of study and discussion from the clinical domain of the mental health field, with also, hopefully, more in the way of longitudinal perspectives (Browning & Duncan, 2005).

Endnotes

Affleck, M.K., & Steed, L.G. (2001). Expectations and experiences of participants in ongoing adoption reunion relationships: A qualitative study. *American Journal of Orthopsychiatry*, 71 (1), 38–48.

Alexander, L., Hollingsworth, L.D., Dore, M.M., & Hoopes, J. (2004). A family of trust: African American parents' stories of adoption disclosure. *American Journal of Orthopsychiatry*, 74 (4), 448–455.

Baden, A.L., & Wiley, M.O. (2007). Counseling adopted persons in Adulthood: Integrating practice and research. *The Counseling Psychologist* (Sage Publications), 35, 868–901.

Baran, A., & Pannor, R. (1990). Open adoption. In: D. Brodzinsky, & M.D. Schechter (Eds.). *The Psychology of Adoption*. Oxford: Oxford University Press, pp. 316–331.

Barroso, R., & Barbosa-Ducharne, M. (2019). Adoption-related feelings, loss, and curiosity about origins in adopted adolescents. *Clinical Child Psychology and Psychiatry*, 24 (4), 876–891.

Bertocci, D., & Schechter, M.D. (1991). Adopted adults' perception of their need to search: Implications for clinical practice. *Smith College Studies in Social Work*, 61 (1), 179–196.

Bettinger, B.T. (2019). *The Family Tree Guide to DNA Testing and Genetic Genealogy* (2nd Ed.). New York: Family Tree Books/Penguin-Random House.

Bowlby, J. (1969, 1973, 1980). *Attachment and Loss* (Vol. 1, 2, 3). New York: Basic Books.

Browning, J., & Duncan, G. (2005). Family membership in post-reunion adoption narratives. *Social Policy Journal of New Zealand*, 26, 156–172.

Buckwalter, K.D., Reed, D., & Mercer, D. (2018). Ghosts in the adoption: Uncovering parents' attachment and coping history. *Families in Society: The Journal of Contemporary Social Services*, 225–234.

Cashen, K.K., Altamari, D. Grotevant, H.D., & McRoy, R.G. (2019). Hearing the voices of emerging adult adoptees: Perspectives on adoption agency practices. *Child Welfare*, 97 (4), 1–22.

Colaner, C.W., & Kranstuber, H. (2010). 'Forever kind of wondering': Communicatively managing uncertainty in adoptive families. *Journal of Family Communication*, 10, 236–255.

Derdeyn, A.P. (1979) Adoption and the ownership of children. *Child Psychiatry and Human Development*, 9, 215–226.

Eldridge, S. (2015). *Twenty Life-Transforming Choices Adoptees Need to Make*. London: Jessica Kingsley Publishing.

Evan, B. Donaldson Adoption Institute. (2010). For the records II: An examination of the history and impact of adult adoptee access to original birth certificates. http://www.adoption institute.org

Farr, R.H., Grant-Marsney, H.A., & Grotevant, H.D. (2015). Adoptees' contact with birth parents in emerging adulthood: The role of adoption communication and attachment to adoptive parents. *Journal of Adolescent Research*, 29 (1), 45–66. https://doi.org/10.1111/famp.12069

Festinger, T., & Jaccard, J. (2012). Suicidal thoughts in adopted vs. non-adopted youth: A longitudinal analysis in adolescence, early young adulthood, and young adulthood. *Journal of the Society for Social Work and Research*, 3 (4), 280–295.

Fisher, F. (1973). *The Search for Anna Fisher*. A. Fields Books.

Fong, F., & McRoy, R. Eds. (2016). *Transracial and Intercountry Adoptions: Cultural Guidance for Professionals*. New York: Columbia University Press.

Garber, K. (2020). Adoptive microaggressions: Historical foundations, current research, and practical implications. In Wrobel, Helder, & Marr (Eds.), *The Routledge Handbook of Adoption*. London & New York: Routledge, pp. 308–320.

Ge, X., Natsuaki, M.N., Martin, D., Leve, L., Neiderhiser, J., Shaw, D.S., Villareal, G., Scaramella, L., Reid, J., & Reiss, D. (2008). Bridging the divide: Openness in adoption and post-adoption psychosocial adjustment among birth and adoptive parents. *Journal of Family Psychology*, 22 (4), 529–540.

Glaser, G. (2021) *American Baby: A Mother, A Child, and the Shadow History of Adoption*. New York: Viking/Penguin Random House LLC.

Godon-Decoteau, D., & Ramsey, P. (2020). Transracial adoptees: The rewards and challenges of searching for their birth families. In G.M. Wrobel, E. Helder, & E. Marr (Eds.), *The Routledge Handbook of Adoption*. London & New York: Routledge, pp. 238–252.

Gordon, D.E., Green, W.F., & Ramsey, P.G. (2014). Transracial adoptees: The search for birth family and the search for self. *Adoption Quarterly*, 17 (1), 1–27.

Greenberg, M., & Littlewood, R. (1995). Post-adoption incest and phenotypic matching: Experience, personal meanings, and biosocial implications. *The British Journal of Medical Psychology*, 68 (1), 29–44.

Grotevant, H.D. (2020). Open adoption. In G.M. Wrobel, E. Helder, & E. Marr (Eds.), *The Routledge Handbook of Adoption*. London & New York: Routledge, pp. 266–277.

Grotevant, H.D., Perry, Y.V., & McRoy, R.G. (2005). Openness in adoption: Outcomes for adolescents within their adoptive kinship networks. In D.M. Brodzinsky, & J. Palacios (Eds.), *Psychological Issues in Adoption: Research and Practice*. Westport: Praeger, pp. 167–186.

Grotevant, H.D., Wrobel, G.M., Von Korff, L., Skinner, B., Friese, S.C., Newell, J., McRoy, & R.G. (2007). Many faces of openness in adoption: Perspectives of adopted adolescents and Their parents. *Adoption Quarterly*, 10 (3–4), 79–101.

Hansen, M.E. (2020). An economic perspective on ethics in adoption policy. In G.M. Wrobel, E. Helder, & E. Marr (Eds.), *The Routledge Handbook on Adoption*. London & New York: Routledge, pp. 36–48.

Henry, D. (2012). *The 3-5-7 Model: A Practice Approach for Permanency Work with Children and Youth*. Pennsylvania: Sunbury Press.

Hindle, D., & Shulman, G. Eds. (2008). *The Emotional Experience of Adoption: A Psychoanalytic Perspective*. London and New York: Routledge.

Homans, M. (2015). *The Imprint of Another Life: Adoption Narratives and Human Possibility*. Ann Arbor: University of Michigan Press.

Howard, J.A. (2012). *Untangling the Web: The Internet's Transformative Impact on Adoption: Policy and Practice Perspective*. New York: Evan B. Donaldson Adoption Institute.

Jackson, K.F., & Samuels, M. (2019). *Multiracial Cultural Attunement*. Washington, DC: NASW Press.

Keum-Cox, S. Ed. (1999). *Voices from Another Place: A Collection of Works from a Generation Born in Korea and Adopted in Other Countries*. Saint Paul: Yeong & Yeong Book Co.

Koskinen, M.G., & Book, M.L. (2019). Searching for the self: Adult international adoptees' narratives of their search for and reunion with their birth families. *Adoption Quarterly*, 22 (3), 219–246.

LaCure, J. (1992). *Adopted Like Me*. Adoption Advocate Publishing Co.

LaCure, J. (1995). *Remembering: Reflections of Growing Up Adopted*. Adoption Advocate Publishing Co.

LaCure, J. (2018). *Finding the Yellow Brick Road: Adoptees' Stories of Truth, Love, and Self-Discovery*. Herndon, VA: Mascot Books.

Lanius, R.A., Vermetten, R., & Pain, C. Eds. (2010). *The Impact of Early Life Trauma on Health and Disease. The Hidden Epidemic*. Cambridge: Cambridge University Press.

Leighton, K. (2013). To criticize the right to know we must question the value of genetic relatedness. *American Journal of Bioethics*, 13 (5), 54–56.

Lifton, B.J. (1979). *Lost and Found: The Adoption Experience*. New York: Dial Press.

Lifton, B.J. (1994). *Journey of the Adopted Self: A Quest for Wholeness*. New York: Basic Books.

Lifton, B.J. (2009). *Lost & Found: The Adoption Experience*. Ann Arbor: University of Michigan Press.

Madden, E.E., Aguiniga, D.M., & Ryan, S. (2020). Birth mothers' options counseling and relinquishment experiences. In: G.M. Wrobel, E. Helder, & E. Marr (Eds.). *The Routledge Handbook of Adoption*. London & New York: Routledge, pp. 219–237.

Marr, E., Helder, E., & Wrobel, G.M. (2020). Historical and contemporary contexts of U.S. Adoption. In G.M. Wrobel, E. Helder, & E. Marr (Eds.), *The Routledge Handbook of Adoption*. London & New York: Routledge, pp. 3–21.

May, T., Lee, R.M., & Evans, J.P. (2018). Healthcare challenges faced by adopted persons lacking family health history information. *Narrative Inquiry in Bioethics*, 8 (2), 103–106.

Merritt, M. (2022). Rediscovering latent trauma: An adopted adult's perspective. *Child Abuse & Neglect*, 130, 1–11.

O'Connor, S.H., Christian, D.R., & Ellerman, M.A. (2016). *Black Anthology: Adult Adoptees Claim Their Space*. Self-published. www.anyaproject.com

Paton, J. (1968). *Orphan Voyage*. New York: Vintage.

Perry, B., & Winfrey, O. (2021). *What Happened to You? Conversations on Trauma, Resilience, and Healing*. New York: Flatiron Books.

Pertman, A. (2011). *Adoption Nation: How the Adoption Revolution is Transforming Our Families – and America*. Boston: The Harvard Common Press.

Pinto, S. (2019). Looked after and adopted children: Applying the latest science to complex biopsychosocial formulations. *Adoption and Fostering*, 43 (3), 294–309.

Riley, D., with Meeks, J. (2006). *Beneath the Mask: Understanding Adopted Teens*. Burtonville, MD: Case Publications.

Roszia, S., & Maxon, A.D. (2019). *Core Issues in Adoption and Permanency: A Comprehensive Guide to Promoting Understanding and Healing in Adoption, Foster Care, Kinship Families, and Third Party Reproduction*. London: Jessica Kingsley Pub.

Sachdev, P. (1992). Adoption reunion and after: A study of the search process and experience of adoptees. *Child Welfare*, 71, 53–68.

Samuels, E.J. (2001). The idea of adoption: An inquiry into the history of adult adoptee access to birth records. In *Rutgers Law Review*. New Brunswick: Rutgers University, The State University of New Jersey, pp. 1–43.

Samuels, E.J. (2013). Surrender and subordination: Birth mothers and adoption law reform. *20 Michigan Journal of Gender and Law*, 20–33, 33–81A.

Sants, H.J. (1964). Genealogical bewilderment in children with substitute parents. *British Journal of Medical Psychology*, 37, 133–141.

Schechter, M.D., & Bertocci, D. (1990). The meaning of the search. In D. Brodzinsky, & M.D. Schechter (Eds.), *The Psychology of Adoption*. Oxford: Oxford University Press, pp. 62–90.

Schooler, J.E., & Atwood, T.C. (2008). *The Whole Life Adoption Book: Realistic Advice for Building a Healthy Adoptive Family*. Colorado Springs: NavPress.

Schore, A.N. (1994). *Affect Regulation and the Origin of the Self: The Neurobiology of Emotional Development*. Hillsdale: Lawrence Erlbaum Associates Publishing (Re-pub. 2016: Routledge).

Schore, A.N. (2001). The effects of secure attachment relationships on right brain development, affect regulation, and infant mental health. *Infant Mental Health Journal*, 22, 7–66.

Schore, A.N. (2002). The neurobiology of attachment and early personality organization. *Journal of Prenatal and Perinatal Psychology and Health*, 16 (3), 249–263.

Schore, A.N. (2003). *Affect Dysregulation and Disorders of the Self*. New York: W.W. Norton.

Schore, A.N. (2013). Relational trauma, brain development, and dissociation. In J.D. Ford, & C.A. Courtois (Eds.). *Treating Complex Traumatic Stress Disorders in Children and Adolescents. Scientific Foundations in Therapeutic Models*. New York: The Guilford Press, pp. 3–23.

Schore, A.N. (2015). *Affect Regulation and the Origin of the Self*. London & New York: Routledge.

Schore, J.R. & Schore, A. (2008). Modern attachment theory: The central role of affect regulation in development and treatment. *Clinical Social Work Journal*, 36, 9–20.

Seligman, M.E.P. (1978). Learned helplessness as a model of depression: Comment and integration. *Journal of Abnormal Psychology*, 87, 165–179.

Seligman, M.E.P. (1992). *Helplessness: On Development, Depression, and Death*. New York: W.H. Freeman.

Sharp, C., & Bevington, D. (2022). *Mentalizing in Psychotherapy: A Guide for Practitioners*. New York: The Guilford Press.

Shier, A.M. (2021). Negotiating reunion in intercountry adoption using social media and technology. *The British Journal of Social Work*, 51 (2), 408–426.

Simmonds, J. (2008) Developing a curiosity about adoption. In D. Hindle, & G. Shulman (Eds.), *The Emotional Experience of Adoption: A Psychoanalytic Perspective*. London & New York: Routledge, pp. 27–41.

Slaton, P. (2012). *Reunited: An Investigative Genealogist Unlocks Some of Life's Greatest Family Mysteries*. New York: St. Martin's Griffin.

Sorosky, A., Baran, A., & Pannor, R. (1978). *The Adoption Triangle*. New York: Doubleday.

Spark, C., & Cuthbert, D. Eds. (2009). *Other People's Children: Adoption in Australia*. Melbourne: Australian Scholarly Publishing.

Strickland, P.A. (2013). *Akin to the Truth: A Memoir of Adoption and Identity*. Idealized Apps, LLC.

Strong-Boeg, V. (2007). Children of adversity: Disabilities and child welfare in Canada from the nineteenth to the 21st century. *Journal of Family History*, 32 (4), 413–432.

Trinder, L., Feast, J., & Howe, D. (2004). *The Adoption Reunion Handbook*. West Sussex: John Wiley & Sons, Ltd.

Triseliotis, J. (1973). *In Search of Origins: The Experiences of Adopted People*. London: Routledge & Kegan Paul.

Triseliotis, J., Feast, J., & Kyle, F. (2005). *The Adoption Triangle Revisited: A Study of Adoption: Search and Reunion Experiences*. London: BAAF.

Verrier, N. (2003). *Coming Home to Self*. Baltimore: Gateway Press, Inc.

Von Korff, L., Grotevant, H.D., & McRoy, R.G. (2006). Openness arrangements and psychological adjustment in adolescent adoptees. *Journal of Family Psychology*, 20, 531–534.

Walton, J. (2012). Supporting the interests of intercountry adoptees beyond childhood: Access to adoption information and identity. *Social Policy and Society*, 11 (3), 443–454.

Wasson, V. (1939). *The Chosen Baby*. Philadelphia: J. B. Lippincott Company.

Welsh, J.A. (2007). Developmental outcomes of internationally adopted children. *Child and Adolescent Social Work Journal*, 24 (3), 285–311.

Whitesel, A., & Howard, J.A. (2013). *Untangling the Web II: A Research-Based Roadmap for Reform*. New York: The Donaldson Adoption Institute.

Wieder, H. (1995/2001). *Handbook on Adoption: A Psychoanalytic View*. San Jose, New York, Lincoln, & Shanghai: Authors Choice Press.

Wolfgram, S.M. (2008). Openness in adoption: What we know so far – A critical review of the literature. *Social Work*, 53 (2), 133–142.

Wrobel, G.M., & Dillon, K. (2009). Adopted adolescents: Who and what are they curious about? In G.M. Wrobel, & E. Neil (Eds.), *International Advances in Adoption Research for Practice*. London: Wiley Blackwell, pp. 217–244.

Wrobel, G.M., & Grotevant, H.D. (2016). *Adoption-Related Curiosity in Emerging Adulthood. (Conference presentation)*. 1–2. Amherst, MA: ScholarWorks@UMass Amherst. https://doi.org/10.7275 R5Z899NN

Wrobel, G.M., & Grotevant, H.D. (2019). Minding the (information) gap: What do emerging adult adoptees want to know about their birth parents? *Adoption Quarterly*, 22 (1), 29–52.

Wrobel, G.M., Grotevant, H.D., Samek, D.R., & Von Korff, L. (2013). Adoptees' curiosity and information seeking about birth parents in emerging adulthood: Context, motivation and behavior. *International Journal of Behavior and Development*, 37 (5). https://doi.org/10.1177/0165025413486420

Zilberstein, K. (2011). Multiple attachment representations in clinical practice: Case study of a six-year-old maltreated child. *Psychoanalytic Social Work*, 18 (1), 23–38.

Zuckerman, J.R., & Buchsbaum, B. (2007). Transference and countertransference paradigms with adoptees. In R.A. Javier, A.L. Baden, F.A. Biafora, & A. Camacho-Gingerich (Eds.), *Handbook of Adoption: Implications for Researchers, Practitioners, and Families*. Thousand Oaks, London, & New Delhi: Sage Publications, pp. 491–495.

APPENDIX

1. Historical accounts regarding adoption practices in the United States can be found in several publications in the popular press (Lifton, 2009; Glaser, 2021) and in scholarly reviews (Marr et al., 2020). They do not, however, address the problem that national organizations representing the fields involved with adoption, particularly social work, have not been willing to endorse or join efforts in adoption reform, particularly regarding the sealed record and the need for better-qualified, highly professional staff in handling adoptive placements.
2. This refers to entitlement to obtain a child regardless of the means, not entitlement to be an authentic parent of an adopted child.
3. The editors encourage our colleagues around the world to consult (online) findings of studies sponsored by the Evan B. Donaldson Adoption Institute. For the purposes of this chapter, we cite from their section "For the Records II" (2010):

   - "The overwhelming majority of birth mothers do not want to remain anonymous to the children they relinquished for adoption, and [they] support . . . access to OBCs." (Original Birth Certificate)
   - "Providing adult adoptees with access to their OBCs does not threaten the integrity of adoptive families or the institution of adoption; indeed, the evidence suggests that the opposite is the case."
   - Regardless of the country or state where the record was never sealed, or where access to OBCs has been restored, "there is no evidence of any of the significant negative consequences critics predict."

4. College counseling services, particularly on large campuses, could consider outreach, such as through the school newspaper, by expressing an interest in assisting adopted students with their special concerns. One option would be the development of a therapy group for adopted students – but only provided the campus therapist is already trained to work from an adoption-specific knowledge base and from a clinical perspective.

PART V

Complexities of Psychotherapeutic Treatment

11
OBSERVATIONS ON CLINICAL PROBLEMS AND THE NEED FOR SHIFTS IN PERSPECTIVES

Doris Bertocci, LCSW, and Linda Mayers, PhD

Introduction

From the prevailing sociological and social work perspectives, the "adoptee" has been viewed as a *child* embedded within the adoptive family and the larger community, as well as within the even larger cultural, sociopolitical, and national context (Marr et al., 2020). The focus of counseling and mental health services has primarily been on *parenting* skills (to help the parents) and on treatment of their adopted children to resolve problematic behaviors (to better "fit into the family"). Medical and mental health professionals have not recognized that the psychology of *being* adopted is about far more than the typically cited issues of traumatic loss and attachment. There has been very limited focus on the adopted person's own development and *internal* experience beyond the childhood years. This pertains especially to the complexities of their personal identity which derive only partly from the adoptive family, usually become prominent concerns in adolescence and young adulthood, and continue to arise intermittently throughout the life span. This chapter emphasizes that very little research has asked the kinds of questions soliciting information that *practicing* clinicians need – or that would justify some researchers' over-generalized conclusions. Overall, there is a significant difference between *clinical topics* as typically identified in the literature, *clinical perspectives* on the multi-layered significance of the topics (and that, in turn, inform differential diagnosis), identification and description of *clinical approaches* to treatment with various supporting case studies, and actual *clinical process* within the treatment. This chapter addresses all four.

The overall consensus of a number of studies has been that "most adoptees seem to be behaviorally and emotionally well-adjusted" (Holmgren et al., 2020, p. 355). This finding of researchers in Finland, along with most research to date, is based on preadolescent subjects, emphasizing those with early histories of severe deprivation, using primarily behavioral criteria and cognitive measures. When inquiry is into the "emotional wellness" of adopted children, such as in surveys and other studies (NSAP/ASPE, 2007–2008), adolescents are typically not differentiated from all "children" under age 18. Further, the questions about adopted subjects have not been designed with the benefit of collaboration with adoption-knowledgeable mental health professionals who have a deeper and more extensive understanding of the actual parameters of such a non-specific term as "emotional wellness." Also, the typical use of parents as informants cannot yield the detailed information that is needed for clinical meaning and use, especially if the adopted subjects are adolescents and young adults.

Mental health practitioners themselves may consider themselves "trauma-informed" or "attachment-informed," but their training has been in a generic framework, without an understanding of how these concepts differ in the case of adopted persons who frequently have complicated early histories and circumstances that do not apply to the non-adopted – and that often are not even included in traditional trauma trainings. Further, many therapists are insufficiently trained generally in early childhood development (the first three years of life), but particularly in the neurobiological and neuropsychological complexities of early trauma. These can include sensory and endocrinological deprivation if separated from the birth mother in infancy (Bergman, 2019), changes or setbacks in brain development very early in life (Perry, 2020), significant anticipatory anxiety that is known in many cases to continue into adulthood, and variants of attachment problems as they pertain specifically to the varied combination of experiences of adopted persons. Severe and protracted trauma within the first three years of life is very different from the trauma of older children referenced in the literature (Merritt, 2022). Of greatest importance, sequelae of this may not be evident until many years later, in adolescence and young adulthood. For these reasons, along with other adoption-specific information that mental health professionals have not been trained to understand, the treatment they provide adopted individuals is usually significantly off the mark. This is partly because they do not know the questions to ask and do not know how to think about the client's answers. There is also the problem in the mental health field generally that, since the latter part of the twentieth century, the importance of including clients' early histories has been de-emphasized in favor of briefer cognitive behavioral, "goal-oriented" approaches. The latter alone is incompatible with the treatment requirements for "special-needs" populations with complicated circumstances, such as adopted persons. But first, mental health practitioners must recognize that adopted persons are a special-needs group, as are their families, and that best practices require that therapists not depend on their conventional training but that they advance their knowledge base so that it is adoption-specific.

The evidence for this need comes from the consistent feedback from innumerable adopted young adults, although presently it is anecdotal because it has been inadequately studied. However, many who have shared with their therapists their previous treatment experiences, of which they typically had many over the years, have stated that these experiences were helpful in only limited ways, while others felt it was actually harmful to them. Regarding the former, adopted adolescents and young adults frequently see therapists "only" for age-appropriate concerns, when neither of them (client or therapist) recognizes the threads that indicate possible unresolved deeper problems with underlying adoption themes. This can be an important opportunity for both. If the therapist is to provide the fuller service the client would most benefit from, he/she needs to consider the significance and timing for pulling those threads. But based on their past disappointing experiences in therapy, many adopted people have stated that they were left doubting that they could benefit from it at all. They attribute this to their therapists having little understanding of the complexities in their lives, such as tending to dismiss the significance of their experience as an adopted person. Many adopted clients have expressed their disappointment that they left all their prior therapies feeling they were never really "heard" (understood) and were therefore unable to make the changes they needed in their lives.

Finally, the authors believe there is a problem with boundaries in both the adoption and mental health fields when "adolescent" is automatically viewed only as an extension of "child," but the actual focus and emphasis of published studies (Waterman et al., 2018), including specific contexts, such as separated adopted twins (Segal, 2021), remain limited to children under age 13, leaving us without the equally important material relating to the years that follow. When the subjects are adopted, this is an example of adolescence being treated as less relevant and less important than earlier childhood. As another observation on the importance of boundaries, although in actual practice there is some overlap, treatment of adopted youth needs to be distinguished from services for foster children (those "in care"), because many of their needs are different. Each topic is a specialty of its own. In welfare adoptions, adoptive placement is typically treated as the final goal, a desired outcome, rather than as the beginning of a new and still challenging part of the life of the child and the family, sometimes warranting specialized services. Practitioners also need to distinguish between two entirely different subgroups: those who were placed for adoption in early childhood and later need treatment, perhaps in adolescence, and those who spent much of their childhoods in foster care, often intermittently living back and forth with a birth parent, and later in adolescence are placed with the extended birth family, legally adopted by the foster family, or placed for adoption with a non-kinship family. Treatment for these subgroups requires their own respective, carefully considered evaluations and modifications.

Adoption-Specific Considerations in Evaluation and Treatment

1. The Alternate Development of the Adopted Individual

The complexities that adopted young adults refer to, in discussing their frustrated experiences in therapy, begin with the adopted person's genetic template for health and personality development deriving from the birth parents – in many cases, people they know nothing about and may never have met. This means they have no point of reference with regard to their genetic and prenatal neurophysiological template or its role in their ongoing physical and personality development and changes over time. For this reason, it is common for adolescents to be anxious about their bodily changes (Chapter 15) and about details that may come up in their medical care that could suggest inheritable vulnerabilities. Therapists should not underestimate the significance and, often, intensity of their concerns.

> *If you don't know anyone you're related to, you have no way of ruling anything out, like cancer or any other disease. But this means that you could be at risk for anything, so there's a lot of anxiety, especially every time your doctor is concerned about a test result.*

Their "genetic factors" may include many forms of giftedness and talent, although the adoption literature tends to reference genetically based characteristics only as "risk factors," an echo of the "bad blood" theme. The developmental template acquired genetically from the birth parents is then integrated with the developmental impact of their early life experience prior to placement (which may or may not include direct contact with a birth parent and, for some, include significant changes and other "adversities"), which must then be integrated internally with adjustments to the adoptive family and their larger social and cultural context. None of this is the experience of people who are not adopted. Bearing all these in mind, the parent-centered perspective derived from the adoption field, social work, and sociological scholarship that, to some degree, has filtered down into the thinking of therapists remains that "at the core of adoption is the desire to create a family" (Esposito & Biafora, 2007, p. 17). By implication, this refers to the legal arrangements made by infertile adult couples in order to acquire a child that is not biologically related to them. This notion minimizes the reality for many midlife adults who have had children by birth and then adopted foster children who continued to be in their care. Overall, this oversimplified "core motive" for what adoption is about, deriving from the adoption culture of the twentieth century, overlooks the complex factors and internal needs underlying the decisions that adults make, such as whether and why to adopt, while it de-emphasizes the other half of the equation, the child her/himself. From the twentieth-century perspective, the child is essentially viewed as the means to the end, namely, parenthood.

The parent-centered focus of the adoption, social work, and sociological fields, and of mental health and their nearly exclusive preoccupation with "the family," has been at the expense of studying in-depth the adopted person's full development, especially with respect to its greatest complexities in adolescence and young adulthood. Therefore, from the perspective of the person who *should have been* the primary concern of the adoption field, at the core of adoption is the human being who arrives in a powerless and entirely vulnerable state, many in the earliest weeks and months of life removed from the neurobiological protections intended by nature, such as the critical postnatal sensory and endocrinological exchanges with the birth mother. Regardless of efforts based on compassion for the child, he/she is still subject to the desires, naïveté, and sociopolitical requirements of many external forces that include the self-interests of adults, cultures, and nations, intertwined with the rigidly narrow, adult-centered focus of family law. The latter refers to the typical legal question within the contexts of both adoption and child custody litigation of "who owns the child" or "who *should* own the child" (Derdeyn, 1979). As stated in an earlier chapter, the legal perspective is fundamentally based on probate (property) law: American family lawyers say there is no need for them to understand the developmental needs of children since "we are lawyers, not psychologists," and many have been heard to scoff at the concept of "the best interests of the child" (Goldstein et al., 1973). They do not recognize or endorse the concept of children's human rights as children (Appendix 2; Chapter 1) in distinction from adult rights. Even if the law hypothetically gives passing reference to what one family court judge vaguely referred to as "the sensitive issues," this still may not result in judicial decisions that are informed or guided by children's unique needs over time, which are very different from adults'. In the United States, judicial dilemmas keep many thousands of children in protracted foster care in deference to the birth mother, who may or may not be able to stabilize her life. The latter is a critical question that requires intermittent *clinical* evaluation, but the judiciary is not trained to know its importance or its capacity to help the court make a better-informed and more rapid decision. The judiciary's negligence in this regard remains, despite all that is known about the child's different time frame *internally* (psychologically) and about the enduring emotional trauma for the child-who-waits, for even brief periods of time.

The fact that the stage of adolescence itself is not generally treated as a clinical specialty of its own likely derives from the original conceptualization of psychiatry up to the mid-twentieth century when the only subgroup other than "adult" was "child." But in the twenty-first century, the psychology of adolescence has come to be recognized as requiring clinical formulations and treatment practices based on the adolescent's significant developmental changes and needs.

However, it needs to be noted that the same applies to the decade beyond adolescence because, in the 20s, there are still significant facets of development that continue to unfold in the brain (Siegel, 2013). This involves further changes in perceptions and meanings ascribed to them, the process of coming to terms with social requirements and a sense of responsibility to others, development of greater capacities for both reflective and critical thinking, and arrival at new understandings of who they have become as persons. Young adulthood is the time for consolidation of personality and its defenses, for re-defining "family" and one's relationship within it, for the challenges of significant life decisions at this part of the life span, and for integrating the different facets of each adopted person's identity, until all become consistent, stable, and consolidated in full adulthood. References to "adopted adults" or to "adulthood" in the literature (Baden & Wiley, 2007; Levy-Schiff,

2016; Darnell, 2017) suggest similar themes, although these studies are still too generalized to help therapists understand the particular internal, integrative processes of *young* adulthood. Overall, and in short, the complexities identified for the adopted individual, from birth through young adulthood, constitute an *alternate* development in many areas of the adopted person's inner experience, requiring *alternate* approaches therapeutically.

In distinction from the social service field's understanding of the fundamentals in the experience of members of the adoption triad, there remain a number of problems in the traditional mental health disciplines, which presently accord no significance or meaning to being adopted. It is considered a minor detail in the history, and treatment proceeds as though they are the same as any other client. Adopted young adults typically report that previous therapists "didn't make much" of their being adopted or even "never brought it up." Such practices undoubtedly derive in part from the adoption culture, which has had the limited mission of recruiting adoptive parents, minimizing any potential problems, and placing children with them. Both the adoption and mental health fields have avoided learning about the developmental complexities for the adopted individual, especially those that follow childhood. This accounts for the continuing inadequate preparation the adoption field provides for adoptive parenting both before and following adoptive placement, about which many parents continue to complain. Over time, this perspective has pervaded the thinking of the health-care fields and limited the focus of research efforts. As one example, for the purposes of this chapter, clinically focused research is needed, not only regarding those whose lives involved "early adversities," but also regarding the developmental *details of* domestically placed adopted adolescents and young adults, along with information about the placement sources, and clinical profiles of adopted patients seen in treatment in different settings. This would involve correlating the six fundamental demographic factors (Chapter 4) with the specific *details of* the early history, including *details of* the treatment history, with the *details of* their current clinical profiles.

2. The Lack of Pre-Placement Information

There are common references in the adoption literature to the problem that, with the exception of most private *agency* placements, there are often insufficient details about the birth family and the circumstances surrounding the placement that were recorded or made available to the adoptive family – information that may be important to the adopted person at a later time. The latter was never a consideration in adoption practice until the 1970s and 1980s, when there arose a groundswell of demand by adopted adults for access to their own birth certificates (naming the birth parents and enabling them to search) and to information from the sources of their adoption. While the "open record" became law in the UK in 1975, presently, only one quarter of states in the United States allow adopted adults unrestricted access (Chapter 1). The problem in the context of treatment is that therapists in the

United States tend to accept at face value that pre-placement material is not available, but without inquiring further, especially if the lack of information becomes problematic for the treatment. There are sometimes means for working with the adoptive family to inquire further from the placement source. If the client/patient has decided to seek more information, it may be helpful, even in the case of adopted young adults, for the therapist to raise the idea of the client and parents together filling out a questionnaire (Appendix 3A), which may stimulate the parents' memories for some details but also provide an opportunity for a mutually shared exchange of information and questions and for the expression of feelings about the disclosure, or about still-unavailable information that the adopted daughter or son wishes to know. Of greatest importance for the treatment, the therapist needs to be mindful of the emotional impact on the adopted client of seeming to have no way to get answers to many of their questions, even to some of the most basic information that non-adopted people take for granted.

> *I wonder if my birth father even knows I exist. My friends have all these photographs of themselves when they were babies and little kids, but I have nothing. All my parents could show me was one of me on a bicycle.*

With the right timing, the therapist may want to explore the meaning to/for the client of "not being able to know," and their attendant fantasies, frustration, and anxiety that may come up at various times in treatment. For those who were placed internationally, they may have been "left at the orphanage," with no way of knowing anything about their birth mother, much less any other information. This lack of information is experienced as an ambiguous but profound loss of a crucial part of themselves (Boss, 2000), for which they usually cannot receive full understanding or empathy from other people in their lives because they have never experienced it. Even under the best of circumstances in the adopted person's current life, as many have expressed, it is unresolvable and another dimension of feeling "disconnected" or "cut off at the knees" early in their life. This is an area in which the therapist's emotional attunement, along with their expressed awareness that the client's predicament is shared by many other adopted persons, can make an important difference in the therapeutic engagement. This is referred to as "clinical empathy" that, through "mutual affective experience" (Main, et al., 2017), enables significant personality change over time. This is not a prerequisite in most cognitive behaviorally based forms of treatment.

3. The Need to Shift from the Perspectives of Child Welfare and Child Psychology to the Psychology of Adolescence and Young Adulthood

Caution is needed when using findings from outcome studies of the overall "psychosocial adjustments of adoptees," because until recently, the vast majority of studies have been limited to families of pre-adolescent children (Brodzinsky & Schechter,

1990; Brodzinsky, 1993; Brodzinsky & Palacios, 2005; Waterman et al., 2018; Wrobel et al., 2020), with the data typically derived from the adoptive parents. In more recent years, focus has expanded to specific developmental difficulties, such as learning problems and ADHD (Lindblad et al., 2010; Roskam et al., 2014); specific ethnic/racial groups and countries of origin (Tessler & Gamache, 2012; Hoffman & Vallejo-Pena, 2013; Riley-Behringer et al., 2014; Kim & Lee, 2020); particular subsets of adoptive families in the United States, such as "special needs" and LGBTQ families (Brodzinsky & Pertman, 2012; Farr & Vazquez, 2020; Johnson et al., 2020); cognitive development and school performance of adopted children (Howard et al., 2004; Van Ijzendoorn et al., 2005; Vinke et al., 2016; Dalen & Therie, 2020); and differences in cognitive performance according to age at adoption and country/area of birth (Odenstad et al., 2008). There have been many studies involving comparisons of a small number of variables, such as adopted vs. non-adopted, domestic vs. international, foster care vs. adopted, typically using non-adopted subjects as controls; family racial composition (Barth et al., 2005; Welsh et al., 2007; Vinke et al., 2016; Dekker et al., 2016); and families formed by different types of adoption compared with each other and with non-adoptive families (Howard et al., 2004). Few studies added other important demographic variables that are an integral part of each topic under investigation (Chapter 4). Particularly needed would be studies of different subgroups of adopted subjects, including adolescents and young adults, with variables such as closed vs. open adoption, age at separation from the birth mother as well as age at actual placement, parents' socioeconomic status and educational level, source of the placement, and information about parents' pre-adoption preparation and also whether, when, and why the family utilized, or had access to, post-adoption services, the nature of such services, and most importantly outcomes of such services. Studies that included information about the adoptive parents have tended to focus on more *external* features, such as "parenting styles" with children (Tan et al., 2012), and on the degree of openness and acceptance of differences in family communication practices (Brodzinsky, 2006; Thomas & Scharp, 2020). The problem with the term "openness" is that the nature of the family's communications with their child about adoption may be confused with open adoption, which relates to the legal arrangements for varying degrees of contact between the adoptive family and the birth parents.

One of the relatively rare and most important American studies to use clinical criteria in studying adoptive parents found that a significant proportion of parents with seriously disturbed very young adopted children had formally diagnosed attachment disorders of their own (Buckwalter et al., 2017). Consistent with this, a study from Spain of "late-placed" children (ages 4 to 7) had similar findings in that the children who demonstrated significant improvement from insecure to secure attachment behavioral patterns had been predominantly placed with adoptive mothers who tested as secure-autonomous through the AAI (Pace et al., 2012, p. 56). That is, the adoptive mothers themselves had significant attachment capacities and resilience. In other words, *attachment needs to be mutual*. These studies support one of the urgent concerns expressed in this handbook having to do with the inadequate skills of many adoption placement workers in parent selection (Chapter 2). Their level of training and the lack of priority given to protecting the child have not been considered in attachment studies involving adopted children. This especially includes adoptions that are welfare-based and "private/independent" adoptions handled by lawyers, that is, the question of skill levels for protection of the child. We also note, however, the inadequate inquiry into the role of adoptive fathers in attachment studies. As an example of the inadequacies of surveys conducted by governmental agencies, the aforementioned NSAP study in the United States combined into one group labeled "private domestic adoptions" those handled through private professional adoption agencies and those handled privately by lawyers. However, these represent opposite ends of the spectrum with regard to protections for the child.

A good deal of study has focused on children and families within the public welfare system and, because of the overlap, combined with foster care populations, including focus on the additional disadvantages for minority families (Barth et al., 2005; Henry, 2012; Jackson & Samuels, 2019). More recently, quantitative studies have focused on adopted adolescents (Reppold et al., 2009; Tessler & Gamache, 2012; Manzi et al., 2014; McConnachie et al., 2021) and young adults (Moyer & Juang, 2011; Oke et al., 2015; Vinke et al., 2016; Levy-Schiff, 2016; Darnell et al., 2017; Sanchez-Sandoval & Melero, 2019; Cashen et al., 2019; Roche & Perlesz, 2000; Despax et al., 2021). However, because of the nature of the studies, few focused on the kind of information that would inform clinical practice or clinical process, such as the modifications needed in evaluation and treatment. Even when the focus includes approaches to helping adopted clients, common references tend to be on cognitively based "supportive strategies" that are fundamental to counseling and social work practice. However, these and various psychoeducational interventions may already be among the skills of some adoption-informed therapists working psychodynamically, which allows exploration of the client's internal life and connecting it with the difficulties for which they seek psychotherapy. Late adolescence and emerging adulthood are critical times to address difficulties with impulse control, judgment, reflective capacities, affect regulation, and incipient characterological problems. These may be special challenges when the client is adopted; on the other hand, many adopted people in this age group are not challenged in this way but seek therapy for the same concerns as their non-adopted peers.

Of particular concern, there are no known studies of the full medical or psychiatric histories of adopted adolescents and young adults, including important details of any treatment. The NSAP study referred to earlier (NSAP/ASPE, 2007–2008) found that adopted children under age 18 are twice as likely as children in the general population to have "special health care needs," but these were not specified in detail other than a reference to asthma which often derives from early pulmonary problems. The report found that for 26% of adopted children, the parents reported "moderate or severe consequences of any of 16 possible medical or psychological conditions." Not only did the report not differentiate between pre-adolescent children and adolescents, but it also did not distinguish between or specify medical from/and psychological conditions and provided inadequate data on the details of these conditions. Despite their significant findings about health-care needs, the report has the effect of minimizing them with its conclusion that the majority of all adopted children "fared well" in health both physically and emotionally. This was based on their limited topical questions about ADHD, depression, anxiety, and conduct problems. Even if their positive conclusions did apply to the alleged majority, there was no expressed concern for addressing the needs of the significant minority. In short, the NSAP's generalized findings, as well as those of most other studies, lack the details that have significance for clinicians in both adolescent medicine and in mental health. More generally, beyond the NSAP study, typical conclusions regarding adopted children "faring well," their "adequate adjustment," "child wellness," "adoption satisfaction," and "positive outcomes" are broad-brush concepts typically used in social work and sociological research, which may have a vested interest interest in getting positive results, but they lack scientific meaning and significance for practicing clinicians. It is this that is needed for psychotherapists, especially those who work psychodynamically, who are interested in the important details of the adopted patient's internal life that are necessary for more accurate differential diagnosis and for development of a suitable adoption-informed treatment plan.

Data from scientific studies and from the developing field of adoption medicine should have continued to be of particular interest and concern to psychiatry, because, from the 1960s to the 1980s, it became so prominent in studies of adopted children (see Dedication). But since then, psychiatry has shifted to focusing extensively and more generally not only on developmental trauma (Van der Kolk, 2015) but also now on *early* developmental trauma (Perry, 2020), although there is limited focus on adopted individuals who might challenge some of their assumptions. Clinical psychology has done a great deal of work in the area of attachment, but except for Steele et al. (2010), there has been limited reference to adopted subjects at any age, whose circumstances are typically different from the non-adopted subgroup with attachment problems represented in the literature (see Foreword). Research on the all-encompassing concepts of "adverse childhood experiences" and "complex trauma" does not actually have much to say specifically about the psychology of *being* adopted, even when the authors have a background in the adoption field (Hendry & Hasler, 2017). As a final consideration for therapists, the multitude of transracial/interracial factors that apply in both domestic and international adoptions must be considered carefully (Fong & McRoy, 2016; Raleigh & Kreider, 2020). These must always be explored in treatment in regard to their meanings to the adopted client, and secondarily to the adoptive family, and we urge more studies that will inform evaluation and treatment of those in adolescence and young adulthood.

Unlike the non-adopted population, the experiences of many adopted persons commonly involve a number of additional difficulties and setbacks that become more significant with age, especially in late adolescence. These include secrecy,

Clinical Problems and the Need for Shifts in Perspectives

distortion, or the absence of important facts in their histories, along with their mounting confusion about their full personal identity. Each of the fundamental demographic factors listed in Chapter 4 represents a significant developmental crossroad that is likely to impact in different ways their self-understanding, their self-esteem, and components of their complex identity. Further, however, the developmental issues of earlier childhood are very different from those of adolescence, when they can become greatly magnified by the complexities inherent in being adopted. For example, the therapist needs to consider whether early trauma may still need to be considered a contributing factor in such problems as social anxiety, specific phobias, or ongoing difficulties with some executive functions that contribute to low self-esteem.

Throughout the adopted person's childhood, the common experience of their parents, when they have concerns about their child's symptoms and/or behaviors, is of their pediatricians giving them the facile advice that their child "will grow out of it" (Appendix 6 in Chapter 4). Those knowledgeable about the development of adopted people into adulthood inform us that this is not at all necessarily true, especially in regard to certain behavioral, medical, psychosomatic, and neuropsychological conditions (Chapter 9), and to the full scope of learning problems that can extend to the college level. What must also necessarily be considered are different facets of the adopted person's development (which may not be consistent with their chronological age), along with their internal emotional life, that, in turn, significantly influences their judgment in the important decisions they will be making at this time in their life. This can be particularly hazardous because, based on anecdotal reports from many parents, their adolescents seem to be much younger emotionally, in some areas at least, than their peers, so that their critical judgment may be impaired to varying degrees. For example, as a young adolescent girl, one of our adopted patients naïvely went along with the suggestion of a troubled friend whom she considered her "blood sister" because of the bond they felt in their both being adopted and ended up going to the apartment of a young man who was a stranger. He raped her. This was her first sexual encounter. She responded to this trauma by becoming, unconsciously, what she had been told her birth mother was, promiscuous and involved with drugs and alcohol. There followed a long period of self-punishment for a bewildering and devastating experience, when in fact the girl's judgment that had led to the trauma had been that of a much younger child simply following a friend's advice.

Over the years, the parents are likely to accept the pediatrician's reassurances without getting a second opinion, as is now available from a physician in adoption medicine. However, the problem in current adoption medicine programs, we believe, is that the vast majority serve only children under age 3, such as those recently arrived from other countries. But there is a great need, we believe, for adoption-knowledgeable psychiatric intervention for adopted adolescents within adoption medicine settings for the reasons discussed in Chapter 9. These include evaluation of the need for medication, such as for significant symptoms of depression or anxiety and possible other related areas of medicine, for example, neuropsychological problems, eating disorders, and endocrinological disorders. But there is also an argument for adoption medicine programs to include clinicians in the mental health field who can provide adoption-knowledgeable services for adopted adolescents, since they are not likely to be available in any other health-care or mental health settings. This is particularly critical in the case of adolescents whose inner turmoil and anger has reached such intensity that it leaves them questioning whether they want to continue living. The common use of the term "suicidal" has little meaning unless skillfully evaluated for the details by an adoption knowledgeable mental health professional (see Chapter 1).

It may not be until the college years that the adopted emerging adult engages in more self-reflection and the struggles heretofore in a dormant state begin to come to the surface. If in college they seek help from a campus counselor or clinician, there will be little or no discussion of the possible relevance of adoption issues, because the mental health field has not been trained to understand their significance or to pose the right questions for the student's consideration. In the actual treatment encounter, therapists are alerted to the fact that many adopted adolescents and young adults report that they learned to "keep a lot inside." This needs to be explored over time in treatment, for example, the vicissitudes of shame, embarrassment, and anxiety, or the deeply ingrained belief that they will not be understood no matter how hard they try. Other examples would include the need for the therapist to explore distorted fantasies that serve to fill the vacuum of missing information, potentially lifelong separation anxiety that is a source of embarrassment, or dysphoria that at times can become major depression, often at the time of a loss of an important relationship or during a difficult life transition. Typically, with age, the adopted person learns more, and thinks more, about certain differences that they have from their peers and from other families. While, for some, envious resentment may become a preoccupation as invidious comparisons are made, with the predictable effect of lowering the client's self-esteem, the adolescent may also become more guarded about what they reveal or share with others, partly because of the odd (to them) reactions they may have already received and therefore anticipate, for example, the "microaggressions" discussed in the literature (Baden, 2016; Garber, 2020), leaving them to experience people as lacking empathy and as being dismissive of what they are trying to express.

Nobody would understand anyway, so I've just learned to live with it.

With some clients, the therapist will want to be alert to some adopted patients' style of communication, perhaps monosyllabic or limited to superficial, concrete facts or events, flat affect, lack of spontaneity, or impaired memory for people and relationships in their past. These could have deeper roots in the early history that is pre-language and pre-memory, and those who survived childcare settings with minimal and inconsistent care may re-enact in therapy the long silences they experienced from early caretakers or "baby homes" (Chapter 15). Such manifestations of early trauma can be subtle and would not necessarily be identified from studies relating to behavioral problems and conduct disorders, school achievement, or "adoption satisfaction," topics and evaluations that permeate the social work research and literature. In adolescence, acting-out behaviors may involve experimentation with alcohol or vaping, illegal substances (perhaps to put themselves in an altered state in order to calm the inner turmoil), high-risk behaviors, or especially if exposed to domestic violence early in their life, self-destructive physical abuse, such as self-mutilation or eating disorders (Fujisawa & Tomoda, 2021), or oppositional behaviors guaranteed to provoke their parents. The latter can be rooted in unconscious fears that they do not have the capacities needed to grow into adulthood and are internally fighting with their sense of helplessness, inadequacy, dependency, and/or low self-esteem. This can be very frightening, and transferentially, it is often acted out in their irritability and defiance and in the way they handle their therapy appointments.

The literature on adopted children emphasizes "externalizing" behaviors and conduct disorders, in large part because young children "act out" their emotions, and it is easier to identify and quantify for research. But a good deal of this changes in adolescence, yet there has been much less in the literature about "internalizing" symptoms, such as intermittent low-grade depression that may account for "lack of motivation" or that can become episodes of major depression and thoughts of suicide (Festinger & Jaccard, 2012), leading in some cases to hospitalization or even death. Missing from this study, and all others on suicidal ideation, were/are questions that clinicians would want to know, such as the full spectrum of thoughts, fantasies, associations, intentions, and any actual plans, and information about their experiences trying to get professional help.

Some adopted adolescents and emerging adults report difficulty in being self-directed and clear-minded in their plans and goals for the future, unable to make decisions, in some cases unconsciously imagining that it would be much easier if they could only know the talents, skills, and interests of their birth parents. Some may eventually articulate this to their therapists, while for others, it remains unconscious. The authors speculate that this could be a form of ego paralysis, a kind of illusion, that their peers, by being born into their families and automatically having specific points of reference, somehow have a much easier time making their decisions. They need their therapist's help in learning to use their developing self-knowledge and self-understanding, that is, themselves, as their best point of reference.

As an example of the importance of details that carry special meanings, therapists should take note of seemingly innocuous details, like tattoos, which today are no longer considered as a form of self-mutilation but rather as a form of self-enhancement or a particular, symbolic, artistic way of representing the self. What is probably most important to understand is the symbolic meaning of the tattoo to the person who has chosen to get something permanently inscribed on their body – a reminder, a memento, a tribute, a statement. Cases have been reported of adopted adolescents wanting to get plastic surgery that actually reflected the parent's wish for them to change a facial feature in order to more closely resemble the parent (but the option of the parent getting the surgery was never a consideration). An adopted young adult male who had felt unloved throughout his childhood and had a history of lying and stealing had a skunk tattooed on his arm with his name underneath; he explicitly referred to himself as a "stinker" and turned his self-definition into a feature of narcissistic pride as he continued to engage in behaviors that got him into trouble (personal communication from a family member). More generally, one of the most important areas to explore with an adopted client is the complexity of their perceptions, feelings, and associations regarding different facets of their body image and parts of their body, undoubtedly associated, at least unconsciously, with the birth parents, along with the details of what each feature means and the degree to which it is valued or devalued (Crook, 2000).

Although it has never been studied and is therefore anecdotal, there appears to be a common pattern with some adopted patients of a rapid attrition rate early in the treatment process when overwhelming terrors or rage starts rising to the surface. However, they are likely to give another reason or leave therapy abruptly in order to avoid giving an explanation when they do not understand it themselves. This may represent the re-enactment of their abandonment, but with the patient being in control of it. It may be a helpful strategy for the therapist to alert the patient to this possible risk at the beginning of treatment and to discuss the possible meanings of impulsive behaviors of this kind. The therapist will also need to evaluate the client's capacity to reflect internally (Sharp & Bevington, 2022) on the underlying meanings of their behavior, as in this instance.

The emphasis in this chapter is that, regardless of the particular intervention with adopted adolescents and adults, it needs to be integrated with dynamic *adoption-informed* treatment, with careful consideration being given to the appropriate timing of each intervention – but most importantly to the *integration* of the fragmented elements of their development. This is because the shorter cognitive behavioral formats, such as life history work, the "brain-based" approaches to treating early trauma, and "attachment-informed" protocols that have insufficiently studied the critical variable of parental emotional attunement, still provide no means for the older adopted patient (adolescent and adult) to engage multiple ego functions for the integration process.

4. Complexities in Sexuality

The complexities of sexuality in the adopted population and within the adoptive family have never been studied or even mentioned in the psychology of adoption until this chapter, again likely because the focus of the adoption field has been primarily limited to families and their young children. It is not until adolescence that issues around sexual development, including gender identity, concerns around fertility (identification with their two sets of parents), and choices of intimate relationships, are likely to become a prominent part of the adopted person's larger questions around personal identity. This is because they are likely to be associated in their minds with the birth parents, for example, unconscious impulses that are sometimes acted upon, resulting in pregnancy/impregnation. The authors believe that these and many other concerns around sexuality are likely more complicated for adopted adolescents and young adults than for their non-adopted peers. Certainly, issues around sexuality are entirely relevant for all others in the triad, but these also remain unstudied and are curiously absent from the familiar "seven core issues" (Roszia & Maxon, 2019). For this reason, from a clinical perspective, the authors regard complexities in sexuality as the eighth "core issue." Further, they are likely to remain the elephant in the room for the adoptive parents unless they are provided an opportunity of their own, with the privacy they, too, need, to discuss various difficult topics with an adoption-knowledgeable family therapist.

Overall, the adoption literature has focused on generic trauma and attachment without the benefit of the small amount of *clinically focused* research on the adopted adolescent/young adult population. But further, we emphasize that, to whatever degree traumatic loss and attachment problems may, or may not, have been significant areas of concern in childhood, they typically become overshadowed by different concerns in adolescence relating to the adopted person's complex identity and by their unique concerns about sexuality, both of which are intimately associated with the mystery of their origins. This becomes painfully evident as they experience changes in their bodies, unfamiliar feelings or irritabilities, conflicted loyalties, difficulties with concentration or with becoming more self-directed in choices of studies and work (e.g., themes of "learned helplessness" deriving from a deeply ingrained sense of powerlessness) and adoption-specific concerns about dating relationships, redefining "family," and conflict around having their own children, regardless of their sexual orientation.

When the adopted child is pubescent and/or adolescent, there may be sexual tensions within adoptive families that arise and that family therapists are not likely to be attuned to. This may be because of their countertransferential difficulty empathizing with certain aspects of the adopted person's inner experience. In a number of cases, adopted patients have revealed to their therapists outright incestuous behaviors, including molestation and rape, by members of the adoptive family who used the lack of a biological relationship as justification. This is the "silent but profound trauma" encountered in the treatment of some adopted patients, and the absence of any references in the adoption and mental health literature has demonstrated the degree to which this subject itself remains entirely unacknowledged and taboo within these fields. For example, some practitioners are known to have asked, "If they aren't related biologically, is it really incest?"

> When I was 11, my older brother, who was also adopted, would keep trying to wear me down as he tried to molest me, and this went on for a couple of years, so I had to lock myself in my room. I never told my parents because I already knew from past

experience that they wouldn't deal with it, and that would have made it even worse. I had a lot of thoughts about running away because I felt trapped having to live there.

These are not uncommon anecdotal themes with adopted adolescents and young adults in treatment or may become clinical themes if therapists know enough to listen for them and approach the topic with great sensitivity.

5. The Need to Consider Recalibrating the Developmental Timeline for the Adopted Client

Our observation from a psychological and psychodynamic perspective is that, along with the unfolding changes in brain development over time, emotional development, some of it biologically programmed, unfolds in a more dramatic way as adolescence is announced with anatomical, physiological, hormonal, emotional, and behavioral changes. Any suspected developmental delays in adopted individuals need to be carefully reviewed in the clinical assessment. We also embrace the recent findings that many facets of neuropsychological development continue to unfold not only throughout adolescence but also well into young adulthood (Siegel, 2013; Galvan, 2017). For example, from a volume of anecdotal information from multiple sources, there is reason to believe that many adopted young adults, disproportionately to non-adopted young adults, may remain several years delayed in leaving home and in stabilizing their lives at a fully adult level. It is our impression that there is a common pattern of "trying out" college courses and jobs into or throughout their 20s, but returning home at intervals to reconstitute, similar to the ways a toddler experiments with new activities and experiences while still needing the security and "re-charging" from the parents. This is the principle of "regression in the service of progression." The challenge for both the therapist and the parents is to appreciate the adoption-normative developmental need for this and to provide the needed supportive resources, while also considering the appropriate timing if and when limits need to be set. The latter would be an important time for the parents to seek adoption-specialized clinical consultation, but it is an important time, too, for the young adult to seek the help of an adoption-informed therapist.

6. Therapists' Observations on the Narcissistic Side of Adoptive Parenting

From all that has been discussed about the larger systemic problems, and also about the six demographic variables that profoundly impact development (Chapter 4), it should be no surprise that, in many cases, the psychology of the adopted adolescent commonly includes doubts, or even suspicion, around what is being hidden or withheld from them, or coming to terms with the likelihood that information they seek may never be available, leaving them with a deep sense of loss that has no resolution (Boss, 2000); coming to terms with the timing of the parents' disclosure of their being adopted, as in the case of "late discovery"; an enduring sense of

Clinical Problems and the Need for Shifts in Perspectives

powerlessness and frustration that is unknown to their non-adopted peers; pockets of low self-esteem and, as a result, sometimes defiant impulses to undermine their best efforts, such as self-sabotage; struggle, for some, with the implications in the adoption narrative that they were "rescued," "lucky," and therefore indebted, with variations on the reverse theme of feeling "undeserving" or "defective"; a realization and resentment in adolescence that their parents seem disappointed with them or are "never satisfied"; anxiety about genetic vulnerabilities to disease, information to which, in some states, provinces, and countries, they are denied access for life, while in fact it typically becomes more important with age.

These, especially in combination, can result in distraction, anxiety, and some level of confusion and conflict throughout their psychosexual development, a neglected area in both research and parenting education because of its limited focus on pre-adolescent children, and the feeling expressed anecdotally by some adopted persons, an area of cognitive dissonance for them, that their parents seemed mostly influenced by familial and cultural pressures and expectations about parenthood but actually demonstrated limited interest in raising them.

It sort of messes with your head until you finally figure it out – and then you have to come to terms with it.

There is a big difference between my parents' behavior with the outside world, saying things about me that are supposed to reflect well on them, and the way they really treat me at home. They tell me I'll never get into a good college, and just because I talked to a guy online, my father called me a slut.

In some cases, the parents wanted a "family lifestyle" in order to "fit into the community" but were not necessarily invested in developing a mutually close relationship with their child. Sometimes this has been because they themselves had never experienced any closeness or affection in their own earlier lives and were limited to focusing on practical details of daily living. In other cases, adopted clients have reported that their parents pursued their careers or interests outside the home as they always had, seeming to leave them on their own to grow up.

My family was wealthy, so I was raised mostly by a series of nannies and babysitters.

It is not uncommon for adopted individuals in treatment to comment that it seemed it was really only their mother who wanted to adopt; it was their father who "just went along with it."

I don't think my father was really interested in children. He used his job as a reason not to be home much – he was never what you'd call "a family man."

When I was in my 20s, my father once commented that he didn't really know me. But he said it in a way that didn't seem to bother him.

Doris Bertocci, LCSW, and Linda Mayers, PhD

> *My mother talked a lot about the limits of what women could do when she was younger. Their only choice was to marry and have children. She would say she "really wanted a career."*

For the adopted daughter or son, difficulties in identity may arise when parents adopt out of the need to "clone" themselves or create a "mini-me," often to the extent, particularly in the case of the male child, of naming the child after themselves, for example, Charles Jr., because of the misguided notion that if they do this, the child somehow is now an extension of them, rather than acknowledged for their own individuality. While this is only one underlying dynamic theme in some cases, and while it is also very common in non-adoptive families, it is likely to take on a different or confused meaning for the adopted person. Adopted people can be especially sensitive about names, their origins and meanings, and many know their original names given when they were born, an important topic for therapy. As demonstrated by a case discussed by Hoksbergen (Chapter 2), in adulthood some choose to change back to their original name, which helps them bridge the divide in order to consolidate – or redefine – their full identity. But it may also represent a rejection of some aspect of their experience of being adopted.

The adopted individual who is questioning what adopting actually meant to their parents may not be aware that, in many countries, the irrational cultural pressures on adults to become parents, but only in the right way, at the right time, and with the right person, apply without regard to the actual needs of anyone. Irrational themes in culture have their own power and, like the law, tend to have a long lifetime – even centuries. However, studies of "parent motives" for adopting would likely benefit from the synergy that could be provided by clinical perspectives that may be able to identify the possible psychodynamic themes underlying the cognitive-only reasons that are typically given at a time the adults are eager to be accepted by the placement source. For example, we know of some adoptive parents who selectively withheld information about significant family or health problems that they knew would become a disadvantage for the child. There are always underlying reasons within the psychology of the adoptive parents, which are not lost on those young adults who have expressed their belief that they were "used to meet somebody else's needs." This perception may be accurate, but it may also be overdetermined.

Here, in the context of *the cumulative effects of numerous narcissistic injuries* that adopted persons have revealed in treatment, therapists would want to be attuned to the clinical significance for their adopted patients of the sub-population of parents who adopted, typically in midlife, as a means of holding a marriage together, sometimes later followed by divorce, in effect representing another abandonment for the adopted person, regardless of their age. Based on a good deal of anecdotal information from adopted clients, this is not uncommon, regardless of whether the parents are heterosexual or same-sex (Goldberg & Garcia, 2015). These researchers interviewed, five years after placement, 190 couples of lesbian, gay/male, and heterosexual parents of children placed under 18 months of age. In total, it was found that 7.9% of couples in all three groups had dissolved their relationship within these five years of parenthood. It might be especially informative if such a study were done after ten years of parenthood, bearing in mind the perception of clinicians who have treated adopted adolescents that parental separation and divorce can be particularly disturbing for them. But once again, clinical perspectives would be most useful in formulating the questions asked in such studies.

There are also complications in some single-parent adoptions, particularly in the case of older women wanting a last chance at parenthood but sometimes lacking the resources they will need to assist in raising the child, especially one that is seriously traumatized. In the case of international adoptions, the adjustments for both parent and adopted "child" are likely to become particularly difficult in adolescence since, as in the case of domestic placement settings, the international adoption organizations see their role as limited to the actual placement without providing – or assisting the parents with finding – adoption-knowledgeable services likely to be needed when the "child" becomes an adolescent. This is left to untrained resources in the community.

There has been insufficient focus by child welfare and social work on the different levels of maltreatment within the adoptive family (Matthews, 2020). A good deal of international research generally has focused on the extremes of "adverse circumstances," such as domestic violence and severe institutional deprivation. But inadequately explored are the far more common forms revealed by adopted clients, such as what appear to be significant limits in the adoptive parents' empathic attunement over time, or other subtle but still significant forms of neglect, the adoptive parents typically described by young adults as "emotionally unavailable." In some families, there may be significant narcissistic problems in one or both parents, such as those referred to in studies as having "authoritarian styles" of parenting, although definitions of the actual behavior and impact on the adopted daughter/son may not be given. Overall, questions on standardized testing protocols are based on the non-adopted population and, more problematic, can involve oversimplified terms and concepts, such as "parent–child closeness" (Loehlin et al., 2010) and "adoption satisfaction" (Nilsson et al., 2011). Clinicians ask different questions and need more in-depth, specific descriptions in order for the data to be useful for assessment and treatment.

7. The Psychology of the Adopted Adolescent and the Potential Role of Family Treatment

Once the adopted person becomes an adolescent, changes need to be considered from the customary treatment approaches with children and their families, in recognition not only of the changes brought on by adolescence but also of the significant emotional vulnerabilities experienced by many adopted adolescents. The usual family therapy model remains applicable, but in a modified way. Treatment no longer only reflects the notion, as suggested in the "adoption competency" model

(Atkinson, 2020; Appendix 5), that the family is the primary agent of "healing," because there are, and in fact there needs to be, additional sources of assistance toward healthy integration and maturation, such as school psychologists and social workers, specialists in learning problems, adolescent medicine (Chapter 9), and adoption-knowledgeable psychotherapists. Most important, at this part of the life span, depending on the clinical profile, the treatment is usually no longer "attachment-focused," although for some there may be residual or subtle forms of anxious attachment requiring clinical skill to identify and address. In adolescence, this is typically reflected in choices of peer and love relationships. They may choose someone as a transitional object as a means of separating from the adoptive parents, although the relationship may also become a developmental setback. While this occurs commonly in non-adopted adolescents, the authors speculate that adopted adolescents may more likely develop a long-standing intense love relationship, described by one adopted adolescent as their being "joined at the hip," that can be especially devastating when the relationship breaks up because of their earlier history of traumatic loss. Anxious attachment may be manifested in social anxiety, conflict with the parents based on struggles with dependency, and concerns about gender identity and intimacy that may become complicated by the parents' reactions to them.

It cannot be assumed that most adoptive parents have the necessary internal capacity, willingness, or resources to work with, as discussed in the "adoption competent" model (Atkinson, 2020). Whatever their strengths may be, adoptive parents are still representatives of their larger community and cultural group, with the same vulnerabilities to illness, social problems, delayed or arrested maturation, personality disorders, financial challenges, national emergencies, or natural disasters (Selman, 2020). However, they are not necessarily open to receiving assistance with their parenting, because for many, it is typically the adopted daughter or son who is perceived as needing treatment. Denial of difficulties and concerns within the family about being "blamed" remain potent barriers.

In treatment planning, in some cases, there may be compelling reasons for the same therapist to see both the adolescent and the parents themselves. Regardless, family therapists may see family treatment as the "core treatment" needed for adoptive families, regardless of the age of the adopted individual. However, the way the family therapist conceptualizes "family" and the adoptive parents' revised concept of "family" may not coincide with the evolving redefinition of "family" in the mind of the adopted adolescent or young adult. Clinicians knowledgeable about the psychology of *being* adopted, however, know the importance of privacy and confidentiality for the adopted adolescent and young adult. They argue that individual treatment for the adopted person serves the important roles, especially complicated for them, of supporting the separation-individuation process and of addressing the mounting questions relating to identity and sexuality "without upsetting the parents." For example, some adopted adolescents have reported feeling they were "overprotected" or, in some cases, infantilized by their parents, but they were still generally eager to experiment with new ideas, plans, and experiences while, at the same time, struggling with anticipatory anxiety that can reach frightening levels, even into adulthood. They may need support and reassurance around relationships and trust at a time of unexpected major changes or losses in the adoptive family, such as divorce, illness, or death. At the same time, the adoptive parents are undergoing their own changes and readjustments, often within the marriage itself, and have the same needs for privacy with their own (separate) therapist. This treatment model would call on the adoptive parents' therapist also to provide family therapy, but in collaboration with the adopted adolescent's therapist.

It is our observation that therapists may more readily feel empathy with the parents' dilemmas, perhaps identifying with them more easily as they describe their views of problems, but without understanding the special circumstances and complex intrapsychic life of the adopted adolescent. It may be more difficult, in this case, to help the parents with this process. This is one argument for the treatment model in which the parents see a separate therapist. This is not "splitting the treatment" but respecting appropriate boundaries for both the adopted patient and their parents. If the adolescent is the only one being seen in treatment, the therapist may be unwittingly colluding with the parents' view of their daughter or son being "the patient" or client rather than the family as well. This is a particular problem in the case of many private practitioners who are inclined to leave out the family component, while there may also be an element of the therapist not recommending consultations for the parents with another therapist in order to remain in control of the treatment.

8. Additional Considerations in Treatment

Emotional attunement of the therapist is needed in any treatment, but the empathic process for the therapist, in the case of the adopted patient, is a particular challenge because much of what they are hearing is outside their personal experience. For example, a therapist may believe they are empathic based on their personal experience with having been adopted by a stepparent, but psychologically, this is very different from growing up adopted in a non-kinship family. One of the most helpful interventions a therapist can provide the adopted client is validation of the reasons for the adopted client's struggles, such as their confusion as they try to redefine who their family is, or frustration about having little information about their birth families. The therapist's exploration is not to be a cognitive exercise using typical (distancing) cliches in the mental health field, and reflected also in a good deal of the literature, such as "sense of self," "life goals," "well-being," "learning who you are," etc. Rather, from a psychodynamic perspective, their expressions of confusion and frustration need to be integrated slowly and sensitively into the empathic relationship that the therapist tries to develop with the client. This needs to be gauged throughout the treatment process in order for the work to have meaning for the client at an emotional level, rather than limited only to the cognitive domain. *A barometer for the authenticity of the therapist's empathy is the degree to which the therapist feels her/his own emotions being stirred, such as feeling "very moved."* Patients' impulses for acting out, such as cancellations of therapy appointments or high-risk behaviors, need to be given immediate and consistent attention, keeping in mind possible adoption themes. The psychodynamic perspective also emphasizes the indispensable use of transference and countertransference (Zuckerman & Buchshaum, 2007; Chapter 15) to guide the treatment, which requires a good deal of advanced training.

9. Clinical Perspectives on the Eight Core Constellations in the Psychology of Being Adopted

The psychology of being adopted, with particular reference to adolescence and young adulthood, makes it necessary to recast the "core issues" identified by the child welfare and adoption fields (Roszia & Maxon, 2019), which, in this context, are actually constellations of multiple overlapping struggles that many adopted persons report, that vary greatly in frequency and difficulty, and that also vary greatly on the degree and extent of the adopted individual's internal resilience.

The clinical perspective of the psychology of *being* adopted conceptualizes eight overlapping constellations of internal experience, many of which may be experienced at one time or another by adolescents and young adults more generally, but which are areas of particular vulnerability for those who are adopted. It is the impact and sometimes intensity of having to struggle with several, or perhaps most, at the same time, that presents the greatest challenge. A Dutch study of international adult adoptees (van der Vegt et al., 2009) confirmed many of the observations in this chapter. They found that children who experienced multiple severe early adversities, although followed by adoptive placement by age 2, had an increased risk of ongoing anxiety, mood disorders, and substance abuse/dependence that could arise *de novo* after childhood and continue into and within adulthood.

Bearing in mind great variations in the severity, chronicity, and cumulative effect over time, the emotional adjustments commonly reported by many adopted adolescents and young adults, especially those seen in treatment, are represented in the following graphic. Since this chapter focuses on topics that may come up with adopted people in treatment, a reminder is needed that these "adjustments" fall into a spectrum of experience that, for many, involve little more than occasional fleeting thoughts.

Eight Core Constellations in the Psychology of Being Adopted

Early Developmental Trauma: neurophysiological brain changes, overwhelmed defenses, separation anxiety, insecure or pathological attachments, alexithymia, impaired mentalization/reflective capacity/concrete thinking impaired cognition/memory dysthymia, intermittent episodes of depression, difficulty conceptualizing the past and future, brief dissociative episodes, delayed or arrested maturation

Clinical Problems and the Need for Shifts in Perspectives

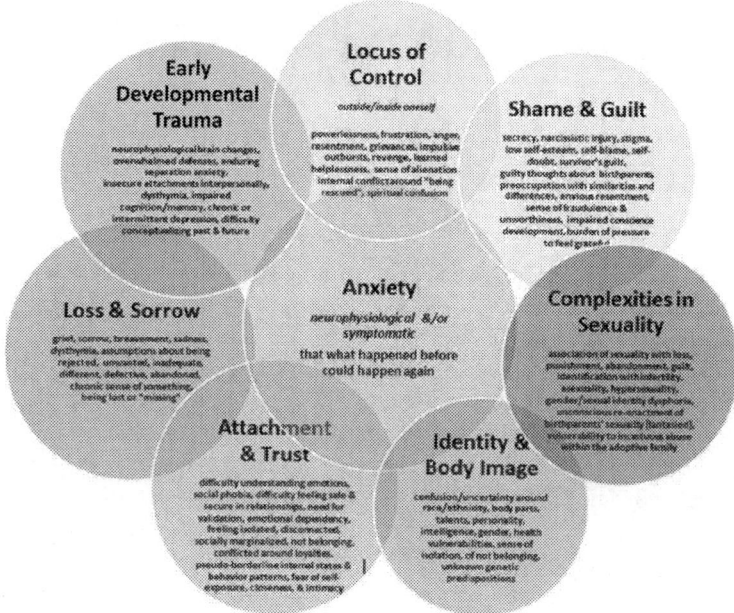

Locus of Control: (outside/inside oneself) powerlessness, learned helplessness, spiritual confusion, internal conflict around being "rescued" and "grateful," sense of alienation, frustration, anger, resentment, grievances, impulsive outbursts

Shame and Guilt: secrecy, narcissistic injury, stigma, low self-esteem, self-blame, self-doubt, sense of fraudulence, survivor's guilt, preoccupation with differences and similarities, envious resentment, impaired conscience development, guilty thoughts about birth parents

Loss and Sorrow: grief, sorrow, bereavement, sadness, dysthymia, assumptions about being rejected, abandoned, unwanted, inadequate, defective, vague thoughts of something being lost or missing, hypersensitivity to future losses

Attachment and Trust: alexithymia, difficulty understanding emotions in self and others, difficulty feeling safe and secure in relationships, need for validation, social phobia, emotional dependency, sense of being isolated and/or disconnected, of not belonging, conflict around loyalties, pseudo-borderline thoughts and internal states, anxiety about self-exposure, closeness, and intimacy

Identity and Body Image: confusion around race/ethnicity and personality development, body features and parts, talents vs. inadequacy, intelligence, gender, unknown health vulnerabilities, unknown genetic predispositions

Complexities in Sexuality: association of sexuality with loss, punishment, abandonment, guilt, identification with infertility, asexuality, hypersexuality, gender/sexual identity dysphoria, unconscious re-enactment of birth parents' sexuality (fantasied), vulnerability to incestuous abuse within the adoptive family, confusion around having children/pregnancy/impregnation, anxiety about parenting

Anxiety: (neurophysiological and/or symptomatic) within the context of all other core constellations, but fundamentally anticipatory anxiety that what happened before could happen again

Copyright Routledge Press/London

Summary

This chapter addresses more specifically particular deficiencies in adoption, pediatric, and mental health practice that reflect inadequate training and understanding, inadequate collaboration in research between allied fields, and lack of advanced adoption-knowledgeable clinical services for adopted adolescents and young adults. Generally, all that has become available in the literature and in various forms and venues of treatment tend to be significantly off-the-mark in attending to the unique needs of this sub-population, needs that are not yet recognized by the traditional mental health field.

Psychodynamically based psychotherapy needs to be distinguished from various cognitive behavioral and "brain-based" treatments, such as use of the neurosequential model, and from other single-issue interventions, such as EMDR for trauma. Each may (or may not) play a legitimate therapeutic role in treatment of adopted adolescents and young adults if carefully chosen for a particular patient at a particular time. However, there is no known research in the use or comparison of different approaches to treating early trauma or anxious attachment with the adopted population. Further, research would need to evaluate the long-term as well as the more short-term benefits. Most importantly, however, any of these approaches need to be understood within the overall larger context of ongoing adoption-informed psychotherapy that is attuned to the process of *integrating fragmented identity*. Clinicians should consider treatment of adopted adolescents and young adults a unique and exceptionally stimulating challenge, provided they are willing to educate themselves and to avail themselves of consultation with qualified specialists who will increasingly become available online. In the process, the therapist will be surprised and greatly enriched by all that they learn about themselves, in fact, much that they probably could not have learned any other way.

Endnotes

Atkinson, A.J. (2020). Adoption competent clinical practice. In G.M. Wrobel, E. Helder, & E. Marr (Eds.), *The Routledge Handbook of Adoption*. London & New York: Routledge.

Baden, A. (2016). "Do you know your real parents?" and other adoption microaggressions. *Adoption Quarterly*, 19 (1), 1–25.

Baden, A., & Wiley, M.O. (2007). Counseling adopted persons in adulthood: Integrating practice and research. *The Counseling Psychologist*, 35 (6), 868–901.

Barth, R.P., Crea, T.M., John, K., Thoburn, J., & Quinton, D. (2005). Beyond attachment theory and therapy: Towards sensitive and evidence-based interventions with foster and adoptive families in distress. *Child and Family Social Work*, 10, 257–268.

Bergman, N.J. (2019). Birth practices: Maternal-neonate separation as a source of toxic stress. *Birth Defects Research*, 111 (15), 1087–1109.

Boss, P. (2000). *Ambiguous Loss: Learning to Live with Unresolved Grief.* Cambridge: Harvard University Press.

Brodzinsky, D. (1993). Long-term outcomes in adoption. *Adoption*, 3 (1), 153–166.

Brodzinsky, D. (2006). Family structural openness and communication openness as predictors in the adjustment of adopted children. *Adoption Quarterly*, 9, 1–18.

Brodzinsky, D., & Palacios, J. Eds. (2005). *Psychological Issues in Adoption: Research and Practice.* California: Praeger Publishers/Greenwood Publishing Group.

Brodzinsky, D., & Pertman, A. (2012). *Adoption by Lesbians and Gay Men: A New Dimension in Family Diversity.* New York: Oxford University Press.

Brodzinsky, D., & Schechter, M.D. Eds. (1990). *The Psychology of Adoption.* Oxford: Oxford University Press.

Buckwalter, K.D., Reed, D., & Mercer, D. (2017). Ghosts in the adoption: Uncovering parents' attachment and coping history. *Families in Society: The Journal of Contemporary Social Services*, 225–234.

Cashen, K., Altman, D., Grotevant, H., & McRoy, R. (2019). Hearing the voices of young adult adoptees: Perspectives on adoption agency practice. *Child Welfare*, 97 (4), 1–22.

Crook, M. (2000). *The Face in the Mirror: Teenagers and Adoption.* Vancouver: Arsenal Pulp Press.

Dalen, M., & Therie, S. (2020) Academic performance and school adjustment of internationally adopted children in Norway. In G.M. Wrobel, E. Helder, & E. Marr (Eds.), *The Routledge Handbook of Adoption.* London and New York: Routledge, pp. 395–406.

Darnell, F.J., Johansen, A.B., Tavakoli, S., & Brugnone, N. (2017). Adoption and identity experiences among adult transnational adoptees: A qualitative study. *Adoption Quarterly*, 20, 155–166.

Dekker, M.C., Tieman, W., Vinke, A.G., van der Ende, J., Verhulst, F.C., & Juffer, F. (2016). *Mental Health Problems of Dutch Young Adult Domestic Adoptees Compared to Non-Adopted Peers and International Adoptees.* California: Sage Publishing, pp. 1–17.

Derdeyn, A.P. (1979). Adoption and the ownership of children. *Child Psychiatry and Human Development*, 9, 215–226.

Despax, J., Bouteyre, E., & Pavani, J.B. (2021). Adoptees' romantic relationships: Comparison with non-adoptees, psychological predictors, and long-term implications of the adoption pathway. *Adoption Quarterly*, 24 (4), 251–276.

Esposito, D., & Biafora, F.A. (2007). Toward a sociology of adoption: Historical deconstruction. In R.A. Javier, A.L. Baden, F.A. Biafora, & A. Camacho-Gingerich (Eds.), *Handbook of Adoption: Implications for Researchers, Practitioners, and Families.* Thousand Oaks, London, & New Delhi: Sage Publications.

Farr, R.H., & Vazquez, C.P. (2020). Adoptive families headed by LGTBQ parents. In G. M. Wrobel, E. Helder, & E. Marr (Eds.), *The Routledge Handbook of Adoption.* London and New York: Routledge, pp. 164–175.

Festinger, T., & Jaccard, J. (2012). Suicidal thoughts in adopted vs. non-adopted youth: A longitudinal analysis in adolescence, early young adulthood, and young adulthood. *Journal of the Society for Social Work and Research*, 3 (4), 280–295.

Fong, R., & McRoy, R. Eds. (2016) *Transracial and Intercountry Adoptions: Cultural Guidance for Professionals.* New York: Columbia University Press.

Fujisawa, T.X., & Tomoda, A. (2021). Shared neural basis for the exposure to child maltreatment and eating disorders. *Academia Letters*, Article 4108, 1–6. https://doi.org/10.20935/AL4108

Galvan, A. (2017). *The Neuroscience of Adolescence*. Cambridge & New York: Cambridge University Press.

Garber, K. (2020). Adoptive microaggressions: Historical foundations, current research, and practical implications. In G.M. Wrobel, E. Helder, & E. Marr (Eds.), *The Routledge Handbook of Adoption*. London and New York: Routledge, pp. 308–320.

Goldberg, A.E., & Garcia, R.L. (2015). Predictors of relationship dissolution in lesbian, gay, and heterosexual parents. *Journal of Family Psychology*, 29 (3), 394–404.

Goldstein, J., Freud, A., & Solnit, A. (1973). *Beyond the Best Interests of the Child*. New York: Free Press.

Hendry, A., & Hasler, J. Eds. (2017). *Creative Therapies for Complex Trauma: Helping Children and Families in Foster Care, Kinship Care, or Adoption*. New York & Philadelphia: Jessica Kingsley Pub.

Henry, D. (2012) *The 3-5-7 Model: A Practice Approach for Permanency Work with Children and Youth*. Pennsylvania: Sunbury Press.

Hoffman, J., & Vallejo-Pena, E. (2013). Too Korean to be white and too white to be Korean: Ethnic identity development among transracial Korean-American adoptees. *Journal of Student Affairs Research and Practice*, 50 (2), 152–170.

Holmgren, E., Raaska, H., Elovainio, M., & Lapinleimu, H. (2020). Behavioral and emotional adjustment in adoptees. In G.M. Wrobel, E. Helder, & E. Marr (Eds.), *The Routledge Handbook of Adoption*. London & New York: Routledge, pp. 353–366.

Howard, J.A., Smith, S.L., & Ryan, S. (2004). A comparative study of child welfare adoptions with other types of adopted children and birth children. *Adoption Quarterly*, 7 (3), 1–30.

Jackson, K.F., & Samuels, G.M. (2019). *Multiracial Cultural Attunement*. Washington, DC: NASW Press.

Johnson, D.E., Eckerle, J., Bresnahan, M., & Kroupina, M. (2020). Adoptees with disabilities or medically involved children: A multidisciplinary approach for preparing parents, assessing the child, and supporting successful family formation. In G.M. Wrobel, E. Helder, & E. Marr (Eds.), *The Routledge Handbook of Adoption*. London & New York: Routledge.

Kim, A., & Lee, R. (2020). A critical adoption studies and Asian American integrativist perspective on the psychology of Korean adoption. In G.M. Wrobel, E. Helder, & E. Marr (Eds.), *The Routledge Handbook of Adoption*. London and New York: Routledge, pp. 120–134.

Levy-Schiff, R. (2016). Psychological adjustments of adoptees in adulthood: Family environment and adoption-related correlates. *International Journal of Behavioral Development*, 25 (2), 97–104.

Lindblad, F., Weitoft, G., & Hjern, A. (2010). ADHD in international adoptees: A national cohort study. *European Child and Adolescent Psychiatry*, 19, 37–44.

Loehlin, J.C., Horn, J.M., & Ernst, J.L. (2010). Parent-child closeness studied in adoptive families. *Personality and Individual Differences*, 48, 149–154.

Main, A., Walle, E.A., Kho, C., & Halpern, J. (2017). The interpersonal functions of empathy: A relational perspective. *Emotion Review*, 9 (4), 1–9.

Manzi, C., Ferrari, I., Rosnati, R., & Benet-Martinez, V. (2014). Bicultural identity integration of transracial adolescent adoptees: Antecedents and outcomes. *Journal of Cross-Cultural Psychology* (Sage Publications), 45, 888–904.

Marr, E., Helder, E., & Wrobel, G.M. (2020). Historical and contemporary contexts of U.S. adoption. In G.M. Wrobel, E. Helder, & E. Marr, (Eds.), *Routledge Handbook in Adoption*. London & New York: Routledge, pp. 3–21.

Matthews, J.A.K. (2020). Maltreatment of adoptees in adoptive homes. In G.M. Wrobel, E. Helder, & E. Marr, (Eds.), *Routledge Handbook of Adoption*. London and New York: Routledge, pp. 321–333.

McConnachie, A.L., Ayed, N., Foley, S., Lamb, M.E., Jadva, V., Tasker, F., & Golombok, S. (2021). Adoptive gay father families: A longitudinal study of children's adjustment at early adolescence. *Child Development*, 92 (1), 425–443.

Merritt, M. (2022). Rediscovering latent trauma: An adopted adult's perspective. *Child Abuse & Neglect*, 130, 1–11.

Moyer, A.M., & Juang, L.P. (2011). Adoption and identity: Influence on emerging adults' occupational and parental goals. *Adoption Quarterly*, 14 (1), 1–17.

Nilsson, R., Rhee, S.H., Corley, R.P., Rhea, S., Wadsworth, S.J., & DeFries, J.C. (2011). Conduct problems in adopted and non-adopted adolescents and adoption satisfaction as a protective factor. *Adoption Quarterly*, 14 (3), 181–198.

NSAP/ASPE (2007–2008). *National Survey of Adoptive Parents/Assistant Secretary for Planning & Evaluation.* www.cdc.gov/nchs/slaits/nsap.htm

Odenstad, A., Hjern, A., Lindblad, F., Rasmussen, F., Vinnerljung, B., & Dalen, M. (2008). Does age at adoption and geographic origin matter? A national cohort study of cognitive test performance in adult inter-country adoptees. *Psychological Medicine*, 38, 1803–1814.

Oke, M., Groza, V., Park, H., Kalyanvala, R., & Shetty, M. (2015). The perceptions of young adult adoptees in India on their emotional well-being. *Adoption & Fostering*, 39 (4), 343–355.

Pace, C.S., Zavattini G.C., & D'Alessio M. (2012). Continuity and discontinuity of attachment patterns: A short-term longitudinal pilot study using a sample of late-adopted children and their adoptive mothers. *Attachment and Human Development*, 14 (1), 45–61. https://doi.org/10.1080/14616734.2012.636658

Perry, B.D. (2020). The neurosequential model: A developmentally sensitive, neuroscience-informed approach to clinical problem-solving. In J. Mitchel, J. Tucci, & E. Tronick, (Eds.), *The Handbook of Therapeutic Care for Children: Evidence-informed Approaches to Working with Traumatized Children and Adolescents in Foster, Kinship, and Adoptive Care*. London & Philadelphia, PA: Jessica Kingsley, pp. 137–156.

Raleigh, E., & Kreider, R.M. (2020). A nationally representative comparison of black and white adoptive parents of black adoptees. In G.M. Wrobel, E. Helder, & E. Marr (Eds.), *The Routledge Handbook of Adoption*. London: Routledge International Handbooks, pp. 135–150.

Reppold, C.T., & Hutz, C.S. (2009). Effects of the history of adoption in the emotional adjustment of adopted adolescents. *The Spanish Journal of Psychology*, 12 (2), 454–461.

Riley-Behringer, M., Groza, V., Tieman, W., & Juffer, F. (2014). Race and bicultural socialization in the Netherlands, Norway, and the USA in the adoptions of children from India. *Cultural Diversity & Ethnic Minority Psychology*, 20 (2), 231–243.

Roche, H., & Perlesz, A. (2000). A legitimate choice and voice: The experience of adult adoptees who have chosen not to search for their biological families. *Adoption & Fostering*, 24, 8–19.

Roskam, I., Stievenart, M., Tessier, R., Muntean, A., & Escobar, M.J. (2014). Another way of thinking about ADHD: The predictive role of early attachment deprivation in adolescents' inattention symptoms. *Social Psychiatry and Psychiatric Epidemiology*, 49, 133–144.

Roszia, S.K., & Maxon, A.D. Eds. (2019). *Seven Core Issues in Adoption and Permanency: A Comprehensive Guide to Promoting Understanding and Healing in Adoption, Foster Care, Kinship Families and Third Party Reproduction*. London: Jessica Kingsley.

Sanchez-Sandoval, Y., & Melero, S. (2019). Psychological adjustment in Spanish young adult domestic adoptees: Mental health and licit substance consumption. *American Journal of Orthopsychiatry*, 89 (6), 640–653.

Schechter, M.D., & Bertocci, D. (1990). The meaning of the search. In D. Brodzinsky, & M.D. Schechter (Eds.), *The Psychology of Adoption*. New York: Oxford University Press, pp. 62–90.

Segal, N.L. (2021). *Deliberately Divided: Inside the Controversial Study of Twins and Triplets Adopted Apart*. Lanham: Rowman & Littlefield.

Selman, P. (2020). Adoption in the context of natural disaster. In G.M. Wrobel, E. Helder, & E. Marr (Eds.), *The Routledge Handbook in Adoption*. London & New York: Routledge, pp. 202–215.

Sharp, C., & Bevington, D. (2022). *Mentalizing in Psychotherapy: A Guide for Practitioners*. New York: The Guilford Press.

Siegel, D.J. (2013). *Brainstorm: The Power and Purpose of the Teenage Brain*. New York: Penguin Group.

Steele, M., Hodges, J., Kaniuk, J., & Steele, H. (2010). Mental representation and change: Developing attachment relationships in an adoption context. *Psychoanalytic Inquiry* (Routledge: T&F Group), 30 (1), 25–40.

Tan, T.X., Camras, L.A., Deng, H., Zhang, M., & Lu, Z. (2012). Family stress, parenting styles, and behavioral adjustment in preschool adopted Chinese girls. *Early Childhood Research Quarterly*, 27 (1), 128–136.

Tessler, R., & Gamache, G. (2012). Ethnic exploration and consciousness of difference: Chinese adoptees in early adolescence. *Adoption Quarterly*, 15, 265–287.

Thomas, L.J., & Scharp, K. (2020). Communications about adoption in families. In G.M. Wrobel, E. Helder, & E. Marr (Eds.), *The Routledge Handbook of Adoption*. London & New York: Routledge, pp. 253–265.

Van der Kolk, B. (2015). *The Body Keeps the Score: Brain, Mind, & Body in the Healing of Trauma*. New York: Penguin Books.

Van der Vegt, E.J.M., Tieman, W., van der Ende, J., Ferdinand, R.F., Verhulst, F.C., & Tiemeier, H. (2009). Impact of early childhood adversities on adult psychiatric disorders: A study of international adoptees. *Social Psychiatry and Psychiatric Epidemiology*, 44, 724–731.

Van Ijzendoorn, M.H., Juffer, F., & Poelhuis, C.W.K. (2005). Adoption and cognitive development: A meta-analystic comparison of adopted and nonadopted children's IQ and school performance. *Psychological Bulletin*, 131, 301–316.

Vinke, A., Dekker, M.C., Tieman, W., Van der Ende, L., Verhulst, F.C., & Juffer, F. (2016). Mental health problems of Dutch young adult domestic adoptees, compared to nonadopted peers and international adoptees. *International Social Work* (Sage Pub.), 1–17.

Waterman, J., Langley, A.K., Miranda, J., & Riley, D.B. (2018). *Adoption-Specific Therapy: A Guide to Helping Adopted Children and Their Families Thrive*. Washington, DC: American Psychological Association.

Welsh, J.A., Viana, A.G., Petrill, S.A., & Mathias, M.D. (2007). Interventions for internationally adopted children and families: A review of the literature. *Child and Adolescent Social Work Journal*, 24 (3), 285–311.

Wrobel, G.M., Helder, E., & Marr, E. Eds. (2020). *Routledge Handbook of Adoption*. London: Routledge Press.

Zuckerman, J.R., & Buchsbaum, B. (2007). "I don't know you": Transference and countertransference paradigms with adoptees. In R. Javier, A. Baden, F. Biafora, & A. Camacho-Gingerich (Eds.), *Handbook of Adoption: Implications for Researchers, Practitioners, and Families*. California: Sage Publications, pp. 491–504.

APPENDIX

1. The "seven core issues" pertaining to the full adoption triad, developed in the 1980s by veterans in child welfare, are loss, rejection, shame and guilt, grief, identity, intimacy, and mastery and control. See Endnotes: Roszia and Maxon (2019).
2. The United States is one of the very few member nations of the United Nations that has refused to ratify the Declaration of the Rights of the Child. The last attempt to address this, during the Clinton administration, was defeated by "conservative right-wing" legislators who dismissed the need because they considered the American Bill of Rights, written for adults, sufficient.
3A. Questionnaire for adopted client and family.

Adoption-Related Background (Non-Kinship Adoption)

1. Name, original name.
2. Age, year of birth, sex, country of birth.
3. Source of the adoptive placement:

    Public welfare/social services department.
    Private/professional adoption agency.
    International placement organization.
    Private/independent adoption (lawyer only).

4. Age when placed in the adoptive home.
5. Closed or open adoption, arrangements for contact with birth family.
6. Caretaking arrangements between birth and placement in adoptive home.
7. What is known about each birth parent? What was the birth father's involvement?

8. What was the extent of the birth mother's medical care throughout pregnancy? Any medical problems before and after giving birth?
9. What reasons did she give for deciding to place for adoption?
10. Current thoughts/wishes about getting more information or for meeting birth relatives, and what would it mean? What information is most desired and why?

3B. Additional questions for the health-care professional/psychotherapist.

11. Full medical, developmental, and social history, beginning with birth mother's pregnancy. Include ages of the adopted person if/when any developmental delays or deviations were noticed; also, was there any professional help in diagnosing and treating them?
12. Any behavioral problems in preschool years, elementary and middle school years (through age 12), and adolescence (ages 13 through 17).
13. School adjustment, current academic status, any learning problems; results of any testing.
14. Full chronological history of psychiatric/psychological care, when and why it was sought, whether and how any aspect of adoption was viewed as a relevant factor in the care. Details of any hospital/IOP/residential care and reasons for the need. What treatment experiences were or were not helpful and why?
15. Any recent and current medical/neuropsychological problems and medical/psychiatric medications.
16. Age and reason for any psychological testing, tests done with findings.
17. At what age was the adopted client first told they are adopted? Content of what was explained? What was their response then, and subsequently over time, to adoption information?
18. What does being adopted mean to them now?
19. Details of relationships within the adoptive family, including siblings and extended family.
20. How significant, and why, is the lack of information about the birth family and details of the early history? What information would be useful for evaluation and treatment now?

4. "Adoption competency" is a concept developed by social service professionals with a background in adoption practice with families and children and is intended primarily for all adoption professionals who work in the child welfare, foster care, and adoption fields. Their "clinical practice principles" (Atkinson, 2020) focus especially on trauma and attachment as it relates to both foster and adopted children, and their model for treatment interventions is "family-based." Versions of the TAC (Training for Adoption Competency) model are much-needed globally for all matters involving placement of children for adoption and its overlap with foster care. Specific countries would need to make modifications

in such trainings to suit their respective needs. At the present time, however, the biggest challenge, particularly in the foreseeable future in Western countries, will be development of advanced clinical trainings for both the mental health field and for developmental psychology, which will require entirely new venues, curricula, and marketing. See also Chapter 4, Appendix 2.

12
NOTES ON THE PSYCHOANALYTIC TREATMENT OF THE ADOPTED PERSON

Christopher F. Deeg, PhD

Introduction: The Question of Modification in the Treatment of the Adopted Person

Do adopted people present a unique psychological organization warranting significant modifications in diagnosis and psychoanalytic technique? Although I have previously answered this question in the negative (Deeg, 2002), I have nonetheless proposed that the issue of adoption constitutes the central dynamic in psychotherapy with adopted people. The adoption of the patient is the core narrative which imbues and is revealed both in the transference and in the associations and fantasies that are the material of the session. These associations, fantasies, and transferences are expressions of the central object relation that consists of adopted self representation connected to birth parent representation by various emotions and combinations of emotions.

Is this a contradiction? The answer to this question lies in the differentiation of the concept of technique versus sensitivity to thematic content. Various authors writing within the psychoanalytic tradition have introduced the need for modifications of basic technique based either on revisions to the identification of what is therapeutic or based on the limitations posed by impediments to ego functioning. The interpersonal school (Greenberg & Mitchell, 1983) and the approach of self-psychology based on the writings of Kohut (1971) are examples of the former. The shift from acquiring an experiential insight to a restorative emotional interpersonal experience fundamentally changes the tenor of interpretations and places the here-and-now experience with the analyst at the top of the ladder. The lived and analyzed transference no longer is viewed merely as the precursor to the patient's expanded insight and ego functioning (see Greenson, 1967, to contrast with this view).

Conversely, the need for changes in technique can be based on the assertion that personality organization and the associated integrity of ego functioning may demand the introduction of new technique or parameters of technique, such as boundary-setting and direct support or restriction of acting out within the treatment (Eissler, 1953; Kernberg et al., 1989).

While not resolving or even addressing the complexities of these issues and the possibility that some of the dichotomies implied by these positions may be false polarities, I would continue to suggest that the story of the patient's adoption itself does not require or necessarily suggest a particular resolution to these theoretical questions. The issue of whether insight alone, or a corrective emotional experience, is the central therapeutic ingredient is not germane to understanding the adoptee in psychoanalytic treatment. Adoption-informed clinicians of either an interpersonal or classical psychoanalytic orientation may work differently with the adoption narrative but still fundamentally address its treatment manifestations. Similarly, being adopted is not a diagnosis, and adopted individuals present with varying levels of ego functioning and therefore do not require a specific deviation from technique.

The Invitation to Therapy and the Adopted Person's Need to Engage the Representation of the Birth Parent

In an earlier paper on treatment of the adopted person (Deeg, 2002), I identified the adopted person's cathexes or internalized connection to the representation of the birth parent as the central dynamic which is revealed in the course of psychotherapy. Prior to that, I have identified the internalized object relation of adopted self to birth parent (the cathexes of the "lost object") as the central feature of the psychology of the experience of being adopted and have traced the development and influence of this object relation throughout the life of the adopted person as it becomes manifest in various defensive and adaptive mechanisms (Deeg, 1989, 1990, 1991). Before turning to a review of transferential manifestations of this object relation, let us examine what brings the adopted person into treatment and what the therapist can offer as a possible benefit.

Often, the adopted person is aware of a desire to "know" the birth parent by acquiring more information, a process which sometimes culminates in a search and possible reunion with the birth parent. Although the fantasies of self and birth parent (usually the birth mother) which underlie cognitions of "interest" or "curiosity" are typically unconscious, I have previously identified this process as an adaptive attempt on the part of the adopted person to consolidate and advance identity formation in a sector of development that is occluded yet prominent (Deeg, 1991).

Psychoanalytic psychotherapy offers the adopted person a venue and a psychological space in which the relationship with the birth parent can be located, cultivated, lived, and ultimately integrated into the rich tapestry of other object relations. Similarly, the self-representation accompanying the object representation of the birth parent can be cathected and allowed to develop and modify in a manner which is consistent with the developmental level of the rest of the personality organization.

The adopted person considering treatment offers a reasonable resistance to this proposition: How can a relationship be resumed in the absence of a real physical person? When the notion that fantasies of the birth parent, both conscious and those that emerge through treatment, are to be given the same working status as reports of interactions with persons populating the patient's external world, the patient may resist for another equally valid intrapsychic reason. The differentiation of internal versus external reality is likely to be partially and transiently blurred while this process ensues, just as other hard-won cognitive maturations are allowed to be set aside by the regression that makes an exploration and reliving of the past possible (Fenichel, 1941, 1945; Greenson, 1967).

The task of the psychoanalytic therapist in treating the adopted person is to facilitate the free and associational expressions of the fantasies of the central object relation of self to birth parent. Most patients will struggle with this as they have a lifetime of experience in considering inner traces of fantasies to be starkly separated from, and "inferior" to, the memory of real experience with a person.

It is probably true that in all psychodynamic therapies, the therapist must gently garner the understanding and trust of the patient in constructing a new conception of fantasy and its role in their lives. The therapist must demonstrate that the retrieval, articulation, and reconstruction of fantasies allow access to feelings and ideas which, although unconscious or at least unarticulated, nevertheless shape daily moods, thoughts, reveries, and human interactions. In a word, fantasy is a gateway, affording a glimpse of the schema which underlay daily conscious feelings of love and hate and their derivatives. Fantasy allows the patient to begin to form a narrative about their object relations.

For the adopted person, the roadblock to this journey is the belief that the absence of the birth parent makes the retrieval and especially the sharing of fantasies regarding the birth parent impossible or ridiculous (Deeg, 2002).

An adopted patient in his early 20s prided himself on being realistic and levelheaded. He abhorred the excessive emotionalism of his adoptive parents and generally avoided intimacy with others both sexually and interpersonally. When the suggestion that he, in fact, had fantasies about his birth mother and that an exploration of these fantasies could be of real practical benefit to him, he scoffed at the idea and said that an exploration of the past was never any use to him. After some exploration of this idea, he ultimately said, "She obviously didn't think much about me; why should I bother to spend any energy on her?" This statement and others like it were the beginnings of a fantasy/narrative in which he was abandoned by a selfish but ultimately daring and iconoclastic mother whom he loathed, longed for, and unconsciously had attempted to shape aspects of his life after.

The resistance of the adopted patient to allowing the birth parent into the treatment room is itself a statement of a fantasy about the birth parent – often a painful one – which deserves invitation, acceptance, and exploration. Despite the natural inclination to avoid pain and, in therapy, the resistance to discussing and experiencing something painful, the therapist offers the adopted patient a unique opportunity, namely, to reopen a relationship, albeit an internalized relationship. This proposition can appeal directly to the adopted person's need and interest in expanding their "knowledge" of the birth parent. To accept this bargain, the adopted patient must allow fantasy to have full therapeutic status alongside memory and perception. From a clinical perspective, the patient must be able to tolerate the regressive dimension of this agreement. The patient must be able to reconstitute normal, daily discriminations between inner and outer reality when the therapeutic hour is finished. To some extent, this is not radically different from the process of psychoanalytic therapy generally, wherein the relation of memory, perception, and fantasy is first challenged and then reconstituted.

The birth parent that enters the therapy in this exchange is the birth parent that constitutes half of the object relation of adopted self to birth parent. In cases where this object relation has been disavowed or is unconscious, the reintroduction or discovery can be startling and possibly overwhelming to the patient who has lived their life up to that point thinking that an event that occurred so long ago has no relation to their current experience, often itself a reflection or derivative of an underlying fantasy of a "dead" birth parent whose absence may be mourned or celebrated, depending on the aggressive or depressive affective valence that colors the object relation.

The Equal Psychological Status of the Birth Parent and the Adopted Self: Both Are Representational

It is a common bias shared by both patient and therapist that the representation of self is more "real" than the object representation, in that it is closer to the "thing-in-itself," namely, the self. The self-representation is typically afforded a tacit or unexamined primacy and is also felt to be closer to experience than the object representation. This bias is predicated on the often-unacknowledged philosophical premise (which is part of an uncritically accepted Western metaphysics; see Derrida, 1974) that underlying the self-representation is a real "self" which is the core of both the psychological and physical essence or being of the person. The representation of the object, on the other hand, is merely an imprint of the "other" and is clearly a copy which does not participate in the being of the other, since the locus of the other is external while the self is considered the very source of interiority.

Returning to the vantage point of deconstructive philosophy and the writings of Derrida (1974), these positions, whether they be tacit and part of a primarily Western cultural tradition or explicitly held by the therapist, are challenged by the idea that the "self" is a metaphysical construct; it is not a reality discovered but a "signifier" in deconstruction terms (signifying other words, not things) or a representation which is constructed as part of a narrative that both embodies and is embodied by experience. In other words, the "self" is not discovered in therapy; it is constructed in a gradual collaboration between the therapist and the patient. In deconstruction terms, the self signifies not a thing but a multiplicity of "selves" which refer to other selves, all of which are linguistic descriptions. Whatever the therapist's philosophical position regarding the "self," the self-representation, as it inhabits psychological theory, is just as constructed and narrative-based as the object representation. There is no real "self" underlying the construction and waiting to be discovered in the treatment room and written about in psychological theory. "Self-representation" (defined as the psychological representation of all the patient's experiences of self in interaction with others) and not "self" is the proper object of study for psychological theory, although the word "self" can function as shorthand for the more cumbersome "self-representation." The term "self" is a philosophical entity essentially equivalent to "soul." "Self-representation," on the other hand, is a psychological term. Self-representation and object representation enjoy equal theoretical and clinical status which, as discussed in the following, enables the adoptee in treatment to work with a representation of a person that they have never actually met, namely, the birth parent.

While these propositions may be somewhat alarming or confusing to the Western mind embedded in the metaphysics that equates the self with the soul, the radical separation of "self" from self-representation affords the therapist treating an adoptive patient with a technical advantage and provides the adoptive patient with a path to including their elusive object-relational partner in therapeutic work. The therapist can earnestly say to the adoptive patient, "Your fantasies about your birth mother or birth father are as 'real' a part of you as the narrative you have of yourself about your childhood or what happened yesterday." The representation of the birth parent is a viable and important part of the patient's inner world, which has both partially determined and is determined by the patient's history. I have attempted to delineate a number of the ways (Deeg, 1990) in which defensive uses of the birth parent representation through various modes of internalization and externalization help to both encapsulate and set the level of the patient's functioning. It is important to note that adopted people who successfully complete a search for their birth mothers often report that not only does the actual person differ from their expectation (an expression of the birth mother representation) but also that the original birth mother representation(s) does not simply vanish when they reunite with their external birth mother. The two are not the same and do not occupy the same psychological "space." I will return to this point later.

The adoptive patient whose depressive register of the loss of their biological mother leads them to the despair in treatment that they can never "correct" the loss and its associated damage can feel some hope that their relationship with the internal birth parent can be redressed and, although the loss cannot be undone, can be understood with the full metal of their adult sensibilities.

The Therapeutic Work with the Adopted Patient

The object relation of adopted self to birth parent is carefully examined in the therapy. To make this possible, the full expression of the object relation is cultivated and facilitated by the therapist's interpretation and support since this expression itself is typically painful and defended against. The therapist plays an educative role in explaining and encouraging the patient to treat their stored and emerging fantasies regarding the birth parent as vital material which needs to be articulated and then associated to, creating an ever-expanding laterality of meaning and connectivity to various aspects of the patient's exterior and interior life. The educative posture of the therapist has consequences for the therapy and for the transference which will pull for feelings toward parental and non-parental educators. This is probably one reason that the transference involving the birth parent typically emerges later (see following text).

The patient's fantasies of birth parent and adopted self, together with the questions, comments, insights, and interpretations of the therapist, form a series of narratives about the patient's adoption. The narratives are co-constructed by two people working collaboratively; they are not edicts passed down to the patient. Often, several narratives emerge as most meaningful or important to a particular patient. The increasing freedom to construct and edit narratives about their adoption increases the laterality of cognitive and emotional response and ultimately enriches the patient's experience of their subjectivity.

Even the most cooperative and psychologically sophisticated adoptive patient will often experience an increasing gradient of anxiety as they allow themselves to report long-held silent birth parent fantasies or to develop these fantasies now as adults. The fantasy material tends to proceed in a centrifugal manner, collecting elements of experience which adhere to each other as they create larger, more encompassing themes and moving with increasing rapidity toward the sense of a center as defenses are interpreted. Patients frequently report a feeling of being swept and inexorably pulled toward something potentially threatening; a feeling of being only partially in control of the treatment may inhabit both the patient and the therapist.

This process may be particularly difficult for the adoptive patient, who has established an idealized representation of the birth mother (Deeg, 2002). As derivatives of aggressive and negative valence begin to emerge from beneath cracks in the shell of idealization, the patient may require active support in facing long-suppressed or repressed feelings and fantasies toward "an abandoner" or hateful maternal image.

The emergence of the central object relation of adopted self to birth parent in the fantasy productions of the patient proceeds in tandem with transferential expressions of the dynamic. I have previously described this process as a binary transference (ibid.), in which elements of the relationship between adopted person and adoptive parents are intermingled with those involving the birth parent image. Since the image of the birth parent has been in part formed from various internalizations of the adoptive parent, differentiation is incomplete and partially mirrors and enacts the lack of information and absence of a lifetime of actual memories regarding the birth parents that the adopted person has grown up without. This loss is mourned in the therapy but is tolerated since the adopted person is now finally able to continue the psychological work that has hitherto been frozen and inaccessible (see following).

In some cases, the transference takes on a predominant theme which can be lived and understood. The adoptive patient is abandoned, rescued, rejected, damaged, or repaired, while the therapist is perceived through a corresponding lens. Unlike my previous paper (ibid.), I have focused here on the centrality of creating a therapeutic space for fantasy rather than on the development of the "binary transference." To a large extent, the success in allowing the transference to unfold, and more particularly, for the patient to be willing to analyze and discuss it, derives from a cultivation of the consideration of fantasy as valid and important material which can be directly experienced yet held in abeyance from a position of optimal psychological distance. The patient allows the binary transference to unfold because they have first overcome their resistance to expressing explicit fantasies about the birth parent. The patient's ego functioning is strengthened by the increasing ability to experience a psychological state and then partially withdraw from it and look at it as they would any external phenomena.

The adopted person's transference is an amalgam of original pre-psychological aspects of the relation of self to birth mother colored by the severance of that relation, projected, and displaced characteristics of the adoptive parents onto the image of the birth parent, and elements of the relationship to the adoptive parents themselves (ibid.). My own term for this, the "binary transference," fails to adequately describe the messy and often-blurred merging of these elements and the manner in which they inhabit the treatment. While the non-adopted patient can often sort out what is the parent and what is the therapist so that an observation like, "You're experiencing me as though I am your father," makes some modicum of sense, the adopted patient can only become aware that there is a transferential process operating "through" them and without their conscious control but typically cannot discern which object or part-object is being projected onto the therapist. The interpretation of transference generally is an assault on the patient's reality testing in that inner process and outer reality become merged. The adopted patient's reality testing is further challenged by not knowing precisely which parent or which mixture of parents is being enacted with the therapist. In addition, the ambiguity underscores precisely what the adoptive patient does not have, namely, a lifetime of memories with a person whom they are deeply emotionally connected to. Support from the therapist is necessary to address both of these very real artifacts of adopted status and being. Often, the ambiguity of the binary transference ushers in a period of renewed mourning for the loss of information and contact which lies darkened in the shadow of the lost object, the birth parent. The patient's frustration with the lack of "information," which is a derivative of a lack of personal memories from which to make sense of the transference, renews the mourning for the lost object and provides the treatment with another opportunity for healing. The adopted patient returns to the questions, "Who is my mother?" and "Who am I?" with a clearer and sadder appreciation of what their adoption has permanently removed from their inner life and identity.

A male adopted adult patient articulated the anxiety and sense of dread that he experienced in thinking about who he was and what kind of person he had become. He said that although he understood most of his major life-determining decisions, was seemingly aware of his goals and values, and could describe his personal characteristics, he always felt that "part of [him] is made up of gaps, blind spots, and black holes that [he] can never really see or understand." The patient also felt that his experience of time was not integrated and that although he was middle-aged, he was seen as an inexperienced and weak boy.

There is a risk of losing the adoptive patient as the loss highlighted by the analysis of the binary transference is focused on. With genuine support and empathy for their plight by the therapist, the adoptive patient can ultimately learn to tolerate (but not fondly) greater degrees of ambiguity. As one patient commented, "I suppose this makes me stronger, but no one would choose to be adopted."

Psychoanalytic Treatment and the Search for Reunion

It is not uncommon for the treatment to reawaken or even generate a desire on the adopted patient's part to actually find the birth mother, father, or other relatives and meet them. Similarly, the patient may enter treatment already interested in that venture or may have already completed a search with varying outcomes. The emergence of fantasies about the birth parents may revive images of self as abandoned and motherless and strengthen frustrated oral needs for nurture, tenderness, acceptance, and on a deeper level, feeding and satiation. Conversely, the adopted person may begin to think of reunion as an opportunity to murder or destroy the birth mother, or to punish her with abandonment, following the talion principle (Freud, 1913).

An adopted young female patient located a woman through social media whose postings and physical appearance made her begin to suspect that she was her birth mother. In addition to discussing the practical aspects of contacting the woman and proposing a reunion, the patient also began developing fantasies about what the actual reunion would be like. Eventually, one fantasy became predominant in which the woman tracked the birth mother down and sat anonymously in a café, watching her with a blank stare and no discernible affect. The patient was killing the birth mother with her stare, and the coldness in her eyes and slight upturned sneer of her lips were weapons secretly attacking, destroying, and finally, punishing the birth mother for the transgression of abandoning the patient.

While work focusing on reunion is extremely helpful in practical terms by allowing the patient to either prepare for the event or recover from a reunion that has occurred and has been disappointing or harmful, other intrapsychic features are prominent. The adopted person eventually becomes aware that the birth mother who is constructed in treatment by an analysis of symptoms, fantasies, and through the transference is not one and the same with the birth parent who is located and is present for the reunion. The birth parent (usually the birth mother)–adopted patient internal object relation is initially split or fractured, and in therapy, this split between all-bad, abandoning mother-abandoned self and reclaimed, idealized mother-"found" nurtured self is integrated and healed. The inner object relation of the birth mother connected to a corresponding self-representation occupies a psychological space that is coexistent with the adopted person's entire life. Reunion with the external birth mother does not simply replace this long-standing dynamic which is embedded within the personality and which has shaped and been shaped by the personality.

While external reunion with the birth parent is often of benefit to the adopted person and can be a springboard for progress in the therapy, it is not a necessary condition for the positive development of the object relation. For lasting change, the birth mother and adopted self representations must be accessed, expressed, and worked through by the patient and therapist working together (ibid.). This is good news for the many adopted patients who cannot either access information about their birth mothers or create opportunities for reunion.

A Specific Countertransference and Its Effect and Role in the Psychotherapy

The identification of the object relation of adopted self to birth parent in all its varieties as constructed from the specific factors of the individual case provides a heuristic structure for the therapy of the adopted person. However, it is important to attempt to not communicate the tacit message to the adopted patient: "your adopted self is welcome here, but not the rest of you." This is particularly problematic for the psychotherapists who themselves are adopted and unconsciously have projected a part of themselves onto the patient and now may wish to psychologically care for or adopt the patient or, if under the sway of their internalized image of the abandoning birth mother, sever the relation to the mother by forcing the adopted patient to experience negative or aggressive feelings either toward them or toward the internalized birth mother. In either case, the full range of the adopted patient's experience, including "non-adopted experience," must be sought, and its expression cultivated. The therapist should seek to convey to the patient that all of them, not just the adopted part, is welcome in the therapy and will be subject to the same endeavor to understand, and same attempt to make conscious.

When the adopted patient begins to experience the therapist as only interested in the issue of adoption, the patient can begin to feel that their freedom and agency are being threatened. This may elicit deeper feelings about the patient's loss of agency which has been "stamped into" the narrative of their life by being an infant subject to the machinery of an institution or subject to the decision of the birth mother to sever their relation. The feeling of "not being in control" or not being fully autonomous may be embedded in depressive, aggressive, or masochistic contexts.

In general, it is a fiction to think that the therapist can work without countertransference, and that the countertransference of the therapist will not affect the therapy and the patient. At some point, the therapist's feelings about adoption and all related factors will enter the therapy – with particular intensity if the therapist is also adopted. The goal is for the therapist to ultimately become aware of this occurrence and consciously decide what to do. For example, if the adopted therapist consistently demonstrates a particular prowess in their knowledge of or sensitivity to adoption issues, the adopted patient may enter a silent collusion with the therapist in which a new, idealized adoption can occur without being examined. When this dynamic is explored, the patient may experience a re-abandonment, but ultimately one that can be discussed and tolerated. When the patient moves away from adoption associations, or when termination of the treatment becomes imminent, the adopted therapist (or non-adopted therapist) may experience an abandonment which, if reflected upon, can deepen their empathy for the patient's experience.

Specific Treatment Issues Surrounding Termination

Termination or the "coming to an end" of any event or process mobilizes feelings and cognitions about the unconscious meanings of the ending, namely, severance, separation, death, birth, or injury (Langs, 1974). It has been noted that a return of symptomology is not uncommon when termination begins to be addressed in the therapy (Dewald, 1966; Firestein, 1969; Kernberg et al., 1989). The adopted patient may experience the ending of the therapy as an abandonment by the birth parent therapist, as punishment from the adoptive parent therapist, perhaps because the latter's infertility has been exposed, or a retribution for their love of the birth parent. The specific factors of the case and the overall gestalt of the transference determine the specific dynamics, but in general, the patient and therapist collaboratively have another opportunity to work through additional feelings and associations about the original loss.

In cases where the adopted patient is beginning a search for the birth parent, a specific resistance to entertaining associations to termination may arise. The patient may express an impatience with merely talking and fantasizing about the birth mother and separation from her and, by association, separation from the therapist. The patient is, in essence, saying, "I've had enough substitution [adoption]. Give me the real thing!" Analysis of this resistance can lead to the fantasy that the inner birth mother is not real or is dead, or that the discovery of the external birth mother will kill or harm the birth mother representation. Wherever the careful articulation and understanding of the resistance take the patient and therapist, the reality of the inner representation of the birth mother in emotional dialogue with the inner representation of the adopted self is confirmed and fortified. The finding of the external birth mother constitutes another, new reality that the adopted patient experiences, and not one that destroys or replaces the lifelong relation to the birth mother image.

As the date of the final session approaches, the patient learns that although physically separated from the therapist, they have access to their memories of the therapy with all its emotional developments and insights. In addition, they take with them an increased access and laterality to their narratives regarding their relationship to the birth parent. The adopted patient, in articulating, co-constructing, and analyzing their inner dialogue with the birth parent, does not "lose" any of the specific fantasies about their birth parents but instead gains a psychological flexibility in cathecting any of a number of narratives that can now be articulated and experienced with the same maturity that characterizes their overall experience of the interpersonal world. This does not wipe away the sadness of the abandoned self in the shadow of the lost object but instead allows this enshrined experience to be viewed in the relative light of conscious experience and the sadness it evokes; it deepens and broadens the tolerance and understanding of the sadness that is a part of the separation inherent in any human relationship.

Endnotes

Deeg, C.F. (1989). On the adoptee's cathexis of the lost object. *Psychoanalysis and Psychotherapy*, 7, 152–161.

Deeg, C.F. (1990). Defensive functions of the adoptee's cathexis of the lost object. *Psychoanalysis and Psychotherapy*, 8, 35–46.

Deeg, C.F. (1991). On the adoptee's search for identity. *Psychoanalysis and Psychotherapy*, 9, 128–133.

Deeg, C.F. (2002). Issues of psychoanalytic technique with adoptees. *Journal of Social Distress and the Homeless*, 11(2), 193–205.

Derrida, J. (1974). *Of grammatology* (G. C. Spivak, Trans.). Baltimore: Johns Hopkins University Press.

Dewald, P. (1966) Forced termination of psychoanalysis. *Bulletin of the Menninger Clinic*, 30, 98–110.

Eissler, K. (1953). The effects of the structure of the ego on psychoanalytic technique. *Journal of the American Psychoanalytic Association*, 1, 104–143.

Fenichel, O. (1941). *Problems of psychoanalytic technique*. Albany, NY: The Psychoanalytic Quarterly, Inc.

Fenichel, O. (1945). *The psychoanalytic theory of neurosis*. New York: Norton.

Firestein, S. (1969). Panel report: Problems of termination in the analysis of adults. *Journal of the American Psychoanalytic Association*, 17, 222–237.

Freud, S. (1913). Totem and Taboo. *Standard Edition*, 13, 154–55.

Greenberg, J., & Mitchell, S. (1983). *Object relations in psychoanalytic theory*. Cambridge: Harvard University Press.

Greenson, R. (1967). *The technique and practice of psychoanalysis*. New York: International Universities Press.

Kernberg, O., Selzer, M., Koenigsberg. H., Carr, A., & Appelbaum, A. (1989). *Psychodynamic psychotherapy of borderline patients*. New York: Basic Books.

Kohut, H. (1971). *The analysis of the self*. New York: International Universities Press.

Langs, R. (1974). *The technique of psychoanalytic psychotherapy*. Northvale: Jason Aronson.

13
FROM FRAGMENTED TO FIRM FOUNDATIONS IN IDENTITY FORMATION

A Neurosequential Approach to the Treatment of Adopted Adolescents and Young Adults with Early Developmental Trauma

Alan John Burnell, OBE, and Jay Vaughan, MBE

Introduction

Family Futures is a voluntary adoption agency (VAA) and an independent foster care agency (IFA) that was set up in 1998, initially as an adoption support agency (ASA). It was co-founded because the majority of placements in foster care or adoption in the UK were older children. Most of these children have been developmentally traumatized (Van der Kolk, 2005). Adoptive parents and foster caregivers of these children were bewildered and overwhelmed as the children in their home were presenting a wide range of difficulties and challenges, such as stealing, lying, aggression, or withdrawn behavior. The children seemed to fail to form secure attachments to their adoptive parents, despite the love and care they were receiving. Family Futures was originally set up as a post-placement assessment and therapeutic service for adoptive families, as there was no effective holistic and long-term therapeutic help available for them. Adoption services were, and are still, functioning predicated on baby placements; they provide limited post-adoption support.

Our therapeutic intervention was developed to address the needs of the children and youth/adolescents who entered placement with an array of early negative experiences. We were a family-based approach so that at the same time as working with children and young people, we were working with the foster or adoptive parents. In the early years of our work, we focused on attachment because this was the key issue and concern. Drawing from attachment theory (Bowlby, 1988), we used the concepts of "internal working models." These include the concept of cognitive or mental models about the self, attachment figures, and the social world; early relational experiences affect beliefs and expectations about later relationships. If the child's early experience involved abuse or neglect by birth parents or other people, their internal working model affects the child's capacity to trust and form close attachments to adoptive and foster parents. They also had no "coherent narratives" (Bowlby, 1988) as to what had happened to them and why; they have an incompleteness to draw on the meaning to past events (Lind et al., 2020). Narrative coherence is intricately linked to psychological well-being (Borelli et al., 2019). To address these issues, we developed a brain-based, sequential, and developmental system that integrates attachment and neuroscience research with sensory, somatic, play-based, attachment, and trauma-focused therapy and narrative: therapeutic life story work (Vaughan et al., 2016). We also worked with their adoptive or foster parents to help them become more attuned to the child. These "life stories" were not just about people and places but the feelings that were attached to those people and places. If these children and youth had any kind of narrative about their past, it was fragmented and incoherent or suppressed and unconscious.

In our practice, we realized that these children had not just experienced a single traumatic event but had multiple pre- and post-birth negative experiences that permeated every aspect of their life and their development. Van der Kolk (2005) described these children's experiences and sequelae as "developmental trauma." Developmental trauma is more holistic, recognizing that every aspect of the child's development is negatively affected by poor and abusive/neglectful parenting that led to the child being taken into public care. Trauma has a negative impact on the capacity to problem-solve and on cognitive processing (Lansdown et al., 2007), as well as having an impact on the brain and nervous system (Levine & Kline, 2006).

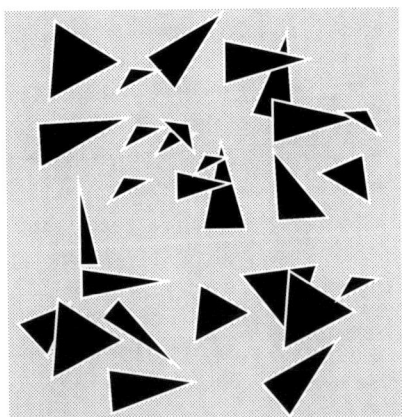

A highly traumatised 7 year old girl, when asked to create a picture of show she felt inside, created the drawing on the left. She cut up pieces of red paper and stuck them on blue. When asked how she felt she said:

"In pieces"

Figure 13.1   In pieces.

Also, trauma affects sensory processing, and many children showed signs of sensory integration disorders (Ayres & Robbins, 2005).

We have five pillars supporting our work – attachment theory, developmental trauma, executive functioning, sensory integration, and bodywork. In order to work effectively with the five areas, we have evolved into an interdisciplinary team that includes social workers, psychotherapists, creative arts therapists, psychologists, occupational therapists trained in sensory integrations, and teachers. We also have consultants, including psychologists, psychiatrists, and a pediatrician/general practitioner.

We developed our approach neurosequentially. Our approach follows the hierarchical sequence of brain and central nervous system development in neonates and infants and directs therapeutic attention to three main areas of brain function – the primitive brain system, the midbrain (limbic), and the higher-order functioning of the cortical brain (Vaughan et al., 2016). We realized that traumatized youth respond to the world from their primitive brain and find it difficult to form midbrain-based attachments as well as coherent reflective memories. Until the person feels safe and regulated, they are not able to move out of a primitive brain response and develop reflective frontal lobe thinking and problem-solving in the limbic and cortical parts of the brain. Dyadic developmental psychotherapy (DDP; Hughes & Baylin, 2012) is an attachment-focused therapy designed to support traumatized children in developing the ability to maintain attachment-based relationships with parents and caregivers (Becker-Weidman, 2012).

A version of Table 13.1 was previously published by Vaughan et al. (2016), "Neurophysiological Psychotherapy (NPP): The development and application of an integrative, wrap-around service and treatment programme for maltreated children placed in adoptive and foster care placements," *Clinical Child Psychology and Psychiatry* 1–14.

Adolescent Identity Integration

With an adolescent who has not had effective therapeutic interventions in childhood, we follow the same neurosequential pattern of therapeutic intervention after a comprehensive interdisciplinary assessment. The assessment includes psychological and sensory processing screening tools, measures of attachment and child–parent interactions, family and child observations, and projective assessments of children, parent, and teacher responses (McCullough et al., 2016; McCullough & Mathura, 2019). The likelihood is that an adolescent's self-image and identity are based upon past experiences with their birth parents and their experience in the child welfare system. The issue for many adolescents is a deep-rooted and sometimes unconscious feeling that they are rubbish, unwanted, and unlovable. They live in a permanent state of fear and anxiety. These feelings can only be addressed by exploring the young person's infancy to understand their adolescence challenges. Using the lens of a neurosequential approach, if a young person is still living with a deep sense of

Table 13.1 Sequential Brain Development

Area of the Brain	Focus	Theme	Interventions
Primitive brain	Trauma responses Physiological regulation Emotional regulation	Fear and stress reduction Emotional and physiological awareness Co-regulation and attunement	• Sleep, diet, and toileting advice • Medication • Somatic and sensorimotor work • Sensory integration • Developmental re-parenting with one-on-one time at home
Limbic brain	Attachment	Developing a more secure attachment Shame reduction Development of conscience and empathy	• Dyadic developmental psychotherapy and creative arts to address trauma re-enactment and support attachment • Theraplay • Developmental re-parenting
Cortical brain	Identity integration	Developing a coherent narrative and reflective capacity.	• Dyadic developmental psychotherapy with a life story focus to help development of a coherent narrative and identity • Facilitated contact • Individual psychotherapy • Identity and self-esteem work • Parent therapy/support • School liaison/interventions • Network meetings • Intensive individual therapy

fear, shame, and with a fight-flight-or-freeze response to any challenge, we begin by dealing with the traumas of infancy in order to help them feel safe and able to be regulated. It is not possible to make sense of one's early traumatic history while still living in a fear state. The first step of any intervention needs to be to support a young person in feeling safe in order to be reflective. Only in this calm, reflective state is it possible to integrate early traumatic experiences. Once a young person has been helped to make sense of their early history and their childhood experiences, their capacity to form attachments will be enhanced. Once they have the capacity to form attachments and to accept love and that they are lovable, they can then begin to build a positive sense of self and form a positive and firm foundation for their identity as adults. A more coherent narrative can then change the internal working models of attachment and provide them with another template for relationships. This reflective capacity enables them to have better executive functioning so they can begin to make sense of the past and begin to think about the future as being different and hopeful. This gives the young person a sense of agency and empowerment that are key to being able to make good decisions about their life and future.

A Case Study: Frankie, Aged 20 Years Old

Frankie kept his hood up and his knees curled in sitting silently on the sofa as far away as he could from his adoptive mother. Frankie did not speak but would snarl and snap one-word responses as the therapist wondered about how he felt about being at Family Futures. He did, however, make it clear he wanted help as things had become so difficult at home and he wanted his adoptive mother there too. Frankie's adoptive mother spoke about how hard things had been at home and the number of police calls as violence had escalated over the winter months. She also told about how much she loved Frankie and wanted to help him. The therapist knew that the police were very close to arresting Frankie on a number of occasions for his assaults on his adoptive mother.

In the individual session, Franke relaxed a little bit and allowed his feet now to touch the floor instead of curling up. The therapist engaged Frankie in thinking about things he enjoyed that made him feel good. Frankie became animated, talking about his love of football and his dreams of a football career, at one point even smiling. Little by little, as Frankie relaxed, the therapist could feel her own body relax too, and the conversation began to flow. Suddenly, in the middle of this ease in the session, Frankie asked if Family Futures could find his birth mother, as he wanted to see her but he did not want his adoptive mother to know. The therapist said how usual this is and wondered about why Frankie would want to keep this normal wish from his adoptive mother. Frankie looked worried and said he did not want to her hurt, but he just needed to know that his birth mother was okay and still alive.

In the coming months, Frankie engaged in dyadic and individual therapy sessions at Family Futures. He, over time, found he could talk to his adoptive mother about his wish to see his birth mother, and she not only could manage not to feel upset about this but was also keen to support him in this happening. Frankie had not had any life story work and only had a limited understanding about why he was adopted, based on his minimal life story book, which said his birth mother loved him but could not care for him. Frankie needed a lot of movement in his therapy sessions to feel able to think, and sessions moved between active, body-based movement sessions and talking sessions. Frankie found that he really liked to hang upside down from the gym suspended equipment, and from here he was able to talk more easily. Frankie also found that the weighted blanket and deep-pressure touch from his adoptive mother helped his body feel calm and his brain work better. Frankie wondered if these techniques would have helped him in school when he was struggling to be still and engage.

As sessions progressed, gone was the silent, hidden young man, and a new, playful, cheeky, and engaging young man emerged. The therapist found that her stress response to sessions reduced, and Frankie's adoptive mother found that police calls became a thing of the past. Frankie even said in one session how much he enjoyed coming and how the play, laughter, and hanging upside down had changed things. Frankie also consistently reported feeling less stressed and less explosive at home.

Frankie was still keen to see his birth mother but also agreed that in small chunks he would do some life story work so he could understand his life story and then think about if he still wanted contact. Frankie was fearful of what he might find out in his life story and used the early sessions to think about his terror about what might be hidden in his past. In one session with his adoptive mother, he bravely said he was worried that he was going to find out that his birth parents had been violent and the police were involved when he was little. Frankie thought he had a memory of being in the back of a police car with a friendly policewoman who gave him some sweets as he was hungry. Frankie shared that he worried he was going to be a violent man and all the attacks he had made on his adoptive mother were evidence he was a bad person.

Frankie's big fear was he would end up on the streets or in prison. Frankie looked anxiously at this adoptive mother, retreating inside his sweatshirt hood a little, as he once more tucked his legs underneath him. Frankie's adoptive mother said, "I love you, Frankie. I have always loved you, even when you lashed out at me. I know you are hurting inside and that sometimes you don't know what to do with all your angry feelings. None of this is your fault; it is because of what happened to you when you were little. We just need to find a way to help you make sense of yourself and your history so you have a chance in life." Frankie's eyes filled with tears, and he moved a little closer to his adoptive mother and took her hand in his.

As the life story work progressed, Frankie counted out the number of times the police had been called when he was with his birth family. Frankie looked ashen when he heard about all the injuries he sustained in the care of his birth parents and the terrible violence he witnessed. There was also in the file history one reference to Frankie being put in the back of a police car whilst the police tried to deal with his birth parents. Frankie smiled from ear to ear and shouted out, punching the air,

"Yes, I was right. There it is – I did remember!" For Frankie, tying together his fragmented memories with the narrative from the local authority case file was a vital part of him feeling he was not a mad or a bad person but a scared little boy with suppressed memories of this time in his life.

In one session, Frankie shared that he had looked at some of the scars from cigarette burns on his arms that were still evident. Frankie said he had always wondered where he got the scars from and had not known who did this to him and worried about it. Frankie talked about his gut-wrenching horror of realizing that somehow in the chaos of his early years, someone hurt him in this way. Frankie then turned to his adoptive mother and said, "I wish I had been born to you, as you would never have done this to me. I have done terrible things to you and you have never hurt me back." Frankie and his mom stayed looking into each other's eyes, both of them with tears streaming down their faces. The therapist suggested that Frankie was saying how much he loved his adoptive mom and how sorry he was that he had hurt her. Frankie whispered, "I love you, Mom, and I am so, so sorry." Frankie's mom wrapped him into her arms and rocked him back and forth, soothing him gently with her words of love and letting him know that she loved him. It was okay, he was safe now, and together they would get through this.

Frankie went on to use both dyadic session with his adoptive mother and confidential individual sessions to process all his feelings about what had happened to him and the scared, frozen little boy who had become an angry young man, not understanding where all his feelings came from.

Frankie still wanted to meet his birth mother, and the local authority got an update about her whereabouts as a first step. Family Futures facilitated contact to support Frankie in this part of the journey. Frankie said that he felt he understood himself more now, and although at times he would still feel the rage inside and even the wish to hurt others and himself, it felt more manageable than it had before. Frankie slowly began to feel better about himself and make some positive choices about his future. Frankie also stopped wearing his hoodie up over his face. It was as if he was risking being seen more now and could make more decisions about what he wanted for his life and what sort of young man he wanted to be.

Conclusion

Identity formation for young people who have been developmentally traumatized in infancy is not an issue that can be taken out of the overall context of the child or young person's neurosequential development, as they are transitioning from trauma to attachment to reflective capacity and a positive sense of self. We need to move towards a model of intervention that is aware of the specific issues for adopted young people who have had traumatic early histories in the care system. Therapy for this population of children cannot be a one-off event but needs to be a lifelong process of supporting them, at key developmental stages, in making sense of themselves and being able to make good choices about their lives. Adolescence is always challenging, but being an adopted adolescent or a child in the care system, with a traumatic history, means that they are going to need help at various times in their life, sometimes with their parents and sometimes without, in individual sessions. The therapy needs to understand the particular challenges for adopted young people and young adults, as for them, the trauma issues and the attachment issues are key, and any approach needs to have an in-depth understanding of these and be able to understand the value of a neurosequential approach to them.

As one young person so eloquently said as an adult looking back at his traumatic history and journey in therapy at Family Futures, it was the therapist and his parent holding on to the **hope** that things could and would be better that kept him going!

Endnotes

Ayres, A.J., & Robbins, J. (2005). *Sensory Integration and the Child: Understanding Hidden Sensory Challenges*. California: Western Psychological Services.

Becker-Weidman, A. (2012). Dyadic developmental psychotherapy: Effective treatment for complex trauma and disorders of attachment. *Illinois Child Welfare Journal, 6*(1), 1–11.

Borelli, J.L., Brugnera, A., Zarbo, C., Rabboni, M., Bondi, E., Tasca, G.A., & Compare, A. (2019). Attachment comes of age: Adolescents' narrative coherence and reflective functioning predict well-being in emerging adulthood. *Attachment & Human Development, 21*(4), 332–351.

Bowlby, J. (1988). *A Secure Base*. London: Routledge.

Hughes, D.A., & Baylin, J. (2012). *Brain-based Parenting: The Neuroscience of Caregiving for Healthy Attachment*. New York: W. W. Norton & Company.

Lansdown, R., Burnell, A., & Allen, M. (2007). Is it that they won't do it, or is it that they can't? Executive functioning and children who have been fostered and adopted. *Adoption and Fostering, 31*(2).

Levine, P., & Kline, M. (2006). *Trauma Through a Child's Eyes: Awakening the Ordinary: Awakening the Ordinary Miracle of Healing*. California: North Atlantic Books.

Lind, M., Vanwoerden, S., Penner, F., & Sharp, C. (2020). Narrative coherence in adolescence: Relations with attachment, mentalization, and psychopathology. *Journal of Personality Assessment, 102*(3), 380–389.

McCullough, E., Gordon-Jones, S., Last, A., Vaughan, J., & Burnell, A. (2016). An evaluation of neurophysiological psychotherapy: An integrative therapeutic approach to working with adopted children who have experienced early life trauma. *Clinical Child Psychology and Psychiatry, 21*(4), 1–21.

McCullough, E., & Mathura, A. (2019). A comparison between a Neurophysiological Psychotherapy (NPP) treatment group and a control group for children adopted from care: Support for a neurodevelopmentally informed approach to therapeutic intervention with maltreated children. *Child Abuse & Neglect, 97*(2019), 104128.

Van der Kolk, B.A. (2005). Developmental trauma disorder: Towards a rational diagnosis for children with complex trauma histories. *Psychiatric Annals, 35*, 401–408.

Vaughan, J., McCullough, E., & Burnell, A (2016). Neurophysiological Psychotherapy (NPP): The development and application of an integrative, wrap-around service and treatment programme for maltreated children placed in adoptive and foster care placements. *Clinical Child Psychology and Psychiatry, 21*(4), 1–14.

14
SIMILARITIES AND DIFFERENCES IN ATTACHMENT REPRESENTATIONS BETWEEN LATE-ADOPTED AND NON-ADOPTED ADOLESCENTS

A Study from Italy

Cecilia S. Pace, PhD; Stefania Muzi, PhD; Fabiola Bizzi, PhD; and Donatella Cavanna

Introduction

It is widely recognized that attachment is a process that has long-life effects on the adaptation of the individual. One of the major ways that attachment impacts subsequent development is conceptualized as "internal working models" (IWMs, Bowlby, 1982, p. 48), particularly representation of the self, the other, and the relationship between the self and the other. The child develops the IWMs during the first years of life within the parent–child relationship, which later become a template for subsequent relationships (Bowlby, 1982; Grossmann et al., 2006, p. 98). If caregivers are continuously sensitive and responsive when the child expresses his/her needs to be nourished, reassured when afraid, and encouraged to explore new situations, the child will generally form a secure IWM of the self as worthy of love and attention (Bowlby, 1982). Securely attached infants show the desire to both connect to others and explore the external physical and emotional environment, and securely attached adults show greater well-being, better emotional regulation, positive social skills, and healthy identity development across the life span

(Irhammar & Bengtsson, 2004). On the contrary, problematic early parent–child relationships predispose the child to developing insecure IWMs. The child may tend to minimize the need for closeness to a caregiver to avoid the caregiver's rejection (avoidant IWM), or the child may show hyperactivation of the attachment system and vigilance to attachment-related stimuli, inhibiting the seeking of continuous proximity because of the uncertainty of the caregiver's availability (ambivalent/resistant IWM). For adults, insecure attachment negatively affects their regulation of emotion, social adaptation, intimate relationships, and parenting abilities (Grossmann et al., 2006). In the most worrisome case, the child fails to organize a unique and coherent attachment strategy, thus demonstrating disorganized/disoriented attachment (Bowlby, 1982). It is characterized by the co-occurrence of avoidant and ambivalent IMWs (Lyons-Ruth & Jacobvitz, 2016) (Appendix 1). A disorganized/disoriented pattern is highly related to frequent attachment disruptions early in life, which can be due to parental loss or abandonment, situations of neglect, abuse, and/or frightened/frightening caregivers (Lyons-Ruth & Jacobvitz, 2016), or prolonged institutionalization early in life. Moreover, the disorganized/disoriented pattern has been related to a higher lifelong vulnerability to psychopathology and psychosocial problems (Madigan et al., 2016; Mikulincer & Shaver, 2012).

Attachment theory is considered useful for understanding and intervening on a wide variety of psychopathological, relational, and identity difficulties (Johnson & Fein, 1991; Raby & Dozier, 2019). Within an attachment framework, "late-placed adopted" (LA) (Appendix 2) children are considered more at risk to develop a disorganized attachment due to the higher incidence of early attachment disruptions (van den Dries et al., 2009; Dozier & Rutter, 2016). Indeed, the first 12–24 months of life constitute the first bonding phase to building an attachment bond with a specific caregiver (Bowlby, 1982) (Appendix 3). Therefore, while babies placed within the first 12 months may develop their first attachment relationship directly with adoptive parents, it may be preceded by neurophysiological attachment to the birth mother and, additionally, other/earlier disrupted attachments. Late-placed adopted children would probably have had at least one postnatal interruption in their early attachment bond with a primary caregiver (van den Dries et al., 2009). The later the children are placed for adoption, the greater the risk for pre-adoption relational traumas (van den Dries et al., 2009). Lastly, late-placed adopted children are also more likely to be identified as having "special needs." This may depend on the number of disruptions and the quality of the care the child had prior to placement. Special needs include complex medical problems, cognitive or physical developmental delays, physical disabilities, and emotional difficulties. Different countries have different criteria used to establish that a child has known or suspected special needs, and these definitions change over time. Adopting a child with special needs requires additional efforts from adoptive families to provide caregiving unique to that child (Mullin & Johnson, 1999), as well as caregiving that can repair negative attachment and behavior patterns already established.

Since the peak of international adoptions (IA) in 2010 (International Adoption Commission [IAC], 2018), Italy became the second-highest receiving country in the world for the number of IA. Most IAs to Italy are late-placed adoptions involving children adopted at ages 4–9 years old (International Adoption Commission [IAC], 2013, 2018). Parents seeking to adopt in Italy must be legally married (Italian laws n. 184/1983, 476/1998, 149/2001). Adoptive parents are generally older than biological ones, and they also have higher levels of education (e.g., 85% high school or higher academic credentials) (Dipartimento Giustizia Minorile e di Comunità, 2019; IAC, 2013, 2018). The main motivation behind the decision to adopt in Italy is the inability of the couple to conceive a child (Santona & Zavattini, 2005). Adoptive parents are described by some researchers as stable and affectionate couples, having clear individual and couple identities, and highly motivated to become a parent (Pace, Santona et al., 2015; Rosnati et al., 2008, 2013). However, from a clinical perspective, the reasons given for adopting might have underlying psychodynamics that are uncovered in clinical work and that may contradict the given reasons.

Meta-analytical evidence from studies of adopted children demonstrate that late-placed adoptees are more likely to show insecure or disorganized IWMs than those adopted before 12 months of age (Juffer et al., 2011; Pace et al., 2014; Pace, Zavattini, et al., 2015; van den Dries et al., 2009). The evidence suggests that the higher incidence of problematic attachments is related to adverse pre-adoption experiences (van den Dries et al., 2009). Furthermore, van den Dries et al. (2009) hypothesized higher attachment insecurity in late-placed adoptees who have lived with their adopted family for only a short time after having lived in pre-adoption dysfunctional relationships or settings. The same meta-analysis also reports higher attachment insecurity in international adoptees than in domestic ones, especially adoptions from Eastern European countries; the differences were explained by the harsher pre-adoptive conditions in the former communist countries (van den Dries et al., 2009). On the other hand, several studies did not find a relationship between age at adoptive placement, length of time in the adoptive home, or type of adoption (intercountry vs. domestic) (Pace et al., 2012, 2019; Veríssimo & Salvaterra, 2006; Vorria et al., 2015). Therefore, the impact of these factors on the attachment of late-placed adopted children is still debated. Moreover, while community/control samples suggest females are more likely to demonstrate attachment security than males, gender does not seem to be a significant factor in the attachment security in late-placed adoptees (Pace et al., 2019; van den Dries et al., 2009). Positive findings from longitudinal studies indicate that a significant relational experience with nurturing adoptive parents can help late-placed adopted children shift from insecure attachment toward secure attachment IWMs, both in the short term and through adolescence (van Ijzendoorn & Juffer, 2006; Beijersbergen et al., 2012; Juffer et al., 2011; Pace & Zavattini, 2011; Pace et al., 2012; Pace et al., 2019; Steele et al., 2008; Steele et al., 2010; Vorria et al., 2015).

Despite the attachment vulnerability of late-placed adopted children, most attachment studies with adopted adolescents reported secure attachment classifications (50–60%), similar to non-adopted, low-risk teenagers' (Bakermans-Kranenburg & van IJzendoorn, 2009; Groza et al., 2012; Groza & Muntean, 2016; Molina et al., 2015; Pace et al., 2015; Pace et al., 2019; Riva Crugnola et al., 2009; Simonelli & Vizziello, 2009; Vorria et al., 2015). In the few studies comparing attachment classifications of late-placed adopted and community/control adolescents, only one study found late-placed adoptees as more likely to be insecure and disorganized than controls (Escobar & Santelices, 2013), while other comparative studies did not find any differences between the groups (Pace et al., 2018; Riva Crugnola et al., 2009; Vorria et al., 2015).

However, it would be misleading to interpret previous results as an absence of attachment in late-placed adoptees during adolescence, as it would ignore the more subtle consequences of unfavorable or adverse childhood experiences of late-placed adopted adolescents that is widely reported by practitioners working with adopted people and adoptive families. In this regard, if comparative studies with adolescents did not reveal any differences in attachment insecurity during childhood, it would be important to avoid, depending solely on the usual attachment classifications. Rather, it is important to focus on specific dimensions of IWMs that predict adolescent's well-being in community/control studies with non-adoptees (Borelli et al., 2019). These concepts that are part of IWMs are narrative coherence, reflective functioning, and affect regulation. Typically functioning adapted adolescents tend to show higher narrative coherence – the ability to access, describe, and discuss their own attachment-related experiences according to Grice's conversational maxims (1975). They can reflect and tell personal memories in truthful, relevant, collaborative, and clear ways. Adaptability in adolescence has been related to higher reflective functioning – the capacity to understand one's own and others' mental states in terms of emotions, desires, wishes, goals, and attitudes (Fonagy et al., 1991; Katznelson, 2014). Securely attached adolescents show different affect regulation strategies to regulate their negative affects. If insecurely attached, they may employ more defensive and potentially ineffective affect regulation strategies, such as anger, idealization, or derogation towards parents (Steele & Steele, 2005). A higher coherence of reflective functioning and a lower level of affective regulation strategies are related to the better well-being of youths (Borelli et al., 2019), but adopted children show vulnerability in these attachment dimensions (Pace et al., 2014). A multilevel assessment of the vulnerabilities of late-placed adopted adolescents would be an important intervention. Given these, this study aimed to answer the following research questions:

1. What is the difference between the quality of attachment of late-adopted adolescent adoptees and those of non-adopted, low-risk peers in Italy?
2. In which attachment-related dimensions do adolescent adoptees seem similar to their peers, and in which ones are they more vulnerable? Included in this

study is an assessment of how attachment vulnerabilities of adolescent adoptees may be related to specific adoption-related variables (children's age at adoptive placement, length of time being adopted, international vs. domestic adoption, sociodemographic data, and control variables (child's age, gender, verbal skills).

Method

Participants

This study involved 98 adolescents (aged 11–18 years); half were late adoptees, and half were a matched group, as described in Table 14.1, which presents the demographic characteristics of the participants.

The first group was composed of 49 adopted adolescents (AG = adopted group), 27 boys and 22 girls, ranging in age between 11 and 18 years (M = 14.57, SD = 2.16). All the adoptees had been placed for adoption after 1 year of age; the average age was 5.3 years (SD = 3 years); therefore, as a group, they are considered late-placed adopted children. They have been living with their adoptive parents for at least 3 years, with an average of 9.2 years (SD = 3.3). About 88% were internationally adopted, coming from Eastern Europe (38%), Asia (20%), South America (18%), or Africa (14%); the smallest percent were domestically adopted (12%). Before adoption, recognizing that information for international adoptees is often inaccurate or incomplete, most (65%) of the adoptees had lived with their family of origin and were removed as a result of maltreatment (35%) or abandonment (25%). Before being adopted, almost all children had been placed in an institutional setting for a period ranging from 6 to 72 months; the average length of institutionalization was 29.6 months (SD = 15.3 months). Most adoptees had siblings (65%), including 17 biological siblings of the adoptee, 12 adopted siblings in the adoptive homes, and 3 biological children born to adoptive parents. More than half of the adoptees were attending middle school, while the others were attending high school, except one adopted person who had already completed high school. At the time of the data collection, 90% of adoptive parents were still married. They ranged in age from 43 to 66 years old and had achieved between 8 and 24 years of education.

The control group (CG) included 49 adolescents, all born in Italy, aged 11–18 years old at the time of data collection; all the control group subjects were raised by their biological parents. They were recruited from middle and high schools and matched for age at the time of the study with the adopted group. Most of the CG participants had biological siblings (81%), two had stepsiblings (4.1%), and two had both biological and stepsiblings (4.1%). At the time of assessment, most of the controls were attending high school (63%). Most of the biological parents were still married and/or cohabiting (73%) and ranged in age from 32 to 61 years old. They had achieved between 5 and 21 years of education.

Table 14.1 Demographics of Participants (N = 98) and Adoption Features of Late-Adoptees

Demographics	Range		Late-Adopted (AG) N (%)	Late-Adopted (AG) M (SD)	Community (CG) N (%)	Community (CG) M (SD)
Age★	11–18		49 (50)	14.6 (2.16)	49 (50)	14.6 (2.16)
Gender	Boys		27 (55)		28 (57)	
	Girls		22 (45)		21 (43)	
Education (type)	Middle school		26 (53)		18 (37)	
	High school		23 (47)		31 (63)	
Family	Parents together		44 (90)		36 (73.5)	
	Parents not together		5 (10)		13 (26.5)	
	Age★	Mother		50.9 (3.8)		48.3 (5.1)
		Father		52.9 (4.5)		51.3 (4.7)
	Education★	Mother		14.6 (4.21)		
		Father		13 (4.81)		
Siblings	No		17 (35)		9 (19)	
	Yes		32 (65)		40 (81)	
Adoption features	Range		N (%)	M (SD)		
Age at adoption★	1–12		49 (100)	5.3 (3)		
Length of adoption	3–17			9.2 (3.3)		
Area of origin	Italy		6 (12)			
	International		43 (88)★★			
	East Europe		17 (34.7)			
	Asia		10 (20.4)			
	South America		9 (18.4)			
	Africa		7 (14.3)			
Reasons	Abandonment		12 (24)			
	Death of biological parent(s)		4 (8)			
	Abuse		17 (35)			
		Severe neglect	10 (20)			
		sexual	1 (2)			
		physical	2 (4)			
		multiple	4 (8)			
	Other difficulties★★★		16 (33)			

(Continued)

Table 14.1 (Continued)

Previous institutionalization	No	1 (2)	
	Yes	48 (98)	
Length (months)	6–7		29.6 (15.3)

Note:
* In years.
** Overlaps with international adoptions.
*** Parental loss or psychopathology or drugs/alcohol abuse or incarceration or early institutionalization for undeclared reasons.

Measures

The Friends and Family Interview (FFI)

The main research tool was the *Friends and Family Interview* (FFI, Steele et al., 2009) used for assessing attachment representations of adolescents. The interview is composed of 27 questions investigating representations of self, favorite teacher, best friend, and family members. The FFIs were transcribed verbatim, and they were assigned to one of the four attachment classifications. Secure-autonomous was determined when the interviewee provided a coherent narrative of his/her attachment experiences, valuing of attachment, could need/missing others, and verbalized low use of defensive affect regulation strategies. Insecure-dismissing was determined when the narrative was poorly coherent due to idealization or derogation of self and/or parents and the interviewee minimized the value of attachment. Insecure-preoccupied was assigned to poorly coherent narratives involving anger or excessive role reversal toward parents (i.e., age-inappropriate excessive desire to please the parents) and/or overwhelmed by attachment experiences. Insecure-disorganized was coded when the narrative reflected the coexistence of incompatible strategies, or a lack of strategy, due to excessive self-derogation or the intrusion of frightening and bizarre content. Scoring was based on the highest score achieved from applying the FFI coding system for the following scales: (1) *coherence*, based on Grice's maxims of good conversation truth (be credible in what you say), economy (provide the right amount of information, neither too little nor too much), relation (provide relevant examples regarding the topic of conversation), and manner (age-appropriate attention and properly educated within the conversation), plus overall coherence that reflects the central tendency of the previous four concepts; (2) *reflective functioning*, in terms of developmental perspective (the interviewee contrasts personal current thoughts and feelings with past attitudes or style of responses), theory of mind (ability to assume the mental perspective of the other), and diversity of feelings (ability to show understanding of both positive and negative feelings within the same significant relationship); (3) *evidence of availability of a secure base/safe haven attachment*, which indicates that a caregiver provides comfort in case of distress and help/encouragement with the exploration (it can be a father, mother, and other significant figure); (4) *evidence of self-esteem*, including social competence (degree of comfort in social activities), school competence (confidence and excitement in schoolwork), and self-regard (like or dislike of the self); (5) *peer relations* (frequency and quality of contact intended as close emotional contact, open discussion of problems in a friendship); (6) *sibling relations* (warmth, hostility, and rivalry with siblings); (7) *affect regulation* (discrepancy between positive evaluation of self or parents and lack of supporting memories), *role reversal* (instances of child taking on "adult" responsibilities or excessive eagerness to please and pacify parents), *anger* (excessive "hot" anger/embarrassment/shame toward parents), *derogation* ("cold" diminishment of the significance of worth of the self or parents), and *adaptive/flexible responses to distress*; and (8) *differentiation of parental representations*. Each subscale is scored on a 4-point scale from 1 to 4, including mid-points (1 = no evidence; 2 = mild evidence; 3 = moderate evidence; 4 = marked evidence), including every single pattern (secure, dismissing, preoccupied, and disorganized), which constitute independently rated scales, each one with a score, of which the one with the highest score corresponds to the final attachment classification assigned to the interview. This double-coding system allows both a categorical and dimensional evaluation of attachment representations.

In this study, 46 of the 98 interviews (47%) were scored by two independent and reliable coders with 98% of agreement on both secure–insecure classifications ($k = .91$, $p < .001$) and on the four-way classification ($k = .92$, $p < .001$), and 100% on disorganized–not disorganized classifications ($k = 1$, $p < .000$). The disagreement between coders was resolved by a third certified and independent coder. The FFI showed good psychometric properties in terms of inter-rater reliability, factor structure, intercountry invariance, content, discriminant, and convergent validity (Pace et al., 2015; Pace et al., 2018; Pace et al., 2020; Psouni & Apetroaia, 2014; Psouni et al., 2019; Steele & Steele, 2005; Stievenart et al., 2012).

The Wechsler Intelligence Scale for Children, IV Version (WISC-IV)

To control for possible confounding effects on attachment narratives due to the differential language competence of adolescents (Pace et al. 2015; Steele & Steele, 2005), participants' verbal skills were assessed using the verbal subtests composing the Verbal Comprehension Index of the Wechsler Intelligence Scale for Children, IV version (VCI-WISC-IV, Wechsler, 2003; Orsini et al., 2012). The VCI is the sum of weighted points in *Similarities*, *Vocabulary*, and *Comprehension* subtests. In the Italian version, Cronbach's α of 0.96 is reported for the VCI; other scales range from 0.69 for comprehension to 0.94 for vocabulary.

Sociodemographic Data Form

A sociodemographic questionnaire was developed by the researchers. The questionnaire was completed by the mothers to collect family data (parents' age of birth, education level, etc.) and information concerning the details of adoption from adoptive mothers, such as children's age on arrival, country of origin, length of adoption, and pre-adoption information.

Procedure

The adoptive families were recruited through the Social Health Service that specializes in adoption work, authorizes intercountry adoption agencies, and promotes associations supporting adoptive families. Among all the adoptive families contacted that were living in urban areas of Liguria, non-adoptive families were part of a large community study on the FFI (Pace et al., 2020), and they were all recruited from middle and high school, each contacted by one of six students belonging to the research team.

The research project had the prior approval of the University of Genoa's Research Ethics Committee, and all participants and legal caretakers signed a voluntary consent form in accordance with the Declaration of Helsinki. The FFI and the VCI-WISC-IV were administered to the adopted adolescents at a university room or at their home, depending on their preference. Most of the data collected from the non-adopted adolescents occurred at school. In both situations, participants were involved in individual sessions lasting around 90 minutes. The sociodemographic questionnaires were independently completed by the mothers.

Data Analysis

Statistical analyses were conducted using the Statistical Package for Social Science (Version 21.0) software. First, we present descriptive statistics and group comparisons on study and control variables for the AG and the CG, through chi-square for categorical variables (gender and FFI classifications distributions) (Appendix 4), and t-test on continuous ones (age, FFI scores). Only in the AG correlations were carried out between FFI scales, demographic variables, and adoption variables using Pearson's r coefficient. All values were considered statistically significant, with $p < 0.05$.

Results

Preliminary Analyses

In comparing adopted and non-adopted adolescents, no difference emerged in sociodemographic and control variables, such as age at the time of the study, gender, number of siblings, education, or verbal IQ (AG: $M = 99.95$, $SD = 13.72$; CG: $M = 105.87$, $SD = 19.45$). No differences were found in verbal IQ between secure vs. insecure FFI classifications both in the AG and in CG. Adoptive parents were less likely to be separated/divorced than biological parents (χ^2, $p = .031$). Adoptive mothers were older than biological ones ($t(92) = 2.81$, $p = .006$). Adoptive fathers had higher education than biological ones ($t(92) = 2.05$, $p = .043$). These data were similar to national Italian statistics on adoptive couples (Pace et al., 2015).

Attachment Classifications in AG and CG

Regarding attachment representations, the FFI's classifications' distribution of the adopted group was 65.3% secure ($n = 32$), 22.7% dismissing ($n = 11$), 4.1% preoccupied ($n = 2$), and 8.2% disorganized ($n = 4$). The distribution of the control group was 67.3% secure ($n = 33$), 20.4% dismissing ($n = 10$), 12.2% preoccupied ($n = 6$), and none disorganized.

Three groups did not differ in their attachment classifications either in the three-way (secure, dismissing, and preoccupied) analysis ($\chi2(2) = 1.90$, $p = .387$) or in the secure–insecure (including dismissing, preoccupied, and disorganized combined for the insecure category) distribution ($\chi2 = .19$, $p = .667$). The presence of disorganized categories only in the adoption group (AG; 8%) suggested a difference on the four-way or organized–disorganized distribution in terms of more disorganization among adoptees. However, the statistical comparison cannot be performed due to the absence of teenagers classified as disorganized in the control group (CG) (Appendix 4).

Attachment Dimensions between the AG and CG: The FFI's Continuous Scales

Table 14.2 presents the comparison of the various FFI (*Friends and Family Interview*) scales. Through scores it was possible to compare AG and CG on levels of disorganization, and the adoptees received higher scores on the disorganized pattern (*t-test*, $p = .04$). The AG also showed less narrative coherence, obtaining lower scores on relation ($p = .02$) and manner ($p = .01$) than the CG. The AG showed less-reflective functioning than community control peers, receiving lower scores on developmental perspective ($p = .02$), theory of mind toward mother ($p = .04$) and teacher ($p < .01$), and diversity of feelings toward self ($p < .01$), mother ($p = .01$), father ($p = .02$), and friend ($p < .01$). Further, the AG showed lower differentiation in representations of parental figures ($p < .01$), together with lower (defensive) use of role reversal toward the mother ($p = .04$) as an affective regulation strategy compared to control peers.

A Focus on Adolescent Adoptees

To deepen the understanding of the AG, we checked whether the FFI classifications and scales were related to (1) age at placement, length of time in the adoptive home, and adoption type (domestic vs. intercountry adoption); (2) sociodemographic variables (gender, age at assessment, number of siblings); and (3) control variables in terms of verbal IQ.

Table 14.2 Mean and Standard Deviation in Attachment Dimension Scores at the Friends and Family Interview (FFI) in an Adoption Group (AG) and a Community Group (CG) of Adolescents (n = 98)

FFI Scales		AG (n = 49)		CG (n = 49)	
		M	(SD)	M	(SD)
Patterns	Secure-autonomous	2.68	(.78)	2.89	(.90)
	Insecure-dismissing	1.81	(.76)	1.70	(.79)
	Insecure-preoccupied	1.46	(.62)	1.50	(.64)
	Disorganized-disoriented★	1.35	(.68)	1.12	(.31)
Coherence	Truth	2.89	(.62)	3.03	(.73)
	Economy	2.62	(.77)	2.88	(.87)
	Relation	2.62	(.72)	2.95	(.67)
	Manner★	3.41	(.68)	3.71	(.48)
	Overall★	2.89	(.60)	3.67	(.61)
Reflective functioning					
Developmental perspective★		2.39	(.80)	2.74	(.65)
Theory of mind	Mother★	2.34	(.81)	2.68	(.84)
	Father	2.28	(.82)	2.43	(.91)
	Friend	2.16	(.79)	2.50	(.94)
	Sibling	2.11	(.89)	2.48	(1.1)
	Teacher★★	2.25	(.93)	2.99	(1.1)
Diversity of feelings	Self★★	2.77	(.74)	3.24	(.61)
	Mother★	2.60	(.73)	3.01	(.87)
	Father★	2.56	(.81)	2.95	(.76)
	Friend★★	2.32	(.82)	2.95	(.81)
	Sibling	2.51	(1)	2.81	(.82)
Secure base/mother		2.71	(.78)	2.50	(.99)
Safe haven/father		2.57	(.88)	2.40	(.88)
Self-esteem	Social competence	3.07	(.68)	3.18	(.68)
	School competence	3.11	(.62)	3.21	(.69)
	Self-regard	2.91	(.64)	2.73	(.54)
Best friendship	Frequency	3.21	(.92)	3.26	(1.1)
	Quality	2.78	(.57)	2.90	(.80)
Sibling relationships	Warmth	2.38	(1.1)	2.75	(.80)
	Hostility	1.86	(1.1)	1.50	(.65)
	Rivalry	1.45	(.88)	1.17	(.37)
Affect regulation strategies (anxieties and defenses)					
Idealization	Self	1.42	(.60)	1.40	(.65)
	Mother	1.69	(.82)	1.65	(.80)
	Father	1.70	(.83)	1.67	(.67)
Role reversal	Mother★	1.22	(.39)	1.45	(.70)
	Father	1.17	(.45)	1.34	(.78)

(Continued)

Table 14.2 (Continued)

FFI Scales		AG (n = 49)		CG (n = 49)	
		M	(SD)	M	(SD)
Anger	Mother	1.37	(.68)	1.38	(.78)
	Father	1.30	(.67)	1.26	(.63)
Derogation	Self	1.22	(.51)	1.32	(.64)
	Mother	1.24	(.57)	1.43	(.80)
	Father	1.26	(.61)	1.32	(.62)
Adaptive response		2.68	(.72)	2.79	(.92)
Differentiation of parental representations★★		2.80	(.88)	3.29	(.73)

Note:
★$p < .05$.
★★$p < .01$.

Both the child's age at adoptive placement and the length of time in the adoptive home did not show correlations with FFI classifications and scales. Domestically adopted adolescents obtained higher scores ($M = 2.17$, $SD = .98$) on the FFI disorganized pattern scale than did internationally adopted ones ($M = 1.24$, $SD = .55$; $t(47) = 3.48$, $p = .001$). None of the sociodemographic variables or the verbal IQ (VCI) were correlated with the FFI classifications and scales.

Discussion

The first question for this analysis was: What is the relationship between attachment representations of adolescent adoptees and those of non-adopted, low-risk peers in Italy? The results of this matched group study found no differences between late-placed adoptees and non-adopted Italian participants in attachment classifications, consistent with several other studies (Pace et al., 2018; Riva Crugnola et al., 2009; Vorria et al., 2015). This suggests that, despite adoptees' pre-adoptive experiences and any ruptures in early attachment relationships, most of them can demonstrate secure attachment representations during adolescence similar to non-adopted adolescents. Although it is not possible to know if attachment security of late-placed adoptees is due to the reparative role of adoptive families or for other reasons (such as late-placed adoptees were already secure when they were adopted), this datum suggests using a salutogenic approach when considering adoptive attachment relationships (Paniagua et al., 2019). A salutogenic approach focuses on factors that support human health and well-being rather than on factors that cause psychosocial problems or illnesses. It is a strength-based approach to development (Antonovsky, 1987, p. 128).

In particular, attachment security represents a strength that adoptees can draw upon when they face the tasks of normative adolescent/early adulthood development that can be more challenging for adopted people. Attachment security may help adopted adolescents in the process of integration between their past (biological and pre-adoptive experiences) and present, in which the family of origin remains a part of the unconscious of the adopted child even if adoptive parents and professionals ignore or minimize it (Kalus, 2016). The ability to integrate two images, the biological parent and adoptive parent, is important in shaping the identity of an adopted person (Kalus, 2016).

Although mainly secure attachment representations were found in late-placed adopted adolescents, a small portion of them showed disorganized attachment patterns; none of the subjects in the control group demonstrated disorganized attachment patterns. The rate of disorganized attachment in this study (8%) appears in line with findings of another late-placed adopted adolescents' study (6%; Vorria et al., 2015) but lower than the rate in another study (> 30%, van den Dries et al., 2009). Time in a stable and restorative adoptive environment may promote a partial recovery in attachment from the negative consequences of pre-adoption traumatic experiences (van den Dries et al., 2009), although the effects may not be uniform in all adopted adolescents.

The second question for this analysis was: In which attachment dimensions do adolescent adoptees seem aligned with their control peers, and in which ones are they vulnerable? Late-placed adopted adolescents had lower scores in different dimensions of coherence and reflective functioning than their matched peers. The lower coherence of late-placed adopted adolescents was expressed in their limited age-appropriate attention and politeness during the interview; they had less of an ability to describe and discuss personal attachment experiences by providing memories and specific events to exemplify the truthfulness of their statements (Steele & Steele, 2005). It is not clear what the reason or reasons are for lower coherence.

Compared to non-adopted peers, late-placed adopted adolescents demonstrated lower differentiation in representations of parental figures and lower use of role reversal toward the mother (which is positive). The struggle to differentiate between the mother and father as a different attachment figure indicates a limit to a nuanced, contextual, and diverse understanding of the complexity of others. Greater differentiation of parental representations allows the adolescent to flexibly rely on the individual parents in different ways, according to their personal needs of the moment. For instance, in case of conflict with one parent, the adolescent could seek comfort from the other parent. Also, adolescents could rely more on the mother for the safe-haven function and the father for the secure-base function (Pace et al., 2020). When there is less parental differentiation, adopted children may perceive lower possible sources of support from either parent.

The lower role reversal toward the mother is a positive indicator that means that late-placed adopted adolescents are less prone than non-adopted peers to show age-inappropriate excessive eagerness to please their mothers or to take on adult responsibilities. This finding suggests that these adoptive mothers were efficient in defining and respecting the parent and child's different roles. The adoptees felt unconditionally loved and accepted by their mothers; they do not feel the need to please them excessively to obtain closeness.

Limitations

This study had several limitations reducing the generalizability of results. They include (1) the heterogeneity of the adoptees regarding age at adoptive placement, length of time with adoptive parents, type of adoption (both international and domestic), and other countries of origin; (2) the absence of measures of adolescents' symptomatology (e.g., emotional and behavioral problems) or of other factors which could have been related to their attachment representations, like dimensions of parental functioning, such as attachment states of mind in terms of parental representations of their own attachment experiences with their attachment figures (Groza & Muntean, 2016); (3) the cross-sectional design that captures a picture of one moment without providing certainty that the results obtained remain valid over time; (4) the lack of any interview protocol inquiring into potential traumatic experiences or difficulties in the adoptive family; and (5) different measures with respective strengths and weaknesses. Indeed, studies on attachment in late-placed adopted children usually used completion tasks, which may be more sensitive in capturing subtle cues of disorganization than the FFI, which can be less efficient than other measures in detecting attachment disorganization (Pace, 2014; Pace et al., 2019, Pace et al., 2020).

Implications

This study has important implications for adoption professionals focusing on attachment as a key issue to better understand and intervene with late-placed adoptees' difficulties (Johnson & Fein, 1991; Raby & Dozier, 2019). Indeed, the focus on the dimension of attachment can help adoption professionals assess areas of possible recovery and vulnerability. The FFI represents a good tool for adoption professionals to use in assessment to collect clinically helpful information in a relatively short time while building a therapeutic relationship with the adopted adolescent (Pace et al., 2020). The assessment process should include determining risk factors (e.g., unresolved traumatic experiences, poor social competence and peer relationships, difficult relationships at school) in different domains of adolescent functioning as well as the presence of strengths to build upon in treatment (Pace et al., 2020). This kind of dimensional evaluation could also contribute to the design and the evaluation of an intervention, checking improvements in targeted dimensions, such as in the reflective functioning (Bastianoni et al., 2020).

The attachment findings of this study suggest a "de-stigmatization" of adoptees as an attachment-vulnerable group, as they were substantially similar to non-adopted peers during adolescence. Professionals and adoptive parents may want to focus on possible relational difficulties of adoptees as part of a typical need of autonomy in adolescence and not only because of past adverse relational experiences.

Furthermore, results of this study may suggest that it may be helpful to study other dimensions, such as coherence and reflective functioning (Borelli et al., 2019). The adoptive caregiver may be the first to provide attachment-related dimensions

(Bizzi et al., 2020), and in this sense, it may be useful to involve adoptive parents in attachment-based programs to improve adolescent–parent attachment by reinforcing parenting skills, by using, for example, the "Connect Parenting Program" (Moretti & Obsuth, 2009) or the "Secure Cycle" program (Kobak et al., 2015). The "Connect Parenting Program" is a manualized ten-week evidence-based program for parents or alternative caregivers of at-risk teens that focuses on the building blocks of secure attachment, including parental sensitivity, cooperation, reflective capacity, and dyadic affect regulation (Moretti & Obsuth, 2009). The "Secure Cycle" program targets both the increase of security in child and parental IWMs, as well as the improvement of parental emotional attunement (Appendix 5) and parent–child dyadic communication skills (Kobak et al., 2015). In the adoption field, clinicians could apply both interventions to identify and help repair attachment ruptures, empathic failures, or misattuned communication in the relationships between late-placed adopted adolescents and their parents.

Endnotes

Antonovsky, A. (1987). *Unraveling the Mystery of Health – How People Manage Stress and Stay Well*. California: Jossey-Bass Publishers.

American Psychological Association. (2007). *APA dictionary of psychology*. Washington, DC: American Psychological Association.

Bakermans-Kranenburg, M.J., & van IJzendoorn, M.H. (2009). The first 10,000 Adult Attachment Interviews: Distributions of adult attachment representations in clinical and non-clinical groups. *Attachment & Human Development, 11*(3), 223–263. https://doi.org/10.1080/14616730902814762

Bastianoni, C., Charpentier-Mora, S., De Gregorio, E., & Bizzi, F. (2020). Exploring adopted adolescents' inner world through the lens of qualitative methodology. *Children and Youth Services Review, 113*, 104973. https://doi.org/10.1016/j.childyouth.2020.104973

Beijersbergen, M.D., Juffer, F., Bakermans-Kranenburg, M.J., & van IJzendoorn, M.H. (2012). Remaining or becoming secure: Parental sensitive support predicts attachment continuity from infancy to adolescence in a longitudinal adoption study. *Developmental Psychology, 48*(5), 1277–1282. https://doi.org/10.1037/a0027442

Bizzi, F., Charpentier-Mora, S., Ensink, K., Cavanna, D., & Borelli, J. (2020). Does Children's Mentalizing Mediate the Role of Attachment and Psychological Maladjustment in Middle Childhood? *Journal of Child and Family Studies*, 1–11. https://doi.org/10.1007/s10826-020-01701-9

Borelli, J.L., Brugnera, A., Zarbo, C., Rabboni, M., Bondi, E., Tasca, G., & Compare, A. (2019). Attachment comes of age: Adolescents' narrative coherence and reflective functioning predict well-being in emerging adulthood. *Attachment & Human Development, 21*(4), 332–351. https://doi.org/10.1080/14616734.2018.1479870

Bowlby, J. (1982). *Attachment and Loss, Vol.1: Attachment* (2nd ed.). New York: Basic Books.

Dipartimento Giustizia minorile e di comunità, servizio statistica. (2019). *Dati statistici relativi all'adozione negli anni dal 2000 al 2018*. www.centrostudinisida.it/Statistica/Analisi/adozione_serie_storiche.pdf

Dozier, M., & Rutter, M. (2016). Challenges to the development of attachment relationships faced by young children in foster and adoptive care. In J. Cassidy, & P. R. Shaver (Eds.), *Handbook of Attachment: Theory, Research, and Clinical Applications* (3rd ed., pp. 667–696). New York: Guilford Press.

Escobar, M.J., & Santelices, M.P. (2013). Attachment in adopted adolescents. National adoption in Chile. *Children and Youth Services Review, 35*(3), 488–492. https://doi.org/10.1016/j.childyouth.2012.12.011

Fonagy, P., Steele, M., Moran, G., Steele, H., & Higgitt, A. (1991). The capacity for understanding mental states: The reflective self in parent and child and its significance for security of attachment. *Infant Mental Health Journal, 13*, 200–216. https://doi.org/10.1002/1097-0355(199123)12:3<201::AID-IMHJ2280120307>3.0.CO;2-7

Grice, H.P. (1975). Logic and conversation. In P. Cole, & J. L. Moran (Eds.), *Syntax and Semantics III: Speech Acts* (pp. 41–58). Cambridge: Academic Press.

Grossmann, K.E., Grossmann, K., & Waters, E. (2006). *Attachment from Infancy to Adulthood: The Major Longitudinal Studies.* New York: Guilford Press.

Groza, V., & Muntean, A. (2016). A description of attachment in adoptive parents and adoptees in Romania during early adolescence. *Child and Adolescent Social Work Journal, 33*(2), 163–174. https://doi.org/10.1007/s10560-015-0408-2

Groza, V., Muntean, A., & Ungureanu, R. (2012). The adoptive family within the Romanian cultural context: An exploratory study. *Adoption Quarterly, 15*(1), 1–17. https://doi.org/10.1080/10926755.2012.661327

Howe, D. (1998). Adoption outcome research and practical judgment. *Adoption & Fostering, 22*(2), 6–15. https://doi.org/10.1177/030857599802200203

International Adoption Commission [Commissione Adozioni Internazionali, CAI]. (2013). Dati e prospettive nelle Adozioni Internazionali. *Rapporto sui fascicoli dal 1° gennaio al 31 dicembre 2013.* www.sitiarcheologici.palazzochigi.it/www.commissioneadozioni.it/dicembre%202018/media/143019/report_statistico_2013.pdf

International Adoption Commission [Commissione Adozioni Internazionali, CAI]. (2018). Dati e prospettive nelle Adozioni Internazionali. *Rapporto sui fascicoli dal 1° gennaio al 31 dicembre 2018.* www.commissioneadozioni.it/media/1619/report-annuale-cai-2018.pdf

Irhammar, M., & Bengtsson, H. (2004). Attachment in a group of adult international adoptees. *Adoption Quarterly, 8*(2), 1–25. https://doi.org/10.1300/J145v08n02_01

Johnson, D., & Fein, E. (1991). The concept of attachment: Applications to adoption. *Children and Youth Services Review, 13*(5–6), 397–412. https://doi.org/10.1016/0190-7409(91)90028-G

Juffer, F., Palacios, J., Le Mare, L., Sonuga-Barke, E.J.S., Tieman, W., Bakermans-Kranenburg, M.J., Vorria, P., van IJzendoorn, M.H., & Verhulst, F.C. (2011). Development of adopted children with histories of early adversity. *Monographs of the Society for Research in Child Development, 76*(4), 31–61. https://doi.org/10.1111/j.1540-5834.2011.00627.x

Kalus, A. (2016). Narratives of identity in adopted adolescents: interview analysis. *Archives of Psychiatry and Psychotherapy, 4*, 35–42. https://doi.org/10.12740/APP/66306

Katznelson, H. (2014). Reflective functioning: A review. *Clinical Psychology Review, 34*(2), 107–117. https://doi.org/10.1016/j.cpr.2013.12.003

Kobak, R., Zajac, K., Herres, J., & Krauthamer Ewing, E.S. (2015). Attachment based treatments for adolescents: The secure cycle as a framework for assessment, treatment and evaluation. *Attachment & Human Development, 17*(2), 220–239. https://dx.doi.org/10.1080%2F14616734.2015.1006388

L. 184/1983 "Disciplina dell'adozione e dell'affidamento dei minori" (1983). https://www.gazzettaufficiale.it/eli/id/1983/05/17/083U0184/sg

L. 476/1998 "Ratifica ed esecuzione della Convenzione per la tutela dei minori e la cooperazione in materia di adozione internazionale, fatta a L'Aja il 29 maggio 1993. Modifiche alla legge 4 maggio 1983, n. 184, in tema di adozione di minori stranieri" (1998). https://www.parlamento.it/parlam/leggi/98476l.htm

L. 149/2001 "Modifiche alla legge 4 maggio 1983, n. 184, recante «Disciplina dell'adozione e dell'affidamento dei minori», nonché al titolo VIII del libro primo del Codice civile" (2001). https://www.parlamento.it/parlam/leggi/01149l.htm

Lyons-Ruth, K., & Jacobvitz, D. (2016). Attachment disorganization from infancy to adulthood: Neurobiological correlates, parenting contexts, and pathways to disorder. In J. Cassidy, & P.R. Shaver (Eds.), *Handbook of Attachment: Theory, Research, and Clinical Applications – Third Edition* (pp. 667–696). New York: Guilford Press.

Madigan, S., Brumariu, L.E., Villani, V., Atkinson, L., & Lyons-Ruth, K. (2016). Representational and questionnaire measures of attachment: A meta-analysis of relations to child internalizing and externalizing problems. *Psychological Bulletin, 142*(4), 367. https://doi.org/10.1037/bul0000029

Mikulincer, M., & Shaver, P.R. (2012). An attachment perspective on psychopathology. *World Psychiatry, 11*(1), 11–15. https://dx.doi.org/10.1016/j.wpsyc.2012.01.003

Molina, P., Casonato, M., Ongari, B., & Decarli, A. (2015). Les représentations d'attachement chez les adolescents adoptés et leurs parents. *Neuropsychiatrie de l'Enfance et de l'Adolescence, 63*(6), 376–384. https://doi.org/10.1016/j.neurenf.2015.04.004

Moretti, M.M., & Obsuth, I. (2009). Effectiveness of an attachment-focused manualized intervention for parents of teens at risk for aggressive behaviour: The connect program. *Journal of adolescence, 32*(6), 1347–1357. https://doi.org/10.1016/j.adolescence.2009.07.013

Mullin, E.S., & Johnson L. (1999). The role of birth/previously adopted children in families choosing to adopt children with special needs. *Child Welfare, 78*, 579–591.

Orsini, A., Pezzuti, L., & Picone, L. (2012). *WISC-IV Italian Edition*. Milano: Giunti OS.

Pace, C.S., Cavanna, D., Velotti P., & Zavattini G.C. (2014). Attachment representations of late-adopted children through attachment narratives: an assessment of disorganisation mentalising and coherence of mind for adoption practice. *Adoption & Fostering, 38*(3), 255–270. https://doi.org/10.1177/0308575914543235

Pace, C.S., Di Di Folco, S., & Guerriero, V. (2018). Late adoptions in adolescence: Can attachment and emotion regulation influence behaviour problems? A controlled study using a moderation approach. *Clinical Psychology & Psychotherapy, 25*(2), 250–262. https://doi.org/10.1002/cpp.2158.

Pace, C.S., Di Di Folco, S., Guerriero, V., & Muzi, S. (2019). Late-adopted children grown up: A long-term longitudinal study on attachment patterns of adolescent adoptees and their adoptive mothers. *Attachment & Human Development, 21*(4), 372–388. https://doi.org/10.1080/14616734.2019.1571519.

Pace, C.S., Di Di Folco, S., Guerriero, V., Santona, A., & Terrone, G. (2015). Adoptive parenting and attachment: Association of the internal working models between adoptive mothers and their late-adopted children during adolescence. *Frontiers in Psychology, 6*, 1433. https://doi.org/10.3389/fpsyg.2015.01433.

Pace, C.S., Muzi, S., & Steele, H. (2020). Adolescents' attachment: Content and discriminant validity of the friends and family interview. *Journal of Child and Family Studies, 29*, 1173–1186. https://doi.org/10.1007/s10826-019-01654-8

Pace, C.S., Santona, A., Zavattini, G.C., & Di Di Folco, S. (2015). Attachment states of mind and couple relationships in couples seeking to adopt. *Journal of Child and Family Studies, 24*(11), 3318–3330. https://doi.org/10.1007/s10826-015-0134-6

Pace, C.S., & Zavattini, G.C. (2011). 'Adoption and attachment theory' the attachment models of adoptive mothers and the revision of attachment patterns of their late-adopted children. *Child: Care, Health and Development, 37*(1), 82–88. https://doi.org/10.1111/j.1365-2214.2010.01135.x.

Pace, C.S., Zavattini G.C., & D'Alessio M. (2012). Continuity and discontinuity of attachment patterns: A short-term longitudinal pilot study using a sample of late-adopted children and their adoptive mothers. *Attachment and Human Development, 14*(1), 45–61. https://doi.org/10.1080/14616734.2012.636658

Pace, C.S., Zavattini G.C., & Tambelli, R. (2015). Does family drawing assess attachment representations of late-adopted children? A preliminary report. *Child and Adolescent Mental Health, 20*(1), 26–33. https://doi.org/10.1111/camh.12042

Paniagua, C., Palacios, J., & Jiménez-Morago, J.M. (2019). Adoption breakdown and adolescence. *Child & Family Social Work*, 24(4), 512–518. https://doi.org/10.1111/cfs.12631

Psouni, E., & Apetroaia, A. (2014). Measuring scripted attachment-related knowledge in middle childhood: The secure base script test. *Attachment & Human Development*, 16, 22–41. https://doi.org/10.1080/14616734.2013.804329

Psouni, E., Breinholst, S., Hoff Esbjørn, B., & Steele, H. (2019). Factor structure of the Friends and Family interview. *Scandinavian Journal of Psychology*, 61(3), 460–469. https://doi.org/10.1111/sjop.12604

Raby, K.L., & Dozier, M. (2019). Attachment across the lifespan: Insights from adoptive families. *Current Opinion in Psychology*, 25, 81–85. https://dx.doi.org/10.1016/j.copsyc.2018.03.011

Riva Crugnola, C., Sagliaschi, S., & Rancati, I. (2009). Qualità dell'attaccamento ed elaborazione delle esperienze infantili avverse in preadolescenti adottati. *Psicologia clinica dello sviluppo*, 13(3), 515–542. www.rivisteweb.it/doi/10.1449/30785

Rosnati, R., Montirosso, R., & Barni, D. (2008). Behavioral and emotional problems among Italian international adoptees and non-adopted children: Father's and mother's reports. *Journal of Family Psychology*, 22(4), 541. https://doi.org/10.1037/0893-3200.22.3.541

Rosnati, R., Ranieri, S., & Barni, D. (2013). Family and social relationships and psychosocial well-being in Italian families with internationally adopted and non-adopted children. *Adoption Quarterly*, 16(1), 1–16. https://doi.org/10.1080/10926755.2012.731030

Santona, A., & Zavattini, G.C. (2005). Partnering and parenting expectations in adoptive couples. *Sexual and Relationship Therapy*, 20(3), 309–322. https://doi.org/10.1080/14681990500142004

Simonelli, A., & Vizziello, G.M. (2009). Ri-costruire gli attaccamenti dopo l'adozione. La qualità delle rappresentazioni delle relazioni nelle famiglie adottive. *Psicologia clinica dello sviluppo*, 13(3), 543–562. www.rivisteweb.it/doi/10.1449/30786

Steele, H., & Steele, M. (2005). The construct of coherence as an indicator of attachment security in middle childhood: The Friends and Family Interview. In K.A. Kerns, & R.A. Richardson (Eds.), *Attachment in Middle Childhood* (pp. 137–160). New York: Guilford Press.

Steele, H., Steele, M., & Kriss, A. (2009). *FFI Scoring System*. New York: Center for Attachment Research at New School University (Unpublished document).

Steele, M., Hodges, J., Kaniuk, J., & Steele, H. (2010). Mental representation and change: Developing attachment relationships in an adoption context. *Psychoanalytic Inquiry*, 30(1), 25–40. https://doi.org/10.1080/07351690903200135

Steele, M., Hodges, J., Kaniuk, J., Steele, H., Hillman, S., & Asquith, K. (2008), Forecasting outcomes in previously maltreated children. The use of the AAI in a longitudinal adoption study. In H. Steele and M. Steele (Eds.), *Clinical Applications of the Adult Attachment Interview* (pp. 427–451). New York: Guilford Press.

Stievenart, M., Casonato, M., Muntean, A., & Van de Schoot, R. (2012). The friends and family interview: measurement invariance across Belgium and Romania. *European Journal of Developmental Psychology*, 9(6), 737–743. https://doi.org/10.1080/17405629.2012.689822

van den Dries, L., Juffer, F., van IJzendoorn, M.H., & Bakermans-Kranenburg, M.J. (2009). Fostering security? A meta-analysis of attachment in adopted children. *Children and Youth Services Review*, 31(3), 410–421. https://doi.org/10.1016/j.childyouth.2008.09.008

van IJzendoorn, M.H., & Juffer, F. (2006). The Emanuel Miller Memorial Lecture 2006: Adoption as intervention. Meta-analytic evidence for massive catch-up and plasticity in physical, socio-emotional, and cognitive development. *Journal of Child Psychology and Psychiatry*, 47(12), 1228–1245. https://doi.org/10.1111/j.1469-7610.2006.01675.x

Veríssimo, M., & Salvaterra, F. (2006). Maternal secure-base scripts and children's attachment security in an adopted sample. *Attachment & Human Development, 8*(3), 261–273. https://doi.org/10.1080/14616730600856149

Vorria, P., Ntouma, M., & Rutter, M. (2015). Vulnerability and resilience after early institutional care: The Greek Metera study. *Development and psychopathology, 27*(3), 859–866. https://doi.org/10.1017/S0954579415000243

Wechsler, D. (2003). *WIeSC-IV Technical and Interpretive Manual.* Washington, DC: The Psychological Association.

APPENDIX

1. IWMs are hypothetical entities that stand for perception, thought, memory, or cognitive operations (American Psychological Association [APA], 2007) derived from repeated interactions with the primary caregivers that become organized into mental schemes. Representations in IWMs concern the *self* as worthy/unworthy of love and caregiving, the *other* as available/unavailable to provide comfort when upset or help and encouragement, and the *significant relationship* as helpful/unhelpful (Bowlby, 1982).
2. Most international literature on adoption considers as late-adopted those children who were adopted after 4 or 5 years of age. Each country has different ages they consider as late-adopted, so there is no uniform definition. In Italy, there is not a specific age range for "late-placed," even if most children were adopted after 6 years of age (IAC, 2018).

   From the attachment perspective (Howe, 1998), all the children who are placed for adoption after the first year of life can be considered as late-adopted, as they have experienced a disruption in their primary attachment bonds to their first attachment figure (often the mother). This was the criterion we used.
3. In animals, imprinting is an instinctive process that occurs during a critical period shortly after birth, when an animal bonds with an "object" (another animal, person, or thing) in order to survive. In attachment theory, the child learns strategies to maintain the proximity to the attachment figure(s) and expectations about a caregiver's responses in the first 24 months of life (Bowlby, 1982). Attachment later becomes embedded in the IWM.
4. Chi-square test provides reliable results with frequency > 5.
5. *Parental attunement* is about empathic capacities that are not usually determined in agency interviews and home visits because this requires advanced clinical skills that most personnel handling adoptive placements do not have (editor's note).

15
COUNTERTRANSFERENCE CHALLENGES IN WORKING WITH ADOPTED ADOLESCENTS

Notes of a Psychoanalyst in Private Practice

Anna Balas, MD

Introduction

According to Paul Brinich, "there is no such thing as an adoptee" (2012). What he means is that being adopted is often compounded by a complex life trajectory of many traumatic events, such as orphanage stays and foster homes or, in other words, absent parents or parent figures, multiple losses of attachment figures, and often, only fragments of information and memory. Each story is different, often with unknown chapters. And the challenge for each individual is to integrate disparate elements of their history, known and guessed or imagined, to forge a solid sense of identity.

The therapist needs to acknowledge the magnitude of the trauma or traumas in the life of the adopted young person, beginning with the fact that the birth mother relinquished them. The therapist needs to contain his/her own feelings when attempting to empathize with the patient's earliest experience. Even though the birth mothers were often forced to relinquish their babies, adopted persons need to contend with the stark fact that their birth mothers did not keep them. The author refers to this as primal abandonment (as imagined by the adopted person). Whether or not the decision was based on actual abandonment, rejection, or incapacity emotionally or financially to raise the child is secondary, and birth mothers' circumstances vary greatly. What we have learned anecdotally is that adopted females are more likely to "understand" (have empathy for) the birth mother's conflict, while adopted males are more likely to assume the abandonment was real. This suggests that the therapist needs to be attuned to possible gender differences in the way being adopted is experienced.

Deeg's chapter in this volume (Chapter 6) emphasizes the implications in the life of adopted persons of feeling such an abandonment by the birth mother while continuing to struggle with the internal residue of the missing object. For most of us, our primal bond is with the mother to whom we are born. However potentially flawed that first maternal attachment may be, which could be only minutes, or hours, or weeks and months, it is the first foundation on which other relationships are built. Some therapists, who are adopted themselves, point out that the profound significance of the final, permanent separation from the birth mother likely constitutes a painful fantasy in the mind of the therapist, accounting for the mental health field's inclination to dismiss the importance of the child's earliest pre-placement experiences. This portends additional countertransference complications. Also, for similar reasons, the adoptive parents often need to downplay the importance of their child's earlier (pre-placement) experiences.

Given the adaptability of human nature, many adoptees are still able to build solid attachments in spite of drastic circumstances at the start of their lives (Pace et al., Chapter 14), although in the case of adopted individuals, there may be specific repercussions throughout life. As therapists, we should consider, and further explore, the dimensions of each adopted patient's resilience. This includes the degree of their flexibility in adapting to change (ego strengths), their capacity to compartmentalize inner turmoil so that intense emotions can be contained within the therapy, to empathize with others' needs and emotions, and to maintain adequate boundaries in their interpersonal relationships.

Treating an adopted adolescent, the therapist needs to be aware of specific added challenges pertaining to the patient's history of adoption. Initially, the therapist may or may not already know that the patient is adopted. Of course, at the outset, the appropriate approach is to listen to the concerns that bring them to consult a therapist and to be ready to meet the patient where they are (Nickman, Chapter 5). Once the therapist learns that the patient is adopted, they need to become especially aware that many adopted people may be reluctant to trust, to commit, and to form an alliance with the therapist. The patient may anticipate uncovering painful and perhaps frightening images or sensations from their early histories that lie in their fragmented memories. At the same time, the therapist also needs to be attuned to the "pull" within the transference of many adopted patients to "return" to the warmth and safety they may continue to crave because of their earliest experiences.

The following are common but challenging themes that the author has experienced in her practice with adopted adolescents and young adults.

Countertransference Themes and Challenges in Empathy

The British psychoanalyst Heinrich Racker (1968) has outlined two countertransference types: complementary and concordant countertransference. The first type is the same as role responsiveness on the part of the analyst – her/his response to the pull of the patient's emotional expressions of their needs. The second, concordant countertransference, is based on the analyst/therapist stepping into the patient's shoes and identifying with facets of their behavior or with personality traits of the patient, that is, transiently experiencing the patient's symptoms. Likewise, in their paper "The Analyst's Reactions to his Patients and Their Parents," Bernstein and Glenn (1988) delineated factors describing the intensity of personal involvement that occurs when working in-depth with children and adolescents. Perhaps this pull is even more intense when they are adopted.

I will begin with my own experience as an immigrant adolescent, starting off in the United States as an "outsider," as a way of connecting with the predicament of an adopted person's challenges during adolescence. However excited I felt about the opportunity to start a new life in the United States, our move included the requirements of adapting to a very different culture and language, while we had to leave behind our old home, friends, grandparents, all that was familiar and comfortable. All turned out well eventually, but one tends to self-protectively play down the magnitude of a challenge while mobilizing efforts to master it. This minimization becomes an important coping style that the clinician needs to recognize and understand in the psychology of the adopted patient – and within themselves. For example, it is not uncommon for adopted patients to be dismissive, perhaps even to show a little irritation, if the therapist "keeps asking about it." While this adaptive response may have great utility at some points in time, it can become an obstacle later on. Thus, the therapist needs to recognize this as a defense and to respect the patient's own pace. Unfortunately, in general practice, typically, therapists do not even think of asking about the patient's adoption history, their feelings about it, or how they believe their development has been affected by it.

If one has more than the usual need to be liked and accepted, an obliging adopted adolescent or young adult can develop a "false self" to please teachers, parents, and peers. Thus, an adolescent will put a lot of effort into seeming happy and cheerful, while to their therapist/analyst, they confess the depth of their despair and loneliness. Keeping between themselves the patient's depth of suffering creates a secret alliance that may contribute to the patient becoming overly dependent on the therapist. This seductive appeal – "You are the only one who gets me!" – needs to be watched so that the therapist does not collude with it out of their own narcissistic need. One approach to reducing the patient's need for a "false self" is to encourage the adolescent to share their genuine feelings with others as well: friends, family members, mentors, or teachers. Often, their terror of the consequences of disclosing personal feelings is much greater than the real consequences of sharing.

Considerations in the Countertransference

1. The therapeutic challenge of handling regression and anger.

While a vulnerable patient invariably requires a sensitive, supportive approach, a certain amount of confrontation is inevitable when a patient's coping style includes avoidant maneuvers. Many can go to great lengths to avoid expressing angry feelings, or even to become aware of anger within themselves: given at least some levels of abandonment anxiety, getting angry at significant people in one's life would seem extremely dangerous. As a consequence, while some adoptees may continually test the adoptive family with misbehavior and provocativeness, my experience is with adolescent adoptees who suppress their anger and get depressed and inhibited instead.

The therapist's task of attempting to repair past suffering and old losses is laborious. Unacceptable angry feelings emerge indirectly in passive-aggressive behavior. For such adolescents and young adults, the tasks of ordinary self-care seem heroic because it separates them from the role of a young child who still needs their parents' presence to protect, reassure, and take care of them. They have to confront the anticipated challenge of going at it alone in the world. If they get paralyzed by depression, then all bets are off and they are back in the infantile position vis-à-vis the parents (and the therapist). It requires consistent patience to nurse them out of such a place.

2. Countertransference with adopted adolescents and young adults, including search fantasies and activated search.

The therapist can facilitate the second individuation of adolescence (Blos, 1962) by using themselves as an alternate parental object and source of identification. While maintaining crucial boundaries, the therapist can guide the adolescent patient through the entanglements of recalled and unrecalled events and emotional reactions in their lives. However, if the therapist is overly invested in getting the young person to like them, or in presenting themselves as exceptionally sensitive, warm, and kind, it can stir loyalty conflicts and guilt in the patient.

Turning to the adolescent patient, he/she may feel guilty about idealizing the therapist and devaluing the parents. This becomes especially complicated when the adolescent is adopted and may harbor secret fantasies about idealized birth parents that then become personified by the therapist, a version of the family romance (Wieder, 1977). The therapist must be especially careful about how this fantasy may interfere with some aspects of the therapist's role. If the therapist is overly standoffish or "formal," it may stir feelings of personal rejection or detachment in the patient, as such tendencies are often already present. If the therapist is too friendly and conceptualizes her/his primary role as "providing support" and warmth, a different kind of threat can emerge within the patient: they may begin to see themselves as weak, vulnerable, and dependent. In each of these scenarios, the patient's engagement in treatment can potentially be compromised, so there needs to be careful exploration and interpretation of their misplaced expectations.

A way of dealing with excessive idealization of the therapist is by disclosing some of her own vulnerabilities. For instance, with a particular patient, the author talked about the challenge and loneliness of finding herself in an English-speaking high school looking to manage with limited language skills. This strategy of limited self-disclosure served to de-idealize the patient's image of the therapist and close the gap between the "successful," non-adopted person and the "flawed" adoptee.

Somewhere in the background float the ghosts of the birth family in the minds of patient, therapist, and adoptive parents. For the patient, the image of the fantasied birth parents is often split into extremes: sometimes it is an idealized pair (as in family romance fantasies of non-adopted children and young people), and at other times demonized, such as images of down-and-out individuals, outcasts with malicious or predatory intent. Therefore, it is frightening to contemplate searching for those unknown figures. And yet they remain the object of longing and understandable musings. What are the ghosts in the mind of the therapist? The therapist might allow their own reverie about missing relatives they were never able to meet. The sadness and longing of such reveries (Ehrensaft, 2005) tap into the sadness and longing of the adopted person for their absent blood kin whom they may have never met, or about whom they have only vague memories. If the therapist can acknowledge and mourn their own missing kin, it enables them to help the patient with their own process of mourning their missing connections.

In the case that follows, the adoptive family was particularly rejecting of the adopted patient. The adoptive mother's own inability to mourn her infertility may have rendered her cruel and vindictive. A young adult patient was adopted through the help of an obstetrician looking for a home for her, as a child born out of wedlock to one of the workers at the clinic. Therefore, the adoptive mother knew something about the child's birth mother. Presumably, the adoptive mother may have felt rivalrous with her from the start, judging from tensions transmitted to her adopted daughter. At the age of 5, this girl asked her adoptive mother whether she would help her search for her birth parents when she got older. This was an unusually precocious age to raise such a concern. The adoptive mother took the request as a rejection, and she became even colder and more distant than before, by way of retaliation. A frequently repeated phrase was, "If I only had my own!" referring to biological children. When the little girl threatened to run away from home, her mother volunteered spitefully to help her pack her little rucksack. Of course, the plan to flee ended in humiliation.

This girl's adoptive parents divorced during her latency, which led to her getting depressed, overweight, and ostracized in school by her peers – with the parents' divorce signifying yet another painful abandonment. Later, as a young woman, she searched for her birth parents as soon as she was of age, further eroding her relationship with her adoptive mother. Through assiduous searching, she was able to find her birth mother. When she was planning to get married, she invited her adoptive mother, her adoptive father, and her birth mother. As a result, the adoptive mother refused to talk to her for many years and, further, vindictively insisted on having the whole of her family cut the daughter off. In reviewing this case, I was reminded that therapists should consider the sources of the adoptive placement, which, in this case, was a private legal arrangement without consideration of the suitability of the placement.

3. Tact and timing.

As analysts and therapists, we always need to be attentive to the need for tact and timing of our interventions. The adopted adolescent or young adult is taking on the challenges and transitions of everyday life, side by side with adoption themes buried within. Usually, no one would know that they were adopted – they don't stand out as "different" in any way. The therapist needs to respect the patient's acknowledged concerns and preoccupations and not intrude with other material, implicitly diminishing the significance of what the patient is trying to convey. And yet the sensitive therapist will also inevitably need to "listen for" adoption-related issues when they arise indirectly. Given that many families may be emotionally invested in avoiding the subject, the young person has trained themselves to keep their adoption thoughts private and often secret. Thus, the therapist needs to communicate their receptiveness to exploring adoption themes as they occur, without being overbearing. This tact allows the young person to develop more flexibility in their associations as they move back and forth between their overriding daily concerns and hints of earlier confusing or painful themes in their lives.

4. The therapist's competitiveness with the parents.

Another issue that arises more prominently during work with adopted adolescents is the therapist's competitive feelings with the parents and the fantasy that they, the therapist, should have been the one to adopt the needy adolescent and would have done a better job than the parents. It is of paramount importance to understand the danger of such situations, given that the patient already has a split loyalty between the adoptive and birth parent, even if it is repressed. Therefore, an overly sympathetic therapist might create difficulties for the patient's relationship with their adoptive parent, a complicated bond to begin with. Sometimes, such situations lead to insoluble impasses in the treatment. But keeping alert to the possibility of an impasse is the best protection. As suggested by Bertocci (Chapters 4 and 11), such themes of competition can be avoided by the parents being seen by another, collaborating therapist.

In another type of challenging situation, a patient resembled her therapist physically much more than she resembled her adoptive parents (Wright, 2009). This became a challenge for both of them, as the fantasy of the analyst being the actual birth mother was stirred up and needed to be interpreted.

5. Trauma's indicators and lasting effects.

Although each adoption story is different, the therapist needs to have some familiarity with understanding trauma and its consequences. In particular, because of the neurobiological complexities, it is essential to distinguish early developmental trauma from the more general developmental trauma developed by Bessel van der Kolk (2005) and for the reasons discussed in Chapter 4. Trauma that occurs pre-language, pre-memory, and pre-consolidation of attachment, or approximately before age 3, is entirely different in its implications for development – and for treatment. The early trauma is more difficult to discern because it has pervasive effects that are embedded in procedural memory, not usually accessible in words, but rather in behavior patterns.

Trauma is defined by object relation theorists as a rupture of attachment bonds to significant figures (Balas, 2019). This definition underlines the profound importance of attachment bonds for a person's well-being and for her/his sense of continuity and belonging in the world. Such disruptions occur in the life of adoptees at least once, when they lose the bond with their birth mother, and perhaps other times throughout their development. Therefore, they have developed coping mechanisms to protect themselves and to ward off further losses, disappointments, and rejections. Specifically with such patients, paying attention to interruptions or other disruptions of the treatment needs to be tracked.

Responding to trauma is complex. In my paper "Challenges to Treatment of Traumatized Individuals" (Balas, 2019) I provide guidelines to such work. In recent times, much is written about the impingement of unfavorable or troubling external events on the lives of patients, whether it is COVID-19, Me Too, Black Lives Matter, the plight of refugees, and yes, even the complexities of being adopted. A good parent looks to strike a balance between shielding a child from bad things and also introducing to the child knowledge about the cruel realities of the external world in piecemeal, manageable bits, according to what is developmentally appropriate and what the child can tolerate based on her/his temperament. Analogously, the good therapist strikes a balance between a supportive, shielding approach on the one hand and exploring painful and unfavorable realities in the life of their patients on the other. The therapist needs to develop empathy with the depth of the patient's pain, which can happen only if the therapist is prepared to tolerate pain within her/himself. Patients use many different means for managing emotional pain: two commonly referred to in the literature are dissociation and withdrawal (Courtois & Ford, 2013).

In general, dissociative states arising from trauma need to be distinguished from states of withdrawal and gazes without smiles. A dissociated person is detached and in an "altered state." They may maintain verbal and visual contact but are cut off from their emotions. They do not understand the therapist's questions about their feelings, may seem threatened, or respond in an "as if" way, but without any internal (affective) engagement. They may state that they feel "empty" or "numb." Courtois and Ford (2013) refer to "a painful sense of not being able to find within themselves any emotions, thoughts, or sense of personal identity and of not feeling 'real' in the world." If they are silent, "it may also be the way a client communicates what it was like during childhood" (ibid., p. 235), such as a "baby home" or orphanage where there was only perfunctory care and little interpersonal contact. The question, however, is how the adopted person can "retrieve or restore their missing sense of self" (ibid., p. 235) if a well-grounded, integrated sense of self was never there in the first place.

In contrast, a withdrawn individual pulls back, appears sullen or depressed, tries to describe a painful "sadness," and is hard to engage altogether. Withdrawal is a sign of depression. It is often accompanied by a sullen demeanor and self-deprecation and self-recrimination. The teenager may sleep all day and refuse to attend school for days or weeks on end. The therapist must be alert to signs of self-injurious behavior, such as cutting, or ingesting pills. With such patients, it is essential to inquire about suicidal thoughts and suicidal impulses.

Dissociation and withdrawal present a challenge to the therapist of an adopted patient, both in recognizing the difference between them and in the therapist's reactions to each. *The clue is often found in the countertransference*: In the case of dissociation, the therapist is perplexed by the affective vacancy, the "flatness," and may become aware of feeling impatient or bored. They may find themselves questioning whether their approach is really effective at all. This can be seen as an example of concordant countertransference, that is, identifying with the patient's affective state. In case of the patient's withdrawal, the therapist is more likely to pick up the hopelessness of their depression.

6. The therapist's inclination to make unwarranted assumptions.

An experienced psychotherapist once commented that she had always assumed that once prospective adoptive parents are screened through the pre-adoption procedures, they must be fundamentally competent to raise a child. A number of psychotherapists, upon learning of the many complexities in being adopted, have stated that they wished they had known about this earlier, because they had always treated adopted patients "the same as anyone else." A director of a trauma program stated that "trauma is basically trauma" so that his program did not see the need to distinguish one kind from another: "the treatment is pretty much the same." Such assumptions prevent the therapist from understanding the reality of the adopted patient's experience, both internally and externally. There are, in fact, many forms, variations, and derivatives of trauma, as there are in the case of struggles with attachment and identity; therefore, there are different approaches for treating whatever applies in each case. Particularly at the outset, the therapist needs to be aware of the assumptions they may be automatically inclined to make. They need to clarify the actual experiences of the patient and, in turn, allow them to guide the course of treatment.

7. Traditional evaluations and diagnoses are not especially useful.

One of the tricky issues in the evaluation and diagnosis, in trying to understand adopted individuals, is the paucity of biological family information. In fact, for many adopted adolescents and young adults, classic diagnostic categories do not seem to apply. It is often challenging, if not sometimes impossible, to determine the origins of their emotional difficulties. Often, there is no family history, no genetic information, no information on the birth mother's pregnancy and delivery or other medical information, little or no information about the birth father, or knowledge about the pre-adoption experiences of their youngest days. Thus, often, much information is missing or deliberately covered up to embellish the pre-adoption record. This problem comes to us in an age (twenty-first century) when neurobiology and epigenetic studies are proliferating in medical science and providing evidence of the significance of all that we are born with – but also of what can or cannot change in the interplay of trauma and resilience.

We find that adopted adolescents typically take longer to separate and develop a firm and cohesive sense of their identity. It is helpful, therefore, to modulate family and personal expectations and to plan accordingly when the adolescents are emotionally younger than their chronological age. For instance, a college experience closer to home may be a wiser choice. On the other hand, there may be situations where the adopted youth has a strong urge to attend school at some distance from home, either to get away from a bad situation and/or to experience "freedom in the larger world." As pointed out by Bertocci (Chapter 11), it has been observed that adopted young adults, often through their 20s, continue to live at home while "saving money," taking college courses, and contemplating their next steps. The therapist should not make the assumption (see no. 6 earlier) that this is "failure to launch," but rather, it may be a necessary stage requiring more time than for a non-adopted peer. But it also suggests the need for professional assistance during this period. The adoptive parents may need some reassurance, but also their own professional consultation, about this reluctance to leave.

Body Image Issues

1. The shock of puberty.

Adolescents and young adults are at the stage of their identity consolidation as they traverse their second separation-individuation vis-à-vis their family. For an adopted adolescent, many dangers lurk at these stages. First of all, any adolescent has to give up much of the comfortable intimacy of childhood and feelings of being protected by parents. The novel entitled *The Member of the Wedding* by Carson McCullers (1946) poignantly illustrates this in-between state of no longer being a child and, at the same time, having not yet found one's identity as an adolescent with a developing body starting to resemble that of an adult while not yet feeling like one.

But for an adopted youngster, there is the added dimension of turning physically into a body that is very unfamiliar, typically not resembling their parents' bodies or that of other family members. The new body and new bodily sensations of more intense sexuality and aggression are likely to stir questions and thoughts about one's biological parents and family: "How did they look as young adults? Does anybody have a nose like mine?" The adolescent's newly discovered fertility, with its palpable potential to reproduce, would also likely raise questions about one's own conception: "How did that unwanted pregnancy get started? What led to relinquishment by the birth mother?" These questions may be like opening a Pandora's box of potential dangers and threats. If the youngster was told that the reason for adopting was parental infertility, the adopted adolescent must also often contend with their identification with the infertile parent, that is, anxiety about the integrity of their own body (Chapter 11).

Another facet of this dilemma is anxiety about the envy within the parents. Envy of the young is already a common parental challenge as adolescents blossom into puberty. However, the added dimension of fertility intensifies the conflict for both the parents and the adolescent, particularly if infertility was their reason for adopting in the first place. These conflicts are likely to affect everyone in the family. Those youngsters who come from a loving family often feel that even letting themselves think about these issues, let alone bring them into the open, is dangerous, potentially hurting their parents. Therefore, they hesitate to disrupt the close bonds with the family, especially at a time when they are expected soon to go into the world by themselves. Leaving home is already a lonely experience for most teens and young adults. Thus, side by side with the spirit of exploration and adventure, anxieties relating to loss and loyalty conflicts raise their ugly heads.

2. Blurred self-concept.

As therapists working with adopted patients, it is important to acknowledge how much our own physical attributes serve as building blocks for developing a solid sense of belonging. This awareness unveils the burden adopted adolescents experience in having no frame of reference within their family for making physical comparisons. This blankness makes it harder for adopted adolescents to integrate their body image.

Here is an example of a creative expression of perplexity about body image. An adopted adolescent, a talented artist, did a series of self-portraits in her favorite medium, oils, for school. These elegant paintings obscured her face, blurring the features. This blurring corresponded to her self-described inability to see herself in the mirror. She said that she knew that she is objectively an attractive, "normal" person, but looking in the mirror, she literally could not see herself (Dalley & Kohon, 2008). She had the same experience of derealization when looking at her hands. It was as if they did not belong to her. As her therapist, I took these symptoms as disguised expressions of her sad and lonely feelings that she did not know anyone who had any of her specific features, in other words, a mother, father, sibling, cousin, grandparent, etc. who, in any way, resembled her. On another occasion, she told me how happy it makes her feel that she has her adoptive father's coloring and that it adds to her feeling close to him. This similarity was an important source of comfort for her.

The foregoing accounts bring home the intensity and poignancy of longings for a blood bond for an adopted youngster, even in the most loving families.

3. The power of blood (biological) ties.

We also see the intensity of this reaction when an adopted individual who has never met a biological relative has a child and, for the first time, encounters a blood relation. This bond is something that they longed for by nature and had usually seen in others all around them but could never obtain for themselves. The therapist needs to acknowledge the depth of such longing in order to appreciate this aspect of the adopted person's sense of disconnection and loneliness – of "always feeling different" over the years. In addition, the absence of their biological family's medical and psychiatric history means the lack of a larger context for knowing their own health risks. This gap, in turn, means that any disease potentially lurks in their bloodstream and genetic makeup. They must live with this underlying anxiety, which, in fact, typically increases with age.

4. Eating disorders and adoption.

As we know from elsewhere, eating disorders are often somatic manifestations of unbearable and unexpressed emotions. With adopted patients who have suffered disruptions of their attachment bonds, one would expect intense undigested emotional states. As a subcategory of eating issues in adopted individuals, I was doing some research on how Eastern European orphanages were run. These "children's homes" were clean and efficiently run. The infants were regularly bathed, fed, and given proper medical care, including vaccinations. They were bathed communally and handled matter-of-factly. The infants were fed methodically and efficiently with a premium on saving time – on average under 12 minutes per infant – so there was no opportunity for dawdling, cuddling, or playfulness. I assumed, therefore, that compliance and passivity were emphasized. An adaptable young baby likely would learn quickly that they should be cooperative about eating and make no fuss. Whatever negative emotions they experienced, it made sense to suppress them promptly and effectively.

Such a model baby would be one to be selected by the director for adoption, one would expect. Picture this type of adaptation of an infant, and later a child, as this young person enters adolescence in a society that prizes initiative and creativity: this adolescent may feel overwhelmed by unstructured expectations, given the way early patterns were laid out in their infancy. So predating the adoption, in the prehistoric era that remains obscure due to the lack of language and verbal memory to communicate these patterns, we see the fallout from early behaviors, lacking conscious awareness of their origins. This fallout may take the form of dissociative states, passivity, lack of initiative, self-isolation, or binge-eating to relieve nonspecific stress, loneliness, and states of emptiness.

5. Conflicts about sexuality.

In the literature about search (attempting to find information and contact with the birth family) and in fiction, there are instances when a young person discovering a blood relation, such as a birth parent or, more likely, a sibling, experiences an irresistible urge to have a sexual encounter. This urge is not really about sex, but it is also not "genetic sexual attraction" (Chapter 11). Rather, it is about the profound longing for intimate ties with a primal relative, a need long suppressed due to the lack of hope that it could ever be fulfilled.

In sorting out one's physical and sexual features, some adopted adolescents lack any firm sense of sexual identity, as in the case of those who announce that they are bisexual. The developing secondary sexual characteristics can be experienced as an alien intrusion, disrupting a safer place of childhood dependency and of softer, more ill-defined features. The new grown-up body may at times be seen as a threat – creating distance from the familiar, adoptive parents and other relatives. Who is this new stranger in the mirror? I suspect that these feelings are also related to early attachment difficulties and the lack of adequate healthy, playful stimulation in infancy. As with other issues, sorting out the etiology of these difficulties of adopted young people, we must contend with many unknowns.

Resurgence of Unresolved Issues from Early Childhood

1. Episodes of regression.

In my experience, adolescence is also a time of resurgence of unresolved challenges from earlier stages of life. Specifically, adopted individuals have suffered losses in infancy and early childhood, in many cases before a time they can consciously remember. How do these early losses impact the young person's later development?

For instance, when in distress, a young woman who spent her first year in an orphanage, or "home for infants" in another country, still lay in bed, facing the wall huddled up. Not surprisingly, this young woman became severely depressed in adolescence. For a while, she stopped going to school, stayed in bed, and turned away from the world. She also gained weight by turning to food as a source of comfort and as a way to avoid dangerous negative emotions. Sometimes the work with the patient was to discuss details of self-care. That kind of concrete interest in the patient's body reflected a reparation of the early absence of a mothering figure, an absence from preverbal days in the orphanage. The same young woman stayed in her comfort zone of passivity, avoiding direct conflict, and generally not taking any initiative. She preferred to spend time soothing herself with warm baths, overeating, and caressing her cat.

After extensive treatment, paradoxically, if given structure, she excelled in school and in visual tasks of significant complexity. She liked to sketch fanciful houses she would like to live in. She continued to do badly with criticism but blossomed when praised, much like a very young child. She had learned long ago that extending herself through physical activity or expressing independent feelings could be dangerous if it drew attention from grown-ups in any way. And so she had made an art of being unobtrusive and of fitting into the family, that is, until her older sibling, who had been very hostile to her over the years, was out of the house.

2. Guilt and shame about one's origins versus pride in one's background.

Therapists need to think about and acknowledge their own narcissistic investment in their own background: family, clan, ethnic, religious, national and racial, and political. But in treating the adopted patient, the therapist must understand how the patient's lack of information about themselves can add up to threats, however subtle, to self-esteem. Only then can both grasp the magnitude of the struggle for an adopted individual, namely, that the theme of pride vs. shame is inevitably prominent. Especially in adolescence and young adulthood, as one is consolidating one's sense of identity and belonging, it is a challenge for the adopted person to feel proud of themselves while feeling tainted by their knowledge that their own birth mother gave them up or was considered unfit to be their parent. At the same time, the birth father and the rest of the biological family all disappeared or were unaware of the patient's existence. The therapist needs to strike a balance between allowing a transient identification with the plight of their patient and, at the same time, not succumb to pity. Pity is a distancing mechanism that places the pitied person in a one-down or inferior position. It may also become an excuse for unfairly reduced expectations of the patient.

Adopted young persons know that their adoptive status is considered a liability by many (Baden, 2016). On the other hand, I have heard expressions of guilt for being the lucky one who was picked from all the needy orphans surrounding them. One of my patients once expressed guilt and gratitude for having a loving home with all her needs met. By contrast, most non-adopted people take their advantages for granted and would not even remark on this distinction.

3. Suicidal impulses and questions about being wanted.

Adolescents and young adults can become suicidal at times. Whether or not this happens due to a biological vulnerability to depression, for the adopted person, there is likely to be a doubt about one's being lovable or wanted. This is profoundly tied to low self-esteem.

Sometimes adopted individuals have difficulty with their birthdays and see no reason to "celebrate" them. It can be a loaded topic that they keep to themselves. They get depressed on the anniversary of the day they were born because it is a reminder that their birth mother was separated from them and may not even have wanted them to be born. To increase adoptees' protective strategies, the therapist needs to dilute the intensity of the patient's attachment to their therapist and extend it into the wider world. This widening of attachments takes place while the adolescent simultaneously struggles with anxiety about the appropriate loosening of the bonds with their parents, the second separation-individuation of adolescence (Blos, 1962). This expansion of close relationships is reminiscent of the normal development of an infant whose world expands with time.

4. Sibling relationships: discrepancies in endowment and envious resentment.

For adopted youth, the issue of siblings looms large. An only child longs for company and wishes that he/she had siblings to share playtime and to help dilute the intensity of the relationship with his parents. If children have siblings, the siblings become their first community. Here they negotiate sharing the love of their parents, sharing possessions and often their living space. Relationships with siblings act also as a vehicle of displacement for conflicts with parents. Therefore, a good parenting situation facilitates good sibling relationships, whereas parental neglect or maltreatment reverberates with the children and how they relate to each other. Siblings occasionally huddle together in distress, but they also may enact resentments against their parents by turning against each other.

Each story of adoption compounds ordinary sibling issues. Unlike children born into a family, when there are several available months for the parents to prepare for a new baby, adopted children can seem to appear suddenly when they "get the call" out of the blue, with everyone expected to adjust as soon as possible. Furthermore, there may be little resemblance in physical features, temperament, or endowment among the new siblings. If some are biologically related to the parents and others are not, there is a differential that needs to be acknowledged and addressed. These are all challenging tasks. Even the best parents are sometimes at a loss adjudicating between their children and addressing their divergent needs.

In my experience of working with several adopted young adults who were exceptionally gifted, their siblings were envious and became physically abusive. One girl's younger adopted, hyperactive, and impulsive brother regularly bashed her head against the wall or the doorframe throughout her childhood. Her parents had been divorced earlier, when she was 6 years old, which she experienced as another abandonment, and her mother favored the otherwise-charming and extraverted brother. My patient felt that there was no recourse but to wait for years, until she could leave her home for good. The brother's ongoing abuse over the years had dire emotional consequences for this young woman: she could not trust men, and she had low expectations from intimate relationships altogether, always hoping for more, always getting disappointed. She unconsciously re-enacted the scenario with her brother symbolically by letting herself be mistreated by men. Only extensive psychotherapy could mitigate those difficulties.

Similarly, a young man adopted internationally had an abusive older sister who beat him when he was little. Later, when they were older, she manipulated their mother into taking sides against him by using emotional blackmail. This young man was much more intelligent and talented than his sister: he also received no protection from his parents. His answer was also to bide his time until he could escape from home by moving away to other families as soon as he could, using any excuse, such as his statement that "he needed to be closer to his athletics practice," and he eventually arranged to live at the home of the coach. Later, in graduate school, he needed intensive treatment to free himself emotionally from his abusive and unnurturing family.

Still on the subject of siblings, the mutual identification typical of siblings who are biologically related to each other is often facilitated by some physical resemblance and shared interests or affinities. Although many of these interests are developed as part of the family culture, there is also a strong innate component, as we know, that is, the "pull" to feel "connected." Thus, children with vastly different backgrounds are less likely to share traits. Another factor at play may be the early experiences of multiple separations and sometimes of early abuse that may likely have led to attachment difficulties in some adopted individuals. Therefore, they may lack the capacity to form close ties with their family members, and it may affect other relationships in their life.

5. Pets: subjects of identification and vehicles for self-soothing.

When an adopted child has no siblings, the wish for a pet is a powerful recurring theme in treatment. I was working with an adopted adolescent of a different race from her parents whose family already owned a little dog. But when the novelty wore off, she insisted on getting one of her own, having seen a stray in the neighborhood. Unexpectedly, during one of my vacations, I received a call that the girl, then almost 14 years old, had suddenly become suicidal. The precipitating event was that her parents had refused to adopt a second animal into the household. As we explored the trigger for this acute crisis, I intuitively guessed that she was identified with the stray dog. Her thoughts went somewhat like this: if nobody had wanted to adopt her as a little toddler, she would have also been homeless, like the poor animal. While in the throes of this fantasy, she experienced her parents as heartless in their decision. This drove her to suicidal despair. As the patient accepted my interpretation and understood her connection with the puppy as representing her infant self, her acute suicidal urge subsided. Yet ancient fault lines existed in the attachment picture, dating back to her infancy.

An adopted college student who lived at home, allegedly for financial reasons, was alone while her divorced mother was tied up with a long business meeting. Taking advantage of the time, the daughter acquired a ferret with a cage and all. Her intensified loneliness, derived from her early trauma, compelled her to "adopt" the ferret on impulse. She would keep its company, letting it run around the room, hoping it would come back to sit in her lap, and would stroke it as much as the pet would tolerate. Even this tactile contact became an indispensable soothing mechanism.

Anna Balas, MD

Parallel Challenges for the Adoptive Parents and Extended Adoptive Family

The mythology of love as the answer for many difficulties is widespread in the parenting communities and even more so among adoptive parents. I call the "love potion" a myth because parents are often unprepared for the complex challenges of raising adopted children. In his paper *Psychoanalytic Perspectives on Adoption and Ambivalence* (1995), Paul Brinich highlights the universal ambivalence of parents toward their children. This ambivalence, and the need to hide it from oneself, is even stronger in adoptive parents. While there is little opportunity in this paper to explore the range of motivations and fantasies of parents who adopt children, it is productive to explore those hopes and compare them with the actual realities that adoptive parents confront as they raise their children. Adolescence and young adulthood are particularly challenging because it is the stage of normal separation and growing away from the family. Leaving home is a physical separation that stirs up anxieties about old attachment wounds and losses. Likewise, for parents, it also stirs up echoes of their pre-adoption loneliness, when they desperately longed for a full family.

It is important to keep in mind that allowing an adolescent to have a therapist is already a big step for many parents. It is easy to feel scrutinized in one's parenting and to worry that the adolescent will attach to another adult or parent figure. If there is not enough trust in the strength of the parent–child bond, then that bond is especially precarious. In an adoptive family, the origin of a physical feature is an authentic mystery, particularly since in the background float the unknown, fantasied birth parents. Consequently, sometimes adoptive families are more inhibited in indulging in "reverie" (Ehrensaft, de Peyer, 2013), fantasizing that usually takes place in families about their children's origins, and therefore also connecting with their future. Consider that much anxiety about the imagined "bad seed" can linger in the air about the unknown birth parents.

Attitudes of the Adoptee's Extended Adoptive Family

Concern about fully belonging to one's adoptive family can lead to anxiety about one's extended adoptive family. In families where the adopted child is welcomed by the extended family, much is positive. The young person feels a solid sense of belonging, being loved and wanted, as do his or her parents by their families.

Just as parents need to work through their disappointment about not having a blood connection with their adopted child, so do the other relatives. One of my patients wanted her grandmother to give her an embroidery of the family tree, only to be told that it was going to be left to "a real grandchild." This was especially hurtful because she was, in fact, her grandmother's favorite. However, her old-fashioned grandmother could not fully accept her as part of her clan. In another family, the grandmother whispered to the new parents that they should be sure to leave the family silverware to a niece or nephew in the biological family.

There are examples of an adolescent searching to strengthen roots and connections but running into different forms of painful rejection from the extended family, whether overt or subtle. An interracially adopted adolescent was painstakingly studying her adoptive family tree. Many members of that extended family were from the Deep South and held strong racial prejudices. Thus, they did not really consider this youngster as belonging to the family clan. Deep within, she was aware of their prejudice, but she needed to deny the painful reality.

Conclusion: The Role of the Therapist

One of the roles of the therapist is to follow the adopted patient's lead as they become involved in ordinary concerns of their age, including loneliness and alienation, while being attuned to adoption-related threads that can be pulled for further inquiry.

The therapist can empathize with the adopted patient's dilemmas and painful feelings while appreciating the parents' own struggles to understand and protect them. Also, the therapist needs to be able to tolerate painful affects, including the patient's need to mourn the losses of what might have been. This allows the young person to function with a wider palette of emotions and freer, healthier options to guide them into their future. Adolescence and early adulthood are excellent times to intervene, before the young people have made irreversible life choices.

Endnotes

Baden, A.L. (2016). "Do you know your real parents?" and other adoption microaggressions. *Adoption Quarterly*, 19 (1), 1–25.

Balas, A. (2019). Challenges of treatment with traumatized individuals from a modern Freudian perspective. In B. Huppertz (Ed.), *Approaches to Psychic Trauma*. New York: Rowman and Littlefield, pp. 253–263.

Bernstein, I., & Glenn, J. (1988). The child and adolescent analyst's emotional reactions to his patients and their parents. *International Review of Psychoanalysis*, 15, 225–241

Blos, P.M. (1962). *On Adolescence: A Psychoanalytic Interpretation*. New York: Simon & Schuster.

Brinich, P.M. (1995) Psychoanalytic perspectives on adoption and ambivalence. *Psychoanalytic Psychology*, 12, 181–199.

Brinich, P.M. (2012). Varieties of adoptive experience. *APS Adoption Conference 2012 LDCEC*.

Courtois, C.A., & Ford, J.D. (2013). *Treatment of Complex Trauma: A Sequenced, Relationship-Based Approach*. New York & London: The Guilford Press.

Dalley, T., & Kohon, V. (2008) Deprivation and development: The predicament of an adopted adolescent in the search for identity. In D. Hindle, & G. Shulman (Eds.), *The Emotional Experience of Adoption: A Psychoanalytic Perspective*. London & New York: Routledge, pp. 225–236.

Ehrensaft, D. (2005). *Mommies, Daddies, Donors, Surrogates: Answering Tough Questions and Building Strong Families*. New York: Guilford Press.

De Peyer, J. (2013) Sequestered selves: Discussion and adoption roundtable. *Psychoanalytic Perspectives*, 10 (1), 149–168.

McCullers, C. (1946). *Member of the Wedding*. New York: Houghton Mifflin Co.
Racker, H. (1968). *Transference and Countertransference*. New York: International Universities Press.
van der Kolk, B.A. (2005). Developmental trauma disorder: Toward a rational diagnosis for children with complex trauma histories. *Psychiatric Annals*, 35 (5), 401–408.
Wieder, H. (1977). The Family Romance Fantasies of Adopted Children. *The Psychoanalytic Quarterly*, 46 (2), 188–200.
Wright, J.L. (2009) The princess has to die: Representing rupture and grief in the narrative of adoption. *Psychoanalytic Study of the Child*, 64, 75–91.

PART VI

Epilogue

An epilogue serves as a bridge between what has already been explored and discussed and what remains to be studied. The idea of establishing connections between what has been found through evidence-based studies and the many speculations about the clinical issues can be conceptualized in a number of ways and are alluded to in many of the chapters of this book. As compared with psychotherapy with non-adopted clients, treatment of adopted clients involves attempts to reconcile several schisms, that is, the unstudied and unresolved gaps of knowledge and the seeming contradictions within health, neurobiology, mental health, and the adoption field itself. An initial question has to do with treatment goals and whether therapists sufficiently explain to adopted clients their options regarding their goals and the means for achieving them.

There is much available in the Adoption literature relating to counseling approaches for various goals, in contrast, most authors for this handbook represent a more in-depth, psychodynamic perspective for helping the adopted client reach a fuller and more cohesive *internal* understanding of themselves and their place in the world. This book explains that such self-understanding, if this is the client's goal, transcends what can be learned through counseling and behaviorally- focused approaches by reinforcing the integrative process enabling significant advances in personality maturation. Further clinical experience demonstrates that such can be achieved within a short term time frame as well as through more open-ended treatment. While these various approaches are still being sorted out, therapists generally have continued to use various forms of treatment developed for non-adopted clients (e.g., trauma and attachment) that, in many ways, do not meet the actual needs of the adopted client, especially when he/she is no longer a young child.

Psychodynamic therapy of the adopted person brings to light a number of theoretical issues: Is the separation of the adopted person from the birth mother necessarily a trauma, whenever it occurs? Are adopted persons more vulnerable to ongoing psychological difficulties due to the original separation from the birth mother? Or later disturbing circumstances? Or the combination? How can we account for the findings that adopted people are often significantly overrepresented in various treatment modalities and facilities while, on the other hand, it is reported that most adopted people do not exhibit or report any psychopathology? One possible way to understand the contention about the "primal wound" is to propose that the experience of being separated from the birth mother at birth or shortly thereafter constitutes an immediate neurobiological trauma which may or may not be ultimately ameliorated by the quality of the subsequent placement with the adoptive family. The problem is that, often, original or early trauma is not clearly differentiated from the trauma of unfortunate events that may follow birth, or very early childhood, such as disruptive foster placements and/or inadequate or even abusive relationships within the adoptive family that the adoption field has historically not acknowledged. But it seems likely that even in the best post-adoptive circumstances, there remains for the adopted person a residue of loss which needs to be addressed in the treatment setting. In writing his perspective for psychoanalytic treatment of adopted persons, Deeg writes that therapy of the adopted person involves establishing the internal connections between the adopted self and the birth parent and all that follows the separation from the birth mother, whenever that occurs. As Bertocci points out, we already know enough to recognize the great need to distinguish between developmental trauma generally and, more specifically, early developmental trauma within the first three years of life. Oddly, this area of specialty and the sub-populations in which it is most likely to be found is inadequately addressed in the overall trauma field. We must also be open to the forthcoming findings from the field of epigenetics which enlighten us to the molecular processes at the interface of nature and nurture, with profound implications for brain plasticity and resilience, for vulnerability to certain diagnoses, and for the potential of psychotherapy to enable permanent change. In short, psychotherapists can no longer dismiss the developmental significance of the first three years of life, but this means that treatment of adopted patients of any age needs to be informed by this area of specialty.

In the editors' view, the treatment of the adopted person presents a unique and relatively rare opportunity to learn about, and work with, some of the most remarkable and daunting mysteries of human development and resilience. Up until now, this has rarely been observed or addressed in either research or the literature, and it is another mystery that the mental health field has, for the most part, basically ignored it. In addition to all the complexities of *being* adopted, brought into relief are many universal issues in human experience that readers will perhaps be able to see for the first time and understand in a new way. This begins on a personal level with contemplating how we define "family", how our perspective on its meanings and importance to us may change over time, and how we understand our place and value within it. Also brought into relief are the many adjustments that adopted people must make regarding fundamental human experiences that they have never had, while the non-adopted world takes these for granted and would not want to live without them.

We hope this handbook will engage increasing numbers of physicians, mental health practitioners, and researchers interested in the psychology of adoption. But we maintain that the psychology of *being* adopted is an essential part of the broader topic. In no way do we minimize the larger context and psychodynamics of adoptive family life, but the emphasis on the latter has been at the expense of learning about the psychology of *being* adopted. We challenge therapists' many assumptions, albeit unwittingly made, because in not understanding the significance of *being* adopted, they limit and misdirect many of their treatment efforts. In support of this observation, we cite in the text a large number of anecdotal reports from adopted people whose voices, until now, have not been represented or heard. Meanwhile, the mental health field continues to focus almost entirely on work with adoptive parents, with the assumption that the adopted person in the family is a child. This book explains at length why the treatment approach needs to be modified when the adopted person is an adolescent or young adult.

We hope that readers will extend themselves to engage their colleagues in open dialogue on the topics we have discussed in this handbook so that they can stimulate new questions but also identify and communicate the topics that they believe need more clinically focused research. One schism has to do with research studies that, to date, have been primarily quantitative, that is, focused on developing empirical support for questions and hypotheses being posed, but often concluding with broad-brush concepts, such as "wellness," that serve primarily academic purposes. But psychotherapists treating adopted patients who want to understand more in-depth about the psychology of *being* adopted in the hope of improving their therapeutic skills are left with little that is applicable specifically to clinical practice and clinical process. It is also pointed out that there are differences in the ways various mental health disciplines conceptualize work at a "clinical" level. The important distinction is made between clinical *topics* identified in the literature, clinical *research* bearing on those topics, and actual clinical *practice* – which introduces the need to develop protocols for "best practices." This handbook is an attempt to bring these perspectives closer together.

In addition to our concerns about the limits and focus of research to date, the book also addresses what we recognize to be serious systemic inadequacies or outright malpractice in the way many *domestic* adoptive placements are handled and enabled legally, sometimes resulting in very flawed, emotionally neglectful adoptive homes. The emphasis in the literature has been on outcomes of *international* adoptions and the impact of institutional neglect, while the continuing problems in domestic adoptions have not been sufficiently studied. They include the serious systemic problem identified by some of the authors regarding the need for more highly professionalized staff and protocols for selecting people wanting to adopt. In particular, we point out that there are different forms and degrees of family neglect that need to be differentiated from each other, that range in the degree to which these problems can be ameliorated, and that vary in their developmental impact on the young person.

There are also puzzling questions about diagnostic and treatment issues. We begin with the problem that most studies to date have focused only on pre-adolescent children. But as in the case of certain medical problems, on the basis of both research and our observations, the full impact of internal trauma can lay dormant until it erupts in adolescence. Lack of awareness of this is the reason that the child-focused research has missed the many difficult complexities that often come in adolescence and young adulthood. Regarding the more disturbed end of the spectrum, the question remains: Why some and not others? Before rushing to the conclusion that "genetic factors" must account for such vulnerabilities, we need also to consider that they may account for the remarkable resilience and other exceptional talents that so many adopted people have demonstrated. A common complaint of adopted adults is that, while they know they worked very hard to earn their distinctions, their parents tend to get more credit than they do, although in the end they admit, "I came this way." Undoubtedly they are right.

These questions highlight the ongoing nature–nurture debate, the results of which, like many other dimensions of adoption, may be unknowable, or at least are likely to remain ambiguous in the foreseeable future. In view of this, studies of neuroplasticity are a crucial area for ongoing evaluation and research, that is, trauma-induced changes in the brain and the capacity to recover over time, as well as studies of the lasting impact of earliest pre-adoption experiences. However, a crucial theme of the handbook is that it is not enough to know about adoption-related trauma and anxious attachment, because the overriding concerns in adolescence and young adulthood are around sexuality and with the adopted person's need to integrate their full identity involving the birth family.

An area of possible disagreement on "best practices" regards the plan for treatment of adolescents, such as the argument from family therapists that the adoptive parents and adopted adolescent primarily need to be seen together in order to help the family work through their difficulties and misunderstandings in order to become a healthier and more cohesive unit. However, a central theme of this book is that *adoption cannot be viewed as being only about the adoptive family*, thus, that the adopted person needs to be understood on their own terms individually, as well as within the context of their life within the adoptive family. The Balas chapter comments on the complexities of countertransference if there is only one therapist. We, the editors, maintain that most importantly, the adopted adolescent deserves to be given a choice.

A number of the clinician-authors in this book contend that there are two fundamentally different approaches to working with adopted clients. Cognitive behavioral approaches and relatively brief, "strengths-based" supportive and psychoeducational interventions involving various family members are within the large domain of counseling and social services. Psychotherapists, especially those whose work is psychodynamically based offer a multilayered clinical approach focusing on the *internal life* of the adopted person and the prospects for more permanent and encompassing change, as well as on the underlying psychodynamics of adoptive family life. The latter is usually missed in quantitative adoption studies. Further, all good psychotherapy is "strengths-based" and "goal-oriented." We are especially concerned by the observed tendency of some fields to dismiss the clinical perspectives of the more traditional mental health fields based on the belief, entirely unfounded, that they "pathologize adoption." Nevertheless, the editors contend that the clinical complexities identified in this handbook require putting aside the proverbial "rose-colored glasses" and facing the internal realities reported by so many adopted adults, regardless of whether treatment was ever involved.

On behalf of vulnerable adopted young people, we emphasize that there is strength in numbers in the needed collaboration between their health-care professionals, especially their psychotherapists, so that they can expand the boundaries of the adoption-specific knowledge base from which we believe they need to work. In particular, we encourage greater collaboration between clinicians and researchers globally, and we hope that this handbook will be just the beginning of a wider interdisciplinary, international dialogue.

INDEX

Note: Page numbers in *italics* indicate a figure and page numbers in **bold** indicate a table on the corresponding page.

AAP (American Academy of Pediatrics) 180, 191
abandonment: anxiety 306; attachment disruption 284, 287; of children in India 156, 159–160; divorce as 97, 250, 307, 316; fear of 59; personal narratives 59, 61, 64; primal 303; psychoanalytic treatment and 271, 273; reenactment of 9, 246; sense/feelings of 112, 118, 125, 135, 304; threats to self-esteem 112; trauma 4, 61, 128
abortion, in India 156–157
abuse: adoption medicine 181, 186; personal narratives 57–58, 63, 65, 67–68, 70; prenatal exposure 186; sexual 67, 181, 191; by siblings 316–317; substance 186–188
academic success, valued in Indian families 163, 165
adolescence: adoptive family narrative 115–118; perspective shift to psychology of 239–246; second individualization of 306
adolescent adjustment 190–191
adolescent development, case studies 116–118
adolescent identity integration 277, 279
adolescents: countertransference challenges 303–319; late-adopted 283–302
adoptee adjustment 82
adoptee voice 57, 163, 167
adoptee vulnerability: anxiety disorders 2, 22, 82–83; dissociation 309–310; eating disorders 22–23, 82, 244, 245, 313; mood disorders 82, 187, 254; neuropsychological development 81, 83, 86, 97, 248; psychic homelessness 44–45
adoption: closed (*see* closed adoption); culture 1, 16–18, 80, 82, 86, 202–203, 207, 210, 236, 238; domestic (*see* domestic adoption); international-transnational (*see* international adoption); interracial/transracial 40, 45, 48, 51, 93–94, 212, 217, 242, 319; kinship 89–90, 96, 154–155, 158; knowledgeable services 4, 12, 20, 103, 244, 251, 255; knowledgeable treatment 244; LGBTQ 27, 94–95, 240; medicine (*see* adoption medicine); non-kinship (*see* non-kinship adoption); open 46, 58, 90–91,

Index

147–148, 238, 240; paths to 4–6, 18, 93, 180, 205; private/independent 5, 18–19, 37, 93, 105, 241; revocation 43
Adoption Act 1952 (Ireland) 157
adoption competence 103, 168, 170, 251–252, 262–263
adoption-informed treatment 7, 10, 242–243, 246, 255
adoption knowledge, Indian-specific 161
adoption-knowledgeable services 4, 12, 20, 103, 244, 251, 255
adoption-knowledgeable therapist/clinician 8, 220, 234, 251
adoption lifebook 113–114
adoption market: forthcoming changes in 23–24; in Netherlands 50
adoption medicine 9, 179–193; adolescent adjustment 190–191; adverse experiences prior to placement 181, **181**; description of 179–180; health-care management 191–192; infectious diseases 182–184; international adoption 179–186, 188, 191; lead exposure 186; parasites 183–184; physician's approach to adoptees 189–190; pre-adoption services 180; prenatal exposures 186–189; school issues 184–186; tuberculosis (TB) 182–183; viral infections, chronic 183
adoption narratives 57–76; adoption systems 68–69; Anne 59–60, 62, 65, 67, 71–73; Birgit 43–44; birth fathers 143–145; Cheryl 59, 61, 63–68, 70–74; Darryl 59, 61, 63, 65–70, 72–73; Frankie 279–281; James 144; John 41; Michael 59–61, 63, 65, 67–68, 70, 72–73; mother loss 61–62; Peter 41–43; recommendations for therapists 72–73; relation to adoptive family 65–68; Robert 144–145; search, contact, and reunion 62–65; self-esteem 69–72
adoption placement organization: naïveté 40, 46, 51–53; in Netherlands 41–42, 50
adoption satisfaction 242, 245, 251
adoption story: components of 107–108; as dynamic 119; fantasy included in 107; openness concerning 163; as opportunity for discussion 111; sharing 158, 163–164; *see also* adoptive family narrative
adoption triad 11
adoptive family: abuse within 67–68; attitudes of extended 318–319; communication 21–22, 111–112; disclosure (*see* disclosure of adoption); Indian 163–168; personal narratives 61–68; placement 91–92
adoptive family narrative 107–120; adolescence 115–118; communication 21–22; differences from adoptee's personal narrative 82; disclosure of adoption 108, 112–115; early adulthood 118–119; effect on development 107–120; family communication patterns 111–112; treatment implications 119
adoptive parents: ambivalence of 318; attitudes toward birth fathers 145; fantasies of 308; generations of, in Netherlands 46, 48–50; love potion myth 318; motives of 249–250; narcissistic side of parenting 248–251; racial and cultural similarities/differences between child and 93–94; same/different gender/sexual identity as adoptee 94–95; therapist competitiveness with 308
adoptive placement information 18–23
age at placement 91–92, 104, 165
alcohol, prenatal exposure (PEA) 186–187
alcohol-related neurodevelopmental disorder (ARND) 186
alternate development 3, 80, 88, 209, 235–238
alternate reproduction 26, 210
alternate sexual development 80
American Academy of Pediatrics (AAP) 180, 191
American Trypanosomiasis 184
amnesia, dissociative 208
anger: at adoptive parent 132; therapeutic challenge of handling 305–306
anxiety: abandonment 306; core constellation 255; separation 9, 61, 244, 254

Index

artificial insemination 23
attachment: anxious 22, 103, 251–252, 255, 324; disorganized 284–286, 289–290, 292, 294–295; disruption of 7, 313; insecure 29, 284–285; neurophysiological to birth mother 92, 284; representations 283–297; to therapist 315; trust and 255; widening of 316
attachment-focused therapy 276–277, 279
attachment-informed 234
attachment inventories 87
attachment security 285, 294–295
attachment theory 276–277, 284
attention-deficit/hyperactivity disorder (ADHD) 105, 185–186; prenatal drug exposure 187–188
attunement: emotional 16, 103, 239, 246, 253, 297; parental 16, 26, 103, 246, 251, 297, 302; therapist 30, 239, 253
autobiographical capacity 111; life story work 276, 280

baby home 24, 96, 144–145, 156–157, 309
behavior problems 182, 192; adjustment in adopted adolescents 190–191
belonging, sense of 41, 107, 217, 255, 309, 312, 315, 318–319
Bernard, Viola 24
Bettelheim, Bruno 138
bias against adoption 108–109
bio-ecological approach 154, 159
biological children 16, 20, 175, 287, 307
birth certificate 202; absence of father's name 139; access to 214, 238; amended 90, 203; denied to Black American slaves 203; original (pre-adoptive) 68, 104, 160, 201, 204, 214; post-adoption 60, 124, 160; sealed records/closed adoption 91, 104
birth circumstances, implications of 159–160
birth fathers 137–150; adopted adolescent's view of 147–148; adoptee's encounters with, and perceptions of 145–147; attitudes toward adoption 140; connectedness and loss 141–143; contact and relationships with adult children 142–145; demographics 140; experiences of adoption 139–140; fantasies about 149; financial support from 18; information gap 80, 109, 148–149
birth mother representation 126–133, 268–269, 273; defensive functions of 129–133; origin/existence of 126–129
birth mothers: attitudes toward birth fathers 145; child's neurophysiological attachment to 92; connection to 124–125; fantasies of 128–133; financial support 53; information about 117; internalized relationship to 125; internalized representation of 126–133; neurophysiological attachment to 92, 284; private adoptions 19; professional assistance to 18; separation from 3, 40, 59, 61–62, 79, 81, 86–87, 128, 216, 221, 304, 322
birth parents: fantasies of 112, 115, 118, 264–266, 268–271, 274, 306; representations 126–133, 264–265, 267–269; *see also* birth fathers; birth mothers
blood (biological) ties 313
body image 22, 71, 84, 96, 246, 255, 311–314
body image issues 255, 311–314; blood (biological) ties 313; blurred self-concept 312–313; conflicts about sexuality 314; eating disorders 313; shock of puberty 311–312; unresolved issues, resurgence of 314–317
bodywork 277
Bohman, Michael 33
boundaries 50, 130, 235, 253, 304, 306
Bowlby, John 138, 204
brain: brain-based treatments 255, 276–277; cortical volume 188–189; early-life stress and 79; impact of trauma 276; plasticity and resilience 322; structural alterations 118, 190; trauma-induced changes 254, 324
brain development 83, 86, 234, 248; arrests in 10; critical ages in 29–30; sequential 277, **278**; in young adults 237
Brent, David A. 45
Brinich, Paul 303, 318

Index

Cadoret, Remi 33
case studies 57–76; adolescent development 116–118; assessing adopted client's development 95–97; identity formation 279–281; internationally placed adoptees in Netherlands 40–45; late disclosure 114–115; search and reunion 42–44; *see also* adoptive family narratives
caste system 156, 163, 165
cathexis 125–127, 131–134, 265
Center for Disease Control (CDC) 210
Chagas disease 184
child custody litigation 17, 203, 237
child labor laws 203
Child Welfare Committee (India) 158, 160
child welfare system 4, 87, 241, 277
chosen, idea of being 66–67
circumcision 113
clinical approaches 21, 39, 98, 233, 324; *see also* therapy; treatment
clinical perspective 233; on complexities in sexuality 247; on core constellations in psychology of being adopted 254–255; inconvenient truths for psychotherapists from 31–32; on parent motives for adopting 250; psychodynamically informed 3, 223–224; on *Three Identical Strangers* 26–28
clinical process 233, 323
clinical social work 10–11
clinical topics identified in the literature 233, 323
closed adoption 79–81, 147–148; Australia 58–60, 68, 71; decline in 148; fantasies of adoptees from 20–21; impact of 81, 85, 88, 96, 120, 212, 214–217; India 158, 162–164; information, lack of 79, 90–91, 147; Ireland 158; open compared 90–91; United States 148, 212
closed records system, Australian 59–60, 68, 71
Clothier, Florence 33
cognitive-behavioral therapy 205, 219
cognitive dissonance 211, 249
Coles, Gary 143
college counseling services 219, 230
commodification of adoption 19, 66, 157–158, 213

communication: adoption-related 148; adoptive family narrative 21–22, 107–120; family difficulties with 22; family patterns 111–112; openness in Indian 163–165
concierge services (alternate reproduction) 23
conduct disorder 185, 210, 245
confidentiality: forced upon birth mothers 205; full 202
connectedness, sense of 217
Connecting Parenting Program 297
Connors Comprehensive Rating Scales 185
contact: with birth fathers 146; personal narratives 63; rejection of 63; *see also* search and reunion
cortical volume 188–189
Council on Foster Care, Adoption, and Kinship Care 180
countertransference 120, 215, 219, 222, 224, 254, 303–319; with adopted adolescents and young adults 306–307; complementary 304; concordant 304–305, 310; considerations in 305–311; dissociation and withdrawal 310; effect and role in psychotherapy 272–273
culture: of adolescents 115; adoption 1, 16–18, 80, 82, 86, 202, 207, 210, 236, 238; connections to 94
curiosity: of adopted persons 10, 149, 167, 209, 265; phases of 149

DDP (dyadic developmental psychotherapy) 277
Declaration of the Rights of the Child 261
defense: functions of birth mother representation 129–133; masochistic 133
demographic factors 28–29, 88–95, 210, 238, 240, 243, 248, 287, **288**, 290–292, 294
demographic subsets of adoptive status 89–95; closed/open adoption 90–91; early/late placement 91–92; kinship/non-kinship 89–90; same/different gender/sexual identity 94–95
devaluation: of adopted parent 131–132; of children 17
development: alternate 3, 80, 88, 209, 235–238; brain (*see* brain

Index

development); case studies of adolescent 116–118; effect of adoptive family narrative 107–120; neuropsychological 81, 83, 86, 97, 248
developmental adjustment 190–191
developmental challenge, fundamental areas of 6–8
developmental delay 184, 187, 248, 284
developmental fault lines 9
developmental screening 191
developmental timeline 248
developmental trauma 276–277
developmental trauma disorder 86
discharge, adoption 73
disclosure of adoption: adoptive family narrative 108, 112–115; case study 114–115; early telling 112; how and when 112–114; impact of 112–114; in India 164; late 112–115; in Netherlands 47–48
discovery: late 59, 62, 84, 114, 248; personal narratives 59, 61–62
dissociation 309–310
dissociative amnesia 208
divorce as abandonment 97, 250, 307, 316
DNA searches 214
domestic adoption: India 157–158, 161–162, 164–166; international placement compared 92–93; kinship 96; Netherlands 46, **47**; religious influence 157; suicide 29, 44; United States 241
donor children 39, 51
drug exposure, prenatal (PDE) 187–199
dyadic developmental psychotherapy (DDP) 277

early adulthood, adoptive family narrative in 118–119
early developmental trauma 6, 8, 16, 30, 57, 82, 86–87, 242, 254, 308–309, 322
early developmental trauma disorder 86
eating disorders 22–23, 82, 244, 245, 313
ego functioning 246, 264–265, 270
ego ideal 132
ego paralysis 245
Eight Core Constellations 254–256
embryos, donated 23
emotional attunement 16, 103, 239, 246, 253, 297

empathy: for birth mother 303; clinical 239; countertransference 303–305; microaggressions and 244; of parents when discussing adoption 115; of therapists 31, 82, 87, 190, 216, 252–253, 271, 273, 303, 309
envy: resentment 316–317; of the young 312
Erikson, Erik 37
eurythmy 128, 130
evaluation, adoption-specific considerations in 235–254
Evan B. Donaldson Adoption Institute 214, 230
executive functioning 277
exploitation 11, 27
externalizing behaviors 29, 187, 190, 245

false self 305
Family Futures 275, 279–280
family law 17–18, 210; adult-centered focus 237; biological fathers 11; property law and 17, 203, 237
family romance fantasy 131, 147–148, 306–307
family therapy 2, 6, 10, 95, 163, 251–252
fantasy 215; in adoption story 107; of adoption workers 214; of adoptive parents 308; birth father 149, 268; birth mother 128–133, 265–266, 268–269, 271; birth parents 112, 115, 118, 264–266, 268–271, 274, 306; countertransference 304, 306–308; family romance 131, 147–148, 306–307; meaning in 206–207, 208, 223, 239, 244; origins of adoptees 21; rescue 120; of self 264–266, 268–269; suicidal 28, 245; tolerance for 129
fathers: birth (*see* birth fathers); as forgotten parents of psychoanalytic thought 137–139; treatment by adoptive 67
fetal alcohol syndrome (FAS) 45, 186
FFI (Friends and Family Interview) 289–292, **293–294**, 294
fight-flight-or-freeze response 279
financial support: birth mothers 53; insufficiency of 40; in Netherlands 46
forced adoptions 27, 38, 53, 59, 224, 303
foster care: adoptive medicine 179–182, 184–186, 188, 191; emphasis on 11; independent foster care agency 275;

misconceptions 81; path to adoption 4; serial placements 83; statistics 181; time in 17–18, 24, 104
Freud, Sigmund 147–148
Friends and Family Interview (FFI) 289–292, **293–294**, 294

GAMA (Guardians and Wards Act) 157
generational differences 22
generations of adoptive parents 46, 48–50; conscious of contradictions 49; economic-realistic 49; open-idealistic 48–49; prepared, optimistic, and demanding 49; traditional closed 46, 48
genetic factors 236, 324
genetic sexual attraction 221–222
Glenn, Jules 33
Gordon, Avery 149
grief: of birth fathers 140–141, 143; for family of origin 190
Guardians and Wards Act (GAMA) 157
guilt 32, 51, 118–120, 133, 141, 167, 207, 218, 255, 306; about one's origins 315; of birth fathers 141

Hague Convention on Intercountry Adoption 5, 158
HAMA (Hindu Adoption and maintenance Act) 157
Hamilton, Alexander 216
health-care management 191–192
helplessness: learned 247, 255; sense of 214, 245
hepatitis B 183
hepatitis C 183
Hindu Adoption and maintenance Act (HAMA) 157
homelessness, psychic 44–45
home studies, pre-placement 18–19
hospitalization 30, 61, 144, 245
human rights 27, 57, 60, 68, 70, 72, 159, 202–203, 213, 237
hypothalamic-pituitary-adrenal (HPA) axis 188

identity: in adolescence 116; body image and 255; denial of 16; development 7; formation 275–282; fragmented 8, 29, 255; integration 255, 277, **278**; search for 133–134; sense of 147, 303, 315; sexual 84, 94, 255, 314; struggle 40, 51, 54
illegitimate child 59, 157
implicit memory 16, 216
imprinting 302
incest 69, 114, 222, 247, 256
independent foster care agency 275
India, adoption in 154–170, 204; adoptee voices 163, 167; age of adoption 165; appraisal of existing services 168; background of 155–157; circumstances at time of birth 159–160; conceptual framework for adoptee well-being 154, *155*; framework for services for adoptee well-being 168–169, *169*; growing up in adoptive families 163–168; influences on well-being of adoptees 159–161; international adoption 157–158, 161–163, 165–166; male child, preference of 156; openness in communication 163–165; record-keeping practices 161–163; school and peer influences 165–166; semi-open records 204; sociocultural beliefs and practice of 156–157; socio-legal scenario impact on services 157–159
infectious diseases 182–184
information: access in kinship adoption 96; adoptive placement 18–23; birth father 80, 109, 148–149; birth mother 117; conflicting and disturbing 119; lack of pre-placement 51, 79, 90–91, 147, 213, 238–239; missing 110; search for origin 62–63; therapist's consideration of 109–110
inner world of adopted persons 124–135
instinct 10, 85, 211, 216, 302
institutionalization: attachment issues 284; countries with history of 109; sleeper effects of 87–88
intercountry adoption *see* international adoption
internal experience 31, 81–82, 149, 209, 224, 233, 254
internalized relation 7, 124, 126, 128–130, 268
internal life 3, 11, 23, 83, 85, 89, 241–242, 325

Index

internal meanings: search and reunion 212; suicidal thoughts/actions 28–30
internal working models (IWMs) 276, 283–286, 297, 302
international adoptees: problems for adoptive parents of 49; suicidal thoughts/actions 44–45
international adoption 4–5; adjustments in adolescence 251; adoptive medicine 179–186, 188, 191; birth fathers 148–149; case studies in Netherlands 40–45; decrease in 53–54, 57, 93, 180; delays in 18; domestic placement compared 92–93; hypothetical case examples 95–96; inadequate handling 19; India 157–158, 161–163, 165–166; information, lack of 51, 213; Italy 285; Netherlands 40–45, **46, 47**, 48, 50, 53; outcomes 39–40; suicidal thoughts/action 29; total recorded worldwide (1990–2019) 40; in United States **52**
interpersonal relationships, impact on 70–72
interracial adoption 40, 45, 48, 51, 93–94, 212, 217, 242, 319
intestinal parasites 183–184
intrapsychic 7, 10, 16, 253, 266, 271
Ireland, adoption in 156–158, 204
IWMs (internal working models) 276, 283–286, 297, 302

Jobs, Steve 216
Joustra Report 49–50
judiciary 17–18, 90, 237
Julian, Megan 87
Juvenile Justice Act (India) 162

kinship adoption: demographics 89–90; in India 154–155, 158; information access 96; preferences for 89–90, 96
Kirk, H. David 33

language of adoption 3, 147
late-adopted adolescents 283–302
late discovery adoptee 59, 62, 248
latent trauma 216
lawyers 5, 12, 18–19, 19, 37–38, 96, 104, 237, 241
lead exposure 186

learned helplessness 247, 255
learning disorders 184–185
legal processes 17–18
LGBTQ families/parents 27, 94–95, 240
lifebook, adoption 113–114
life story work 276, 280
Lifton, Betty Jean 62
limbic system 30
locus of control 214, 255
loss: birth father 141–143; mother 61–62; overt and covert 108; traumatic 6, 29, 40, 86, 149, 233, 247, 252
lost object 126, 129, 132, 222, 265, 270, 274

malnutrition 179, 181, 183
Mann, J. John 45
masochism 131, 133, 214, 272
maternal stress, prenatal 189
maternal undernutrition 189
McCullers, Carson 311
McDormand, Frances 216
medical passport 109, 123
Medical Termination of Pregnancy Act (India) 156
medicine *see* adoptive medicine
memory: fragmented 113, 281, 304; implicit 16, 216
mental health practitioners, inconvenient truths for 87–89
mentalization 103
microaggressions 109, 166, 168, 192, 215, 244
mirroring 65–66, 71, 103, 216
mood disorders 82, 187, 254
mother-and-baby home 144–145, 156–157

narcissism 27, 41, 129–130; adoptive parenting and 248–251; narcissistic supplies 132–133; pride 246; regulator 130; therapist's own 205–206, 222, 315
narcissistic injury 21, 32, 125, 207, 211, 250
narrative: adoption 57–76; adoptive family 107–120
narrative coherence 276
National Institute of Mental Health (NIMH) 210
National Survey of Adoptive Parents (NSAP) 234, 241–242
nature-nurture debate 24–26, 37, 324

Index

neglect: adoptive medicine 179, 181–182; cultural and institutional 22; personal narratives 57–58

Netherlands 39–56, 213, 254; case studies from clinical practice 40–45; generations of adoptees 50–51; generations of adoptive parents 46, 48–50; international adoption 40–45, 45, **46**, **47**, 48, 50, 53; non-relative adoptions of Dutch-born children 45, **47**

Neubauer, Peter 24–25, 27–28

neurobiological changes/impact 16, 37, 81, 83, 87, 234, 308, 322

neurobiology: protections by nature 237; research/studies 3, 27, 29, 79, 217, 311

neurocysticercosis 184

neurophysiological attachment to birth mother 92, 284

neuropsychological based problems 9, 37, 81, 87, 210, 234, 244

neuropsychological development 81, 83, 86, 97, 248

neuropsychological response/excitement 222

neuropsychological testing 105

neurosequential approach 87, 275–282

neurosequential model 10

NICHQ Vanderbilt Assessment Scales 185

NIMH (National Institute of Mental Health) 210

non-kinship adoption 84; alternate development 80, 84, 88, 96, 216; clinical observations 233, 235; demographics 89–90; factors for therapist to consider 79–83; incomplete narrative 107; in India 154–155; questionnaire 261–262; suicide 28

non-relative adoptions of Dutch-born children 45, **47**

normative crises of adoption 190

NSAP (National Survey of Adoptive Parents) 234, 241–242

object relation 124–126, 128, 264–269, 271–272

open adoption 46, 58, 90–91, 147–148, 238, 240

oppositional behaviors 245

oppositional defiant disorder 185

origin information, search for 62–63

orphanages 129, 160, 166, 181–182, 239, 303, 309, 313–314

orphan trains 203

parasites 183–184

parent-centered perspective 236

parent–child closeness 251

parenting styles 159, 163, 218, 240, 251

parents' rights 213

PDE (prenatal drug exposure) 187–199

PEA (prenatal exposure to alcohol) 186–187

permanency of disadvantages 90

personal ads 5

pets 317

placement: age at 91–92, 104; early vs. late 91–92

placement agency: follow-up, lack of 20; in India 161–162, 169

Plomin, Robert 20, 37

policy and practice, changing nature of 108–109

populations of adopted children 180–182

post-adoption services 18–19, 37, 145, 159, 180, 202, 204, 213, 275

postnatal development 37, 83

posttraumatic stress disorder (PTSD) 45, 61, 69, 185

pragmatic language disorder 185

prejudice 59, 108–109, 165, 319

premature birth 60–62

prenatal drug exposure (PDE) 187–199

prenatal exposures 186–189; alcohol (PEA) 186–187; drug (PDE) 187–188; stress 188–189

prenatal exposure to alcohol (PEA) 186–187

present tense, adoptive status as in 81

pride in one's background 315

primal abandonment 303

primal wound 3–4, 127, 322

Pringle, Mia Kellmer 138

private adoption agencies 4, 12, 19, 104, 205, 238

private/independent adoptions 5, 18–19, 37, 93, 105, 241

probate (property) law 17, 203, 237

property: children as 26; inheritance of 108

property law 17, 203, 237

psychic homelessness 44–45

Index

psychoanalytic conception of psychology of adoption 124–135
psychoanalytic treatment: birth parent fantasies 264–266, 268–271, 274; birth parent representations 126–133, 264–265, 267–269; countertransference, effect and role of 272–273; countertransference challenges 303–319; invitation to therapy 265–267; modification of 265–267; object relation 124–126, 128, 264–269, 271–272; search for reunion 271–272; self-representations 264–265, 267–268, 271–273, 283, 289; termination, issues surrounding 273–274; transference 264, 269–271, 273
psychodynamic therapy 219, 266, 321
psychodynamic training 11, 103, 210, 221
psychological parenting 16, 26
psychological testing 87, 93, 221
psychology: of adoption 11, 15, 28, 33, 58, 124–135, 205, 223, 246, 322; of being adopted 2–4, 6–7, 15, 20, 58, 82, 89, 206, 210, 220, 225, 233, 242, 252–255, 322–323
psychotherapeutic treatment 10, 231–325; adoption-informed 255; countertransference, effect and role of 272–273; dyadic developmental psychotherapy (DDP) 277
psychotherapists: adoption-knowledgeable 251; adoption narratives 58, 72–73; adoptive placement information, relevance of 18–23; best practices 220–221; common themes for 214–222; inconvenient truths for 31–32; non-kinship adoption, factors to consider in 79–83; self-disclosure by 223–224; unwarranted assumptions 310
psychotherapy *see* psychotherapeutic treatment
PTSD (posttraumatic stress disorder) 45, 61, 69, 185
puberty 84; precocious 191; shock of 311–312

questionnaire, non-kinship adoption 261–262

Racker, Heinrich 304
RAD (reactive attachment disorder) 7
randomness, role of 19–20, 25
rape 69, 114, 133, 243, 247
reactive attachment disorder 45
record-keeping, in India 161–163
reflective functioning 286, 289, 292, **293**, 295–296
reflective thinking 118, 279
regression 248, 266, 305–306; episodes of 314–315; therapeutic challenge of handling 305–306
rejection 261, 303, 319; avoidance 284, 309; of difference 48; of experience of being adopted 250; personal narratives 62–65; secondary 63–64; sensitivity to 221; as severe narcissistic injury 125
representations: attachment 283–297; birth mother 126–133, 268–269, 273; birth parent 126–133, 264–265, 267–269; parental 290, 292, 295–296; self 124, 127, 133–134, 264–268, 271–273, 283, 289
rescue fantasy 120
resentment, envious 316–317
reunion: with birth fathers 142, 144–147; sustaining 63–64; *see also* search and reunion
role reversal 289–290, 292, **293**, 295
root search 160–161, 163

Salvation Army 63, 68
Schechter, Marshall 33
school issues 184–186; attention-deficit/hyperactivity disorder (ADHD) 185–186; experiences of adoptees in India 165–166; learning disorders 184–185
sealed records 25–26, 38, 58, 104, 201–204, 211, 230
search 201–225; the American experience with 210–214; background for mental health professionals 203–206; clinical/psychodynamic perspective 206–207; common themes for psychotherapists 214–222; countertransference 306–307; DNA searches 214; implications for health and mental health 206–210; sociological

Index

perspective 209; therapeutic responses to client's search 222–225; who searches and why 214–216
search and reunion 9–10; in adolescence 116; birth fathers 146–147; case studies 42–44; doctors as confidant 192; genetic sexual attraction 221–222; in India 160–161; internal meanings 212; literature informing clinical practice 212; personal narratives 62–65; psychoanalytic treatment 271–272
second individuation process 30
secrecy 26, 60, 112, 156, 158, 162, 166; *see also* closed adoption; sealed records
Secure Cycle program 297
self, sense of 31, 69, 134, 253, 279, 281, 310
self-concept, blurred 312–313
self-destructive behavior 29, 245
self-disclosure, by therapists 223–224, 307
self-esteem 9; of birth fathers 141; ego ideal 132; personal narratives 69–72
self-mutilation 245
self-representation 124, 127, 133–134, 264–268, 271–273, 283, 289
self-soothing 317
self-worth 69–71
sensory integration disorders 277
sensory processing disorder 185
separation anxiety 9, 61, 244, 254
separation from birth mother 3, 40, 59, 61–62, 79, 81, 86–87, 128, 216, 221, 304, 322
sexual abuse 67, 181, 191
sexual attraction, genetic 221–222
sexual development, alternate 80
sexual identity 84, 94, 255, 314
sexuality: complexities in 246–247, 255–256; conflicts about 314
shame 32, 44, 59, 80, 141, 144, 156–157, 167, 222, 255, 279, 315
sibling relationships 316
social work, professionalized 104, 205, 221
somatic dissociative process 84
Sorosky, Arthur 33
sorrow 255
special needs, children with 48, 181, 234, 284
splitting 112, 128–129, 132
state laws 211, 213–214

stepparents, adoption by 4, 81, 89, 253
stigma 64, 95, 108, 114.156, 158, 164, 168, 192, 255, 296
stranger adoption 157–158, 162
stress: posttraumatic stress disorder (PTSD) 45, 61, 69, 185; prenatal exposures 188–189; toxic 179
substance abuse 186–188
suicidal thoughts/actions 11, 25, 28–32, 245; internal meanings 28–30; international adoptees 44–45; personal narratives 61, 64
surrogates 23, 27, 49
systemic dysfunction 3, 27
systemic factors 15–38; adoption market 23–24; adoptive placement information 18–23; inconvenient truths 31–32; legal processes 17–18; randomness, role of 19–20; suicide 28–31

TAC (Training for Adoption Competency) 262
Taenia solium 184
talion principle 271
TB (tuberculosis) 182–183
therapists: adoption-informed 33, 114, 241–265; adoption narratives 58, 72–73; adoptive placement information, relevance of 18–23; attachment to 315; best practices 220–221, 324; competitiveness with parents 308; idealization of 120, 306; non-kinship adoption, factors to consider in 79–83; patient dependence on 305–306; self-disclosure 223–224, 307; training 3, 6–7, 10–12, 31, 54, 58, 88, 103–105, 205–206, 221, 234; unwarranted assumptions 310; *see also* psychotherapists
therapy: attachment-focused 276–277, 279; best practices 220–221, 324; dyadic developmental psychotherapy (DDP) 277; family 2, 6, 10, 95, 163, 251–252; importance of distinctions and timing 218–220; invitation to 265–267; modifications to 265–267; psychoanalytic treatment 264–274; responses to client's search 222–225;

tact and timing need for 308; termination, issues surrounding 273–274; *see also* psychotherapeutic treatment

Three Identical Strangers (film) 25–28
time, internal sense of 30
Toussieng, Povl 33
trafficking, child 5, 27
training: psychodynamic 11, 103, 210, 221; therapist 3, 6–7, 10–12, 31, 54, 58, 88, 103–105, 206, 221, 234; trauma 205, 234
Training for Adoption Competency (TAC) 262
transference 120, 219, 254, 264, 269–271, 273, 304
transference dyads 88–95
transracial adoptions 93–94; *see also* interracial adoption
trauma: definition 309; developmental 276–277; early developmental 6, 8, 16, 30, 57, 82, 86–87, 242, 254, 308–309, 322; impact of 276–277; indicators and lasting effects 308–310; latent 216; neurobiological 87, 322; as ongoing 73; primal 128; response to 309; separation from birth mother 62; training 205–206, 234; traumatic loss 6, 29, 40, 86, 149, 233, 247, 252
trauma-informed 234
traumatic loss 6, 29, 40, 86, 149, 233, 247, 252
treatment: adoption-informed 7, 10, 242–243, 246, 255; adoption-specific considerations 235–254; brain-based 256, 276–277; family therapy 2, 6, 10, 95, 163, 251–252; neurosequential approach 275–282; preliminary considerations 83–87; psychoanalytic (*see* psychoanalytic treatment); psychotherapeutic 10, 231–325; *see also* psychotherapeutic treatment; therapy
treatment modifications 265–267
trust 255
tuberculosis (TB) 182–183

United States: American experience with search and reunion 210–214; closed adoption 148, 212; intercountry adoption **52**
unwed mothers, in India 156–158, 160

Verbal Comprehension Index (VCI) 290–291
Verrier, Nancy 40
viral infections, chronic 183
visual recognition 217

Wechsler Intelligence Scale for Children, IV Version (WISC-IV) 290–291
well-being: conceptual framework for adoptee in India 154, *155*; definition 154
Wieder, Herbert 33
Winnicott, Donald 138
withdrawal 309–310

young adulthood: adolescent adjustment 190–191; countertransference with 306–307; perspective shift to psychology of 239–246

Printed in the United States
by Baker & Taylor Publisher Services